FRONTIERS IN NEUROENDOCRINOLOGY

VOLUME 4

Frontiers in Neuroendocrinology

Volume 4

Edited by

Luciano Martini, M.D.
Professor and Chairman
Institute of Endocrinology
University of Milan
Milan, Italy

William F. Ganong, M.D.
Professor of Physiology
Chairman, Department of Physiology
University of California
School of Medicine
San Francisco, California

Raven Press ▪ New York

Made in the United States of America

International Standard Book Number 0–89004–033–8
Library of Congress Catalog Card Number 77–82030

Raven Press, Publishers
1140 Avenue of the Americas
New York, N.Y. 10036/U.S.A.

Preface

This book is the fourth in a series of volumes surveying the frontiers of the new and rapidly expanding science of neuroendocrinology. Neuroendocrinologists are concerned not only with neural control of endocrine secretion, but also with the effects of hormones on the brain and behavior, and with the broader problem of the interactions between the brain and the internal environment. The field was reviewed in a comprehensive two-volume survey published ten years ago (*Neuroendocrinology*, L. Martini and W. F. Ganong, eds., Academic Press, New York, Volume I, 1966; Volume II, 1967). The present series is designed to update the initial survey by publishing, at intervals of approximately two years, a collection of papers reviewing the areas of neuroendocrinology in which there have been advances, innovations, and controversies. The first three volumes in the *Frontiers in Neuroendocrinology* series were published by Oxford University Press; one in 1969, one in 1971, and one in 1973. The present volume, Volume 4, again surveys selected active areas.

Striking developments since the appearance of *Frontiers in Neuroendocrinology, 1973* include the identification and synthesis of a third hypothalamic hormone, somatostatin, continued rapid progress in clinical neuroendocrinology, and the development of techniques that have made it possible, for the first time, to visualize the cells producing the hypothalamic hormones. It has also become possible to localize hypothalamic hormones, catecholamines, and related enzymes to various small pieces of tissue. Three of these subjects are considered in separate chapters in the current volume, and others are discussed as part of more general reviews in other chapters. Rapid publication has made it possible to combine the features of review monographs and journal articles. The contributors are experts in their fields, and they have been encouraged to include not only published data but also, where pertinent, the results of their own current research. This should make the book of particular value to investigators engaged in research in neuroendocrinology and other aspects of neurobiology. This volume should also be of interest to psychologists, psychiatrists, neurophysiologists, biochemists, and all those concerned with any of the multiple facets of the interaction between the brain and the endocrine glands.

Luciano Martini, M.D.
William F. Ganong, M.D.

Contents

1. Distribution of Hypothalamic Hormones and Neurotrans-
   mitters Within the Diencephalon 1
   *M. J. Brownstein, M. Palkovits, J. M. Saavedra, and
   J. S. Kizer*

2. Localization of Hypothalamic Hormones by Immunocytochemical Techniques 25
   Earl A. Zimmerman

3. Mode of Action of Hypothalamic Regulatory Hormones in
   the Adenohypophysis 63
   *Fernand Labrie, Georges Pelletier, Pierre Borgeat, Jacques
   Drouin, Louise Ferland, and Alain Belanger*

4. Unit Responses in Preoptic and Arcuate Neurons Related
   to Anterior Pituitary Function 95
   Robert L. Moss

5. Brain Regulation of Growth Hormone Secretion 129
   Joseph B. Martin

6. Regulation of Prolactin Secretion 169
   Robert M. MacLeod

7. Secretion of Corticotropin-Releasing Hormone *In Vitro* 195
   Mortyn T. Jones, Edward Hillhouse, and Janet Burden

8. Clinical Neuroendocrinology 227
   G. M. Besser and C. H. Mortimer

9. Development of Hormonal Secretion by the Human Fetal
   Pituitary Gland 255
   Selna L. Kaplan and Melvin M. Grumbach

   Subject Index 277

Contributors

Alain Belanger
Medical Research Council Group in
   Molecular Endocrinology
Centre Hospitalier de l'Université
   Laval
2705, Boulevard Laurier
Sainte-Foy, Québec, Canada G1V 4G2

Gordon M. Besser
The Medical Professorial Unit
St. Bartholomew's Hospital
London EC1A 7BE, England

Pierre Borgeat
Medical Research Council Group in
   Molecular Endocrinology
Centre Hospitalier de l'Université
   Laval
2705, Boulevard Laurier
Sainte-Foy, Québec, Canada G1V 4G2

Michael J. Brownstein
Laboratory of Clinical Science
National Institute of Mental Health
National Institutes of Health
Bethesda, Maryland 20014

Janet Burden
Sherrington School of Physiology
St. Thomas's Ilospital Medical School
Lambeth Palace Road
London SE1 7EH, England

Jacques Drouin
Medical Research Council Group in
   Molecular Endocrinology
Centre Hospitalier de l'Université
   Laval
2705, Boulevard Laurier
Sainte-Foy, Québec, Canada G1V 4G2

Louise Ferland
Medical Research Council Group in
   Molecular Endocrinology
Centre Hospitalier de l'Université
   Laval
2705, Boulevard Laurier
Sainte-Foy, Québec, Canada G1V 4G2

Melvin M. Grumbach
Department of Pediatrics
University of California
San Francisco, California 94143

Edward Hillhouse
Sherrington School of Physiology
St. Thomas's Hospital Medical School
Lambeth Palace Road
London SE1 7EH, England

Mortyn T. Jones
Sherrington School of Physiology
St. Thomas's Hospital Medical School
Lambeth Palace Road
London SE1 7EH, England

Selna L. Kaplan
Department of Pediatrics
University of California
San Francisco, California 94143

J. S. Kizer
Laboratory of Clinical Science
National Institute of Mental Health
National Institutes of Health
Bethesda, Maryland 20014

Fernand Labrie
Medical Research Council Group in
   Molecular Endocrinology
Centre Hospitalier de l'Université
   Laval
2705, Boulevard Laurier
Sainte-Foy, Québec, Canada G1V 4G2

Robert M. MacLeod
Department of Internal Medicine
University of Virginia School of
   Medicine
Charlottesville, Virginia 22901

Joseph B. Martin
Departments of Neurology and
   Experimental Medicine
Montreal General Hospital
1650 Cedar Avenue
Montreal, Québec, Canada H3G 1A4

C. H. Mortimer
The Medical Professorial Unit
St. Bartholomew's Hospital
London EC1A 7BE, England

Robert L. Moss
Department of Physiology
University of Texas Health Science
   Center at Dallas
Southwestern Medical School
Dallas, Texas 75235

M. Palkovits
Semmelweis Medical University
Tüzoltó-ú 58
Budapest, Hungary

Georges Pelletier
Medical Research Council Group in
   Molecular Endocrinology
Centre Hospitalier de l'Université
   Laval
2705, Boulevard Laurier
Sainte-Foy, Québec, Canada G1V 4G2

J. M. Saavedra
Laboratory of Clinical Science
National Institute of Mental Health
National Institutes of Health
Bethesda, Maryland 20014

Earl A. Zimmerman
Department of Neurology and
The International Institute for
   the Study of Human Reproduction
College of Physicians and Surgeons
   of Columbia University
630 West 168 Street
New York, New York 10032

Frontiers in Neuroendocrinology, Vol. 4,
edited by L. Martini and W. F. Ganong.
Raven Press, New York © 1976.

Chapter 1

Distribution of Hypothalamic Hormones and Neurotransmitters Within the Diencephalon

M. J. Brownstein, M. Palkovits, J. M. Saavedra, and J. S. Kizer

*Laboratory of Clinical Science, National Institute of Mental Health, Bethesda, Maryland 20014;
and Semmelweis Medical University, Tüzoltó-ú 58, Budapest, Hungary*

During the course of the last few years two hypothalamic-releasing hormones and one release-inhibiting hormone have been purified, characterized, and synthesized (Bøler et al., 1969; Burgus et al., 1969; Baba et al., 1971; Matsuo et al., 1971; Vale et al., 1972; Brazeau et al., 1973; Rivier et al., 1973). The synthetic peptides have been used to develop sensitive radioimmunoassays. Similarly, significant advances have been made recently in assaying neurotransmitters and their biosynthetic enzymes. At the same time new microassays were being developed, a simple and reproducible method for removing hypothalamic nuclei from the brain was devised (Palkovits, 1973). The convergence of these neuroanatomical and biochemical techniques has enabled quantitative neuroendocrinological and neuropharmacological studies to be undertaken in discrete areas of the hypothalamus. These studies have thus far been centered around two main problems: (1) What are the roles of individual nuclei of the hypothalamus? (2) How do transmitters regulate the synthesis and release of neurohormones by cells of the hypothalamus?

To date, the amount of information collected is relatively small. Regional distributions of luteinizing hormone-releasing hormone (LRH), thyrotropin-releasing hormone (TRH), and somatostatin have been determined. Areas of the brain involved in regulating the release of LH, TSH, and growth hormone (GH) from the anterior pituitary have been better delineated. The levels of several putative neurotransmitters have been measured in the hypothalamus before and after lesioning specific areas of the brain. Consequently the nature of the innervation of many hypothalamic nuclei is now partially understood. Metabolic studies of biogenic amines after endocrine manipulations have provided new data about the identity of nuclei involved in regulating the anterior pituitary and about the role of amines in effecting neuroendocrine changes.

MICRODISSECTION

Two problems had to be solved for a microdissection procedure (Fig. 1–1) to be developed: (1) the morphological features and topographical localization of the hypothalamic nuclei had to be determined; and (2) a simple and reproducible method for removing the nuclei had to be devised.

Nuclei are areas of the brain which have a greater density of nerve cells than the surrounding tissue. In order to define the size, shape, and location of the hypothalamic nuclei of the rat, serial frontal sections of the brain 10 μ in thickness were cut, stained with Luxol fast blue and cresyl violet, and magnified and projected onto a grid. The number of cells lying within each square of the grid was tabulated. (Only those cells in which the nucleolus could be observed in the plane of the section were counted.) Drawings were prepared of each of the serial sections, and a grid identical in scale to the first one was superimposed on these drawings. Different cellular packing densities were indicated by different colors; each square of the grid was assigned a color according to the number of cells it contained. The nuclei stand out from the surrounding areas of hypothalamic tissue in drawings such as those described. The sizes and shapes of the nuclei can be ascertained by studying each of the serial sections in turn (Palkovits, 1975).

Many of the hypothalamic nuclei are composed of morphologically distinct subdivisions. It has been found that cells in any given area of the brain can be classified according to the shapes and volumes of their nuclei (Palkovits and Fisher, 1968). The latter are either elongated or spherical, and large or small.

In order to study the cellular constitution of the hypothalamus the serial sections were projected again, and the diameters of the nuclei of the cells were measured square by square. The neurons were categorized into four groups: those with (1) small, elongated nuclei; (2) small, spherical nuclei; (3) large, elongated nuclei; and (4) large, spherical nuclei. Each group was represented by a color, and the colors were used to fill squares of a grid overlying a drawing of one section of the hypothalamus. Using this "dot diagram" method (Palkovits and Fisher, 1968) to distinguish among different types of cells, it has been possible to partition several of the hypothalamic nuclei. The ventromedial nucleus, for example, can be divided into anterior, medial anterior, lateral anterior, medial posterior, and lateral posterior parts.

$\rightarrow$

FIG. 1–1. Microdissection technique. A: Frozen frontal section of the brain at the anterior hypothalamic level from which the anterior hypothalamic nucleus, suprachiasmatic nucleus, supraoptic nucleus, and medial forebrain bundle have been removed. CO, optic chiasm, CI, internal capsule. B: Frontal section of the brain at the anterior hypothalamic level stained with Luxol fast blue and cresyl violet. The locations of the anterior hypothalamic nucleus (NHAd, NHAd, NHAv), suprachiasmatic nucleus (NSC), supraoptic nucleus (NSO), periventricular nucleus (NPE), and medial forebrain bundle (MFB) are shown. CO, optic chiasm. F, fornix. Circles drawn around these nuclei indicate the size of the punch used to remove them. The large punches have an inside diameter of 500 μ, and the small ones 300 μ. C: Scale drawing of the hollow needle or punch used for microdissections.

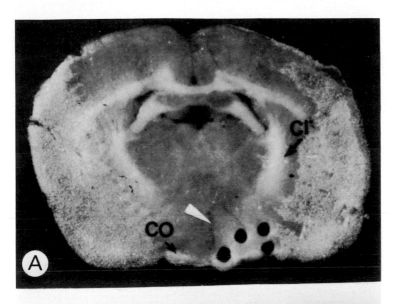

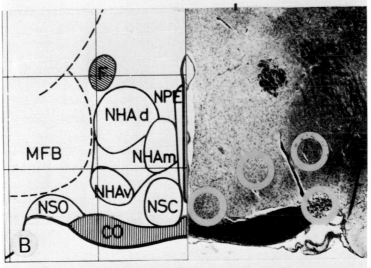

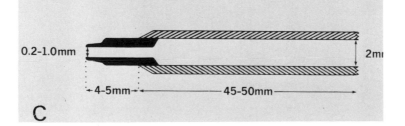

When the size, shape, and location of the hypothalamic nuclei were known, it became possible to dissect them from the brain reproducibly, quickly, and simply. The rat was decapitated and the brain quickly removed, mounted on a chuck, and frozen on Dry Ice. Freezing the brain ensures the stability of the substances subsequently measured. After they were frozen, the brains were serially sectioned in a cryostat at $-10°C$. The sections were 300 μ thick, and the individual hypothalamic nuclei were removed from the sections with hollow needles or "punches" (Palkovits, 1973). The sections were kept frozen on Dry Ice and viewed under a stereomicroscope during the dissection procedure. The tissue pellets were blown from the lumen of the punch onto the tips of a microhomogenizer.

Since the hypothalamic nuclei themselves cannot be seen on the frozen sections, they were removed by reference to landmarks that can be visualized, e.g., the third ventricle and optic chiasm. A detailed description of the localization of the hypothalamic nuclei appears elsewhere (Palkovits et al., 1974a; Palkovits, 1975). In all, 33 subdivisions of 16 hypothalamic nuclei can be removed from sections of the brain. Descriptions of nuclei of the brainstem (Palkovits et al., 1974b), limbic system (Palkovits et al., 1974c), thalamus (Brownstein et al., 1975a), and preoptic area (Saavedra et al., 1974a) are also available, and detailed studies of the distributions of several neurotransmitters have been undertaken in these areas (Brownstein et al., 1974a, 1975a; Palkovits et al., 1974b,c; Saavedra et al., 1974b; Kobayashi et al., 1975).

LOCALIZATION

Neurotransmitters

Catecholamines

The distribution of dopamine, norepinephrine, and phenylethanolamine N-methyltransferase (epinephrine) appear in Fig. 1–2 and 1–3. The results presented in Fig. 1–2 agree well with those obtained by use of fluorescence histochemical techniques (Dahlstrom and Fuxe, 1964; Fuxe, 1964, 1965; Carlsson et al., 1962a,b; Fuxe and Hökfelt, 1966, 1969, 1970; Björklund et al., 1970; Loizou, 1972; Jacobowitz and Palkovits, 1974). Thus histo-

$\longrightarrow$

FIG. 1–2. Distribution of norepinephrine (A), dopamine (B), dopamine-β-hydroxylase (C), and tyrosine hydroxylase (D) in the hypothalamus. ■ > ▨ > ▥ > ▤. A, anterior ventromedial nucleus. CA, anterior commissure. M, mesencephalon. MB, mamillary body. MFB, medial forebrain bundle. NDM, dorsomedial nucleus. NHA, anterior hypothalamic nucleus. NHP, posterior hypothalamic nucleus. NIST, nucleus interstitialis striae terminalis. NPE, perventricular nucleus. NPF, perifornical nucleus. NPMD, dorsal premamillary nucleus. NPMV, ventral premamillary nucleus. NPOM, medial preoptic nucleus. NPV, paraventricular nucleus. NSC, suprachiasmatic nucleus. NSO, supraoptic nucleus. NVM, ventromedial nucleus. OC, optic chasm. P, pituitary. S, preoptic suprachiasmatic nucleus. TH, thalamus.

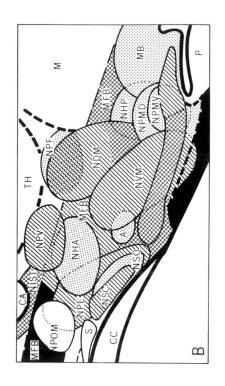

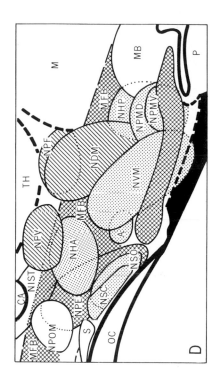

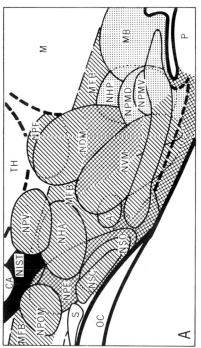

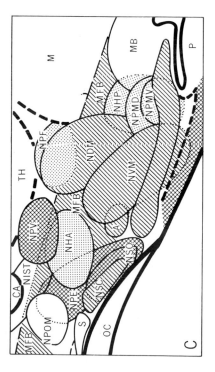

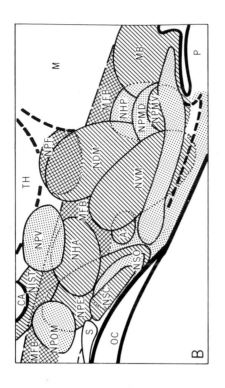

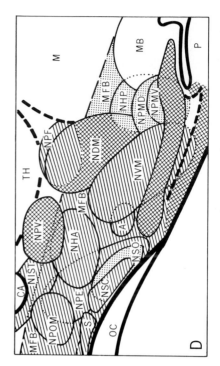

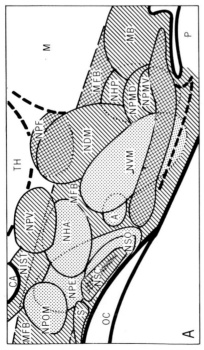

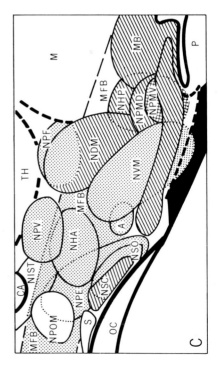

chemical data complement the data obtained by use of microassays. Although the latter provide quantitative information, they have one distinct short-coming: When a molecule is measured in an extract of tissue, its site of synthesis and storage remains a mystery. One cannot say whether it was present in nerve cell bodies, axons of passage, nerve terminals, or extraneuronal structures. Thus the histochemical studies must go hand in hand with biochemical pursuits.

Norepinephrine

Norepinephrine (Fig. 1–2, Tables 1–1 and 1–2), which appears to be present in axons of cells located in the brainstem is highly concentrated in the periventricular nucleus (34 ng/mg protein), retrochiasmatic area (48 ng/mg protein), dorsomedial nucleus (39 ng/mg protein), and the median eminence (30 ng/mg protein), as reported by Palkovits et al. (1974a). Within certain nuclei the norepinephrine concentration differs from subdivision to subdivision (Palkovits et al., 1974a). For example, there is nearly three times as much norepinephrine in the ventral part of the dorsomedial nucleus as in its dorsal part, and the rostral parts of the arcuate nucleus are much richer in norepinephrine than the dorsal parts.

The distribution of dopamine-β-hydroxylase, the enzyme that converts dopamine to norepinephrine, parallels that of its product (Saavedra et al., 1974c). The activity of tyrosine hydroxylase, on the other hand, is highest in nuclei that contain large amounts of dopamine (Saavedra et al., 1974c). In spite of this, tyrosine hydroxylase must be present, to some extent, in noradrenergic and adrenergic neurons of the hypothalamus.

The effect of locus ceruleus lesions on norepinephrine levels in some hypothalamic nuclei has been studied by Kobayashi and his colleagues (Kobayashi et al., 1974). Such lesions cause no changes in the concentrations of norepinephrine in the medial forebrain bundle and dorsomedial nucleus but produce falls of 38.5% and 42.5% in the paraventricular and periventricular nuclei, respectively. Bilateral mesencephalic knife cuts that transect the ventral noradrenergic bundles result in a complete loss of dopamine-β-hydroxylase (and, by implication, norepinephrine) from the medial basal hypothalamus (J. Kizer and D. Jacobowitz, *personal communication*). Similarly, hypothalamic deafferentiation with a Halász knife (Halász, 1969) results in a total loss of dopamine-β-hydroxylase from the median eminence and the arcuate, ventromedial, and dorsomedial nuclei (M. J. Brownstein, M. Palkovits, M. L. Tappaz, J. M. Saavedra, and J. S. Kizer, *in preparation, a*). Based on the above studies, it is safe to say that practically all of the

---

←

FIG. 1–3. Distribution of serotonin (A), tryptophan hydroxylase (B), histamine (C), and phenylethanolamine-N-methyltransferase (D) among nuclei of the hypothalamus. ■ > ▨ > ▧ > ▨. See legend to Fig. 1–2 for explanation of abbreviations.

TABLE 1–1. *Biogenic amines in the hypothalamus of the rat*

Region	Norepinephrine[a] (ng/mg protein)	Dopamine[a] (ng/mg protein)	Serotonin[b] (ng/mg protein)	Histamine[c] (ng/mg protein)
Periventricular nucleus	33.5 ± 3.3	7.1 ± 0.9	10.9 ± 4.1	3.7 ± 0.4
Supraoptic nucleus	23.6 ± 5.0	3.7 ± 0.6	9.5 ± 2.8	3.0 ± 0.6
Paraventricular nucleus	51.0 ± 6.4	10.0 ± 1.5	13.5 ± 3.1	2.4 ± 0.5
Anterior hypothalamic nucleus	16.2 ± 4.6	5.0 ± 0.9	10.2 ± 2.3	3.3 ± 0.8
Suprachiasmatic nucleus				
Internal	20.5 ± 4.0	8.5 ± 2.4	37.2 ± 4.7	
External	29.2 ± 3.9	9.5 ± 1.3	17.0 ± 1.3	
Retrochiasmatic area	48.0 ± 7.9	15.1 ± 1.1	15.9 ± 2.3	
Arcuate nucleus				
I	35.9 ± 3.4	28.2 ± 3.7		
II	18.9 ± 3.0	18.7 ± 4.4		
III	21.2 ± 4.1	12.0 ± 2.6	36.4 ± 9.8	6.2 ± 0.7
IV	12.5 ± 1.1	7.1 ± 2.1		
V	12.0 ± 1.5	7.0 ± 1.7		
Ventromedial nucleus (anterior)	16.1 ± 1.8	5.7 ± 0.8		
Anterior medial	16.3 ± 2.6	6.0 ± 1.1		
Anterior lateral	22.5 ± 2.0	7.0 ± 1.1	8.5 ± 3.9	3.6 ± 0.8
Posterior medial	38.2 ± 3.6	10.0 ± 1.1		
Posterior lateral	17.9 ± 2.0	5.1 ± 0.5		
Dorsomedial nucleus				
Dorsal	21.8 ± 3.3	8.5 ± 0.7		
Ventral	54.6 ± 12.9	11.9 ± 2.4	13.6 ± 5.3	4.0 ± 0.5
Perifornical nucleus	17.9 ± 3.8	6.0 ± 1.1	30.0 ± 10.9	2.2 ± 0.6
Dorsal premamillary nucleus	14.2 ± 4.2	3.9 ± 1.2	22.9 ± 8.8	2.9 ± 0.5
Ventral premamillary nucleus	16.3 ± 6.2	3.4 ± 0.9	18.3 ± 8.2	8.1 ± 0.8
Hypothalamic nucleus (posterior)	13.9 ± 2.2	4.3 ± 1.0	24.5 ± 7.6	4.6 ± 0.7
Medial forebrain bundle (anterior)	16.9 ± 1.9	6.1 ± 0.9	21.6 ± 5.8	2.7 ± 0.5
Medial forebrain bundle (posterior)	20.2 ± 2.7	11.0 ± 1.5	30.7 ± 8.0	
Median eminence	29.5 ± 4.0	65.0 ± 6.1	15.3 ± 3.2	17.8 ± 2.2

[a] Palkovits et al., 1974c.
[b] Saavedra et al., 1974d.
[c] Brownstein et al., 1974b.

norepinephrine present in the hypothalamus is contained in axons and nerve terminals arising from cell bodies in other areas of the brain, but not all of these cell bodies are present in the locus ceruleus. Other groups of cells (e.g., those in the "locus subceruleus," A1, A2, A4, and A5) have been postulated to play a part in providing noradrenergic innervation to the hypothalamus. Recent studies in our laboratory have given no support to the idea of such a role for the A2 area (area of the vagal nuclei); lesions there caused no change in tyrosine hydroxylase or dopamine-β-hydroxylase levels in hypothalamic nuclei (J. M. Saavedra, M. Palkovits, J. Zivin, and M. J. Brownstein, *in preparation*).

Dopamine

Dopamine (Fig. 1–2, Tables 1–1 and 1–2) was measured in many areas of the brain where it could not be detected using fluorescence histochemical

TABLE 1–2. Levels of enzymes involved in the synthesis of neurotransmitters in the rat hypothalamus

Region	Tyrosine hydroxylase[a] (nmoles product/ mg protein/hr)	Dopamine- β-hydroxylase[a] (nmoles product/ mg protein/hr)	Phenylethanolamine N-methyltransferase[b] (pmoles product/ mg protein/hr)	Tryptophan hydroxylase[c] (nmoles product/ mg protein/hr)	Choline acetyltransferase[d] (nmoles product/ mg protein/hr)
Periventricular nucleus	4.55 ± 0.70	4.19 ± 0.45	4.2 ± 0.3	0.44 ± 0.05	8.0 ± 0.9
Supraoptic nucleus	0.92 ± 0.14	1.83 ± 0.36	8.3 ± 1.1	0.31 ± 0.04	5.2 ± 1.3
Paraventricular nucleus	3.14 ± 0.82	3.55 ± 0.82	7.7 ± 0.8	0.32 ± 0.05	15.0 ± 2.5
Anterior hypothalamic nucleus	1.46 ± 0.20	0.68 ± 0.08	7.4 ± 0.3	0.68 ± 0.12	5.9 ± 1.3
Suprachiasmatic nucleus	1.83 ± 0.33	0.79 ± 0.14	5.0 ± 0.9	0.55 ± 0.08	5.6 ± 0.7
Arcuate nucleus	4.33 ± 0.43	0.83 ± 0.32	4.3 ± 0.7	0.29 ± 0.04	10.3 ± 2.0
Ventromedial nucleus	1.83 ± 0.61	1.00 ± 0.33	3.6 ± 0.5	0.43 ± 0.07	8.3 ± 1.6
Dorsomedial nucleus	2.10 ± 0.32	3.06 ± 0.93	8.4 ± 1.2	0.47 ± 0.07	10.9 ± 3.2
Dorsal premamillary nucleus	0.42 ± 0.10	0.51 ± 0.09	11.1 ± 0.8	0.24 ± 0.02	4.1 ± 0.5
Ventral premamillary nucleus	0.90 ± 0.20	0.58 ± 0.13	4.0 ± 1.0	0.33 ± 0.07	4.9 ± 1.4
Posterior hypothalamic nucleus	1.46 ± 0.30	0.59 ± 0.06	13.7 ± 1.3	0.35 ± 0.05	5.1 ± 1.0
Perifornical nucleus	4.50 ± 0.71	0.46 ± 0.07	7.9 ± 0.8	1.16 ± 0.17	8.1 ± 1.6
Medial forebrain bundle					
Anterior	5.70 ± 1.04	0.88 ± 0.16	11.1 ± 0.9	—	6.2 ± 0.5
Posterior	7.20 ± 0.80	0.83 ± 0.18	—	1.13 ± 0.19	5.3 ± 1.2
Median eminence	18.03 ± 1.04	1.26 ± 0.31	19.5 ± 0.6	.41 ± 0.03	15.6 ± 3.0

Results represent the mean ± SEM for groups of six to eight animals.

[a] Saavedra et al., 1974b.
[b] Saavedra et al., 1974c.
[c] Brownstein et al., in preparation a.
[d] Brownstein et al., 1975ba.

methods. Dopamine levels are particularly high in the median eminence and arcuate nucleus and moderately high in the suprachiasmatic nucleus, paraventricular nucleus, medial part of the ventromedial nucleus, dorsomedial nucleus, and the posterior part of the medial forebrain bundle (Palkovits et al., 1974a). Part of the dopamine found in the hypothalamus is present in cell bodies in the arcuate and periventricular nuclei (Dahlstrom and Fuxe, 1964; Fuxe, 1965; Fuxe and Hökfelt, 1966, 1969, 1970; Björklund et al., 1970). The suprachiasmatic nucleus may also contain dopaminergic cell bodies (Lidbrink et al., 1974). Axons arising from dopaminergic cell bodies in the arcuate nucleus terminate in the external layer of the median eminence. Dopamine present in areas of the hypothalamus other than the arcuate nucleus and median eminence may be in axons and nerve terminals of hypothalamic or extrahypothalamic origin. Furthermore, some dopamine is probably present in noradrenergic axons. Deafferentation of the basal hypothalamus has no significant effect on its dopamine content but reduces its norepinephrine content markedly (Weiner et al., 1972). This may mean that extrahypothalamic dopaminergic cell bodies provide no significant input to the hypothalamus, but studies of individual nuclei must be done in order to state this with confidence.

Epinephrine

Although it has been known for two decades that epinephrine (Fig. 1–3, Table 1–2) is present in the brain of mammals, it was only recently found to exist in specific neuronal pathways. Hökfelt and his colleagues (1973) described an immunohistological technique for visualizing phenylethanol-N-methyltransferase (PNMT). This enzyme was present in cell bodies in the A1 (lateral reticular nucleus of medulla) and A2 regions and in axons and nerve terminals in the medial basal hypothalamus. PNMT activity was found to be high in regions where it was visualized immunohistochemically (Saavedra et al., 1974d). Moreover, epinephrine was generally present in high concentrations in areas rich in PNMT (Koslow and Schlumpf, 1974). Deafferentation of the hypothalamus causes a substantial reduction in the activity of PNMT in the median eminence and arcuate nucleus (M. J. Brownstein et al., *in preparation, a*). Lesions of the A2 region, on the other hand, do not appear to influence the PNMT level in the medial basal hypothalamus (J. M. Saavedra et al., *in preparation*). Thus another group of cell bodies—perhaps the A1 group—must supply this region with its adrenergic input.

Serotonin

Serotonin (5-HT) is considerably more difficult to visualize using fluorescence histochemical techniques than are the catecholamines. In the hypothalamus 5-HT (Fig. 1–3, Tables 1–1 and 1–2) can be seen consistently in the suprachiasmatic nucleus. Weak yellow fluorescence is seen in several other nuclei but not in the median eminence (Fuxe and Hökfelt, 1969). The 5-HT level in the suprachiasmatic nucleus—especially in its central portion—is high (Saavedra et al., 1974a). Similarly, the medial forebrain bundle, which contains serotonergic fibers traveling through the lateral hypothalamus to more rostral areas, is rich in 5-HT (Saavedra et al., 1974a).

Like dopamine, 5-HT was found in many places where it could not be visualized (Saavedra et al., 1974a). It is present in relatively high concentrations in the arcuate nucleus and in moderate concentrations in the preoptic area, premamillary nuclei, posterior hypothalamic nucleus, and median eminence.

Tryptophan hydroxylase was found in the highest concentrations in areas of the hypothalamus that are rich in serotonergic axons (e.g., medial forebrain bundle). Its presence in the median eminence and in all of the hypothalamic nuclei confirms the idea that 5-HT is synthesized there (M. J. Brownstein, M. Palkovits, J. M. Saavedra, and J. S. Kizer, in preparation, b).

Cells of the raphe nuclei appear to provide the medial basal hypothalamus of the rat with the major part of its serotonin. Serotonergic fibers destined to terminate in the tuberoinfundibular area form a compact bundle in the mesencephalon, just above the interpeduncular nucleus, prior to entering the hypothalamus (M. Palkovits, M. J. Brownstein, J. M. Saavedra, D. Jacobowitz, and J. S. Kizer, in preparation). Knife cuts which cause complete deafferentation of the hypothalamus also cause more than half of the 5-HT in the arcuate nucleus, ventromedial nucleus, and median eminence to disappear. Knife cuts which do not reach the base of the brain caudally have a less profound effect (M. J. Brownstein et al., in preparation, a).

Histamine

There are no histochemical techniques currently available for the visualization of histamine (Fig. 1–3, Table 1–1) or its biosynthetic enzyme histidine decarboxylase. Therefore it is impossible to say with certainty whether histamine is intra- or extraneuronal in the mammalian central nervous system (CNS). The fact that it can be shown to be present in synaptosomes is in favor of the existence of histaminergic nerves (Carlini and Green, 1963; Kataoka and De Robertis, 1967; Kuhar et al., 1971). However, it is difficult to eliminate the possibility that histamine enters the synaptosomes in the course of their preparation. Transecting the medial forebrain bundle causes histamine and histidine decarboxylase to fall by 20% and 40%, respectively, in areas rostral to the lesion, e.g., the septum and cerebral cortex (Schwartz et al., 1974). This also favors the idea of histaminergic nerves in some areas of the brain.

Against the theory that histamine is present in nerve cells in the brain, especially in the hypothalamus, are two facts: (1) There are mast cells in the CNS which almost certainly contain histamine. (2) Other extraneuronal elements may contain histamine. However, two glial clones have been proved not to contain histamine and histidine decarboxylase (Garbarg et al., 1975).

The highest level of histamine in the hypothalamus was found in the median eminence (Brownstein et al., 1974*b*). Mast cells, present in the median eminence of the rat, may contain some or all of the histamine found there. The parenchyma of the hypothalamus is said to be essentially devoid of mast cells, however. The basal and posterior hypothalamic nuclei are richer in histamine than the rest (Brownstein et al., 1974*b*).

Histamine was measured in three nuclei—the arcuate, ventromedial, and dorsomedial—and in the median eminence after total isolation of the medial hypothalamus. There were no changes in histamine levels from the control values in these areas as a result of the surgical procedure (M. J. Brownstein et al., *in preparation, a*). Other areas of the brain do not appear to contribute histaminergic nerves to the medial hypothalamus. Whether histamine in the hypothalamus is in hypothalamic neurons or in mast cells remains to be seen.

Acetylcholine

Two types of assay suitable for the determination of acetylcholine (Fig. 1–4, Table 1–2) in small samples of tissue are currently available: the enzymatic-isotopic assay (Goldberg and McCaman, 1973) and the mass fragmentographic technique (Hanin and Schuberth, 1974). Neither has been applied extensively to the mammalian CNS. Koslow et al. (1974) determined the level of acetylcholine in seven nuclei of the rat brain, among them the anterior hypothalamic nucleus, which had 0.97 nmoles of acetylcholine per milligram of protein.

Unlike its product, choline acetyltransferase is simple to measure. The level of this enzyme correlates well with the amount of acetylcholine found in discrete regions of the nervous system. The distribution of choline acetyltransferase within the hypothalamus has been described (Brownstein et al., 1975*a*). The choline acetyltransferase level was highest in the median eminence. The medial forebrain bundle was also rich in the enzyme, as were the premamillary nuclei. In general, the distribution of choline acetyltransferase follows maps of cholinergic pathways in the CNS based on histochemical localization of acetylcholinesterase (Koelle 1954, 1966; Shute and Lewis, 1961, 1967; Jacobowitz and Palkovits, 1974).

Surgical isolation of the medial hypothalamus does not produce any change in choline acetyltransferase activity in the median eminence but causes re-

FIG. 1–4. Localization of choline acetyltransferase (A), LRH (B), TRH (C), and somatostatin (D). ■ > ⊠ > ▨ > ▨. See legend to Fig. 1–2 for explanation of abbreviations.

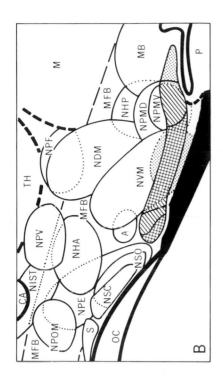

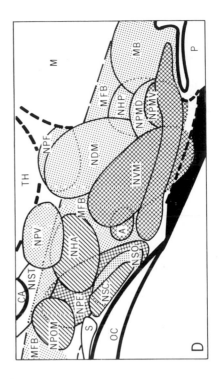

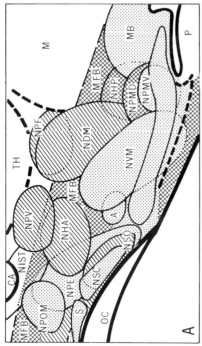

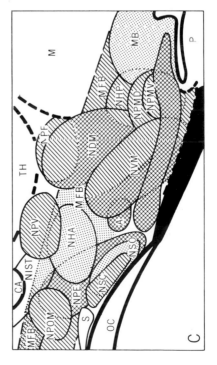

ductions of 38% in the arcuate nucleus, 29% in the ventromedial nucleus, and 69% in the dorsomedial nucleus. Apparently there are cholinergic cell bodies in the medial hypothalamus—perhaps in the arcuate nucleus or ventromedial nucleus—which send their axons to the median eminence. Cholinergic nerves with their cell bodies outside of the "island" seem to terminate in the dorsomedial nucleus (M. Brownstein et al., *in preparation, a*).

γ-Aminobutyric Acid

The distribution of γ-aminobutyric acid (GABA) and other amino acids that may serve as neurotransmitters in the CNS has not been determined. Glutamic acid decarboxylase, the enzyme which converts glutamic acid into GABA, has been assayed in the hypothalamic nuclei. The anterior hypothalamic nucleus, suprachiasmatic nucleus, paraventricular nucleus, dorsomedial nucleus, and medial forebrain bundle were relatively rich in glutamic acid decarboxylase (M. J. Brownstein, M. L. Tappaz, and M. Palkovits, *in preparation, c*).

Biologically Active Peptides

Arginine Vasopressin, Oxytocin, and Neurophysins

George and Jacobowitz measured arginine vasopressin levels in the nuclei of the rat hypothalamus by use of radioimmunoassay (*personal communication*). As expected, the median eminence and supraoptic nucleus have very high levels of this peptide (440 and 40 ng/mg protein, respectively), and the paraventricular nucleus contains 24 ng/mg protein. Areas of the brain through which fibers bearing vasopressin proceed from the supraoptic nuclei to the median eminence also have substantial amounts of this material. Thus the suprachiasmatic nucleus, retrochiasmatic area, and arcuate nucleus contain vasopressin in amounts of 20 to 70 ng/mg protein; other areas of the hypothalamus contain less than 1 ng/mg protein.

According to Zimmerman and his colleagues, the distribution of arginine vasopressin in the cow is qualitatively similar to that in the rat (Zimmerman et al., 1974). Arginine vasopressin (measured either by bioassay or radioimmunoassay) was present in the paraventricular nucleus in a concentration that was almost half that in the supraoptic nucleus, which had 480 ng/mg protein. Approximately the same amounts of oxytocin were found in the supraoptic and paraventricular nuclei. Neurophysin I was also found in the same concentration in both of the magnocellular nuclei. Neurophysin II, on the other hand, was concentrated in the supraoptic nucleus and thus seems to be associated with vasopressin.

Releasing Hormones and Release-Inhibitory Hormones

Luteinizing Hormone-Releasing Hormone

The concentration of radioimmunoassayable LRH (Fig. 1–4, Table 1–3) is high in the median eminence (29 ng/mg protein) and in the arcuate nucleus (3 ng/mg protein), according to Palkovits et al. (1947d). Other hypothalamic nuclei—the ventromedial, supraoptic, and suprachiasmatic nuclei—have small amounts of this releasing hormone. This distribution agrees reasonably well with the results of studies that employed bioassay methods (Crighton et al., 1970). The medial preoptic nucleus seems to contain very little LRH, but both Wheaton and his colleagues (1975) and Kordon (*personal communication*) found it in the organum vasculosum, which contains approximately 1.5 ng/mg protein—25 to 50 times more than the surrounding tissue (J. Kizer, M. Palkovits, and M. Brownstein, *in preparation*). The data cited above are complimented by immunohistological studies demonstrating LRH in cell bodies of the arcuate nucleus and in axons and tanycytes of the median eminence and organum vasculosum (Chapter 2).

Since both LRH and dopamine seemed to be present in cell bodies of the arcuate nucleus and nerve endings of the median eminence, we wondered whether they were in the same or different neurons. Injections of 6-hydroxy-

TABLE 1–3. *Luteinizing hormone-releasing hormone (LRH), thyrotropin-releasing hormone (TRH), and somatostatin in the rat hypothalamus*

Region	LRH[a] (ng/mg protein)	TRH[b] (ng/mg protein)	Somatostatin[c] (ng/mg protein)
Medial preoptic nucleus	<0.05	2.0 ± 0.1	14.0 ± 2.5
Periventricular nucleus	<0.05	4.2 ± 0.7	23.7 ± 9.0
Suprachiasmatic nucleus	Trace (<0.1)	1.8 ± 0.2	8.0 ± 0.6
Supraoptic nucleus	Trace (<0.1)	0.9 ± 0.2	3.2 ± 0.6
Anterior hypothalamic nucleus	<0.05	0.8 ± 0.3	8.6 ± 1.5
Lateral anterior nucleus	<0.05	0.7 ± 0.2	4.9 ± 1.1
Paraventricular nucleus	<0.05	2.6 ± 0.7	4.4 ± 1.8
Arcuate nucleus	2.9 ± 0.8	3.9 ± 0.9	44.6 ± 6.1
Ventromedial nucleus			14.6 ± 2.1
Lateral part	0.6 ± 0.5	3.0 ± 0.6	
Medial part	Trace (<0.1)	9.0 ± 3.3	
Dorsomedial nucleus	<0.05	4.0 ± 0.8	5.4 ± 2.1
Perifornical nucleus	<0.05	2.0 ± 0.7	3.8 ± 0.7
Lateral posterior area	<0.05	1.2 ± 0.5	3.5 ± 0.7
Posterior hypothalamic nucleus	Trace (<0.1)	1.8 ± 0.2	3.8 ± 0.8
Dorsal premamillary nucleus	<0.05	1.5 ± 0.2	4.3 ± 0.7
Ventral premamillary nucleus	<0.05	1.3 ± 0.3	17.3 ± 4.4
Median eminence	22.4 ± 2.2	38.4 ± 8.3	309.1 ± 60.8

[a] Palkovits et al., 1974a.
[b] Brownstein et al., 1974a.
[c] Brownstein et al., 1975b.

dopamine into the third ventricles of rats caused dopamine and norepinephrine to fall 80% to 85% in the arcuate nucleus and median eminence.
The drug, which is specifically toxic for catecholaminergic nerves, did not
cause the LRH level to decrease. Thus LRH does not seem to be in the
same medial basal hypothalamic cells as dopamine (Kizer et al., 1975).

Thyrotropin-Releasing Hormone

Unlike LRH, TRH is not confined to a few areas of the hypothalamus; in
fact, it is not confined to the hypothalamus at all. It is present in significant
amounts in the spinal cord (R. Utiger, *personal communication*), brainstem, mesencephalon, preoptic area, septum, basal ganglia, and cerebral
cortex (Brownstein et al., 1974c; Jackson and Reichlin, 1974; Oliver et al.,
1974; Winokur and Utiger, 1974).

Within the hypothalamus, TRH is concentrated in the median eminence
(Brownstein et al., 1974c; Krulich et al., 1974). It is found in large amounts
in the ventromedial nucleus (especially the medial part), arcuate nucleus,
periventricular nucleus, and dorsomedial nucleus (Brownstein et al., 1974c).
The location of cell bodies which synthesize TRH remains unknown. It may
be that TRH is present in axons and nerve terminals in many parts of the
brain other than the median eminence. In this case, TRH may act as a
neurotransmitter or modulator of neuronal firing patterns in addition to
acting as a releasing hormone. Just as acetylcholine and serotonin are no
longer called "Vagusstoff and enteramine," perhaps TRH should no longer
be referred by a name with a functional connotation.

Somatostatin

The tetradecapeptide somatostatin is found in high concentrations in the
brain (Brownstein et al., 1975 b), pancreas (A. Arimura, *personal communication*), and stomach (A. Arimura, *personal communication*). In the
nervous system it is present in the hypothalamus as well as beyond the limits
of the hypothalamus. Its manifold actions are being explored, and it must
have functions in addition to inhibiting GH release from the anterior
pituitary.

The highest concentration of somatostatin measured in the brain was in
the median eminence. High levels were also found in the arcuate, periventricular, ventral premammillary, and ventromedial nuclei. The location and
nature of the cells which synthesize and store somatostatin remain to be
determined.

Somatostatin-like activity has been estimated by bioassay in extracts of
hypothalamic nuclei (Vale et al., 1974), and a distribution was similar to
that obtained by radioimmunoassay. There was one important difference
between the results of the bioassay and immunoassay studies: bioassayable

somatostatin-like activity was relatively low in the ventromedial nucleus. Perhaps there is as much GH-releasing hormone (GRH) in the ventromedial nucleus as there is GH release-inhibiting hormone (GIH; Krulich et al., 1971).

Catecholamines and Stress

Dopamine, norepinephrine, and tyrosine hydroxylase levels were measured in several hypothalamic nuclei of rats after stressing the animals (Palkovits et al., 1975). This was done as a screening procedure in hopes of finding the site(s) of action of catecholamines in the stress response. The norepinephrine and dopamine levels were significantly and acutely decreased in one nucleus (the arcuate nucleus) after cold, formalin, and immobilization stresses (Fig. 1–5). Repeated immobilization (for five consecutive days) caused the tyrosine hydroxylase activity to increase in the arcuate nucleus but not in the median eminence. Chronic formalin and cold stress did not alter tyrosine hydroxylase levels. Failure of stressful stimuli other than immobilization to increase tyrosine hydroxylase may reflect insufficient repetition of the stress, the brevity of each stress period, or the interval between the final exposure to stress and killing.

Catecholamines and Neuroendocrine Control Mechanisms

Tyrosine hydroxylase and dopamine-β-hydroxylase were assayed in the medial preoptic area, periventricular nucleus, paraventricular nucleus, arcuate nucleus, ventromedial nucleus, dorsomedial nucleus, medial forebrain bundle, and median eminence of rats 9 days after adrenalectomy, thyroidectomy, or gonadectomy (Kizer et al., 1974). Following gonadectomy (Fig. 1–6) there was a significant rise in tyrosine hydroxylase activity only in the median eminence; treatment with testosterone partially reversed this increase. Thyroidectomy also caused tyrosine hydroxylase in the median eminence to rise above the control value. The increase in tyrosine hydroxylase in the median eminence was accompanied by increases in the dorsomedial, arcuate, and periventricular nuclei. However, although thyroxine caused the tyrosine hydroxylase in the median eminence to fall significantly below the control value within 12 hr, tyrosine hydroxylase activity in the other areas fell only to control values. Adrenalectomy produced a significant decrease in tyrosine hydroxylase in the median eminence. The administration of dexamethasone to adrenalectomized animals caused tyrosine hydroxylase to increase to a level greater than that measured in untreated adrenalectomized rats.

The activity of dopamine-β-hydroxylase did not change in response to any of the endocrine manipulations described above. The activities of tryptophan hydroxylase (J. Kizer, M. Palkovits, J. Saavedra, and M. Brownstein, *in preparation*) and choline acetyltransferase also seem not to change in hypo-

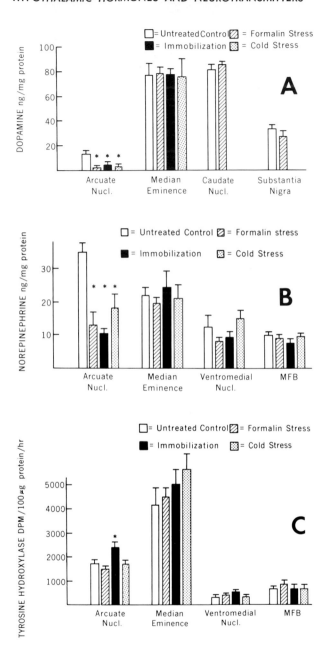

FIG. 1–5. Effect of stress on catecholamine and tyrosine hydroxylase levels. Bars represent mean values, and brackets represent standard errors of the mean. Asterisks indicate statistically significant differences between treated and control groups. MFB, medial forebrain bundle. A: Effect of acute formalin, immobilization, and cold stresses on dopamine levels. B: Effect of acute formalin, immobilization, and cold stresses on norepinephrine levels. C: Effect of chronic formalin, immobilization, and cold stresses on tyrosine hydroxylase levels. (From Palvokits et al., 1975.)

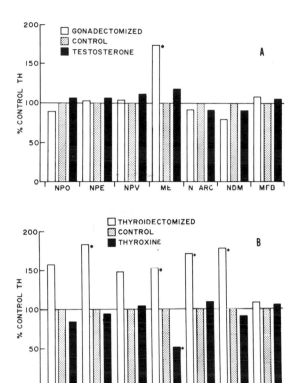

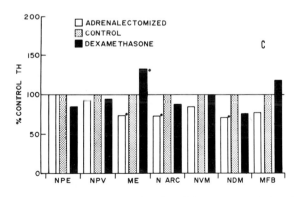

FIG. 1–6. Changes in the activity of tyrosine hydroxylase following removal of endocrine glands. Bars represent average values of tyrosine hydroxylase activity expressed as percent of control for each nucleus. Asterisks denote statistically significant differences between treated and control groups. A: Effect of gonadectomy and testosterone replacement (100 μg daily) on tyrosine hydroxylase activity in the medial preoptic nucleus (NPO), periventricular nucleus (NPE), paraventricular nucleus (NPV), median eminence (ME), arcuate nucleus (N ARC), dorsomedial nucleus (NDM), and medial forebrain bundle (MFB). B: Effect of thyroidectomy and thyroxine replacement (20 μg) on enzyme activity in the NPO, NPE, NPV, ME, N ARC, NDM, and MFB. C: Effect of adrenalectomy and dexamethasone replacement (100 μg daily) on enzyme activity in the NPE, NPV, ME, NARC, NVM (ventromedial nucleus), NDM, and MFB. (From Kizer et al., 1974.)

thalamic nuclei after endocrine manipulations. Furthermore, ventral bundle lesions that cause noradrenergic nerves to disappear from the hypothalamus do not block any of the alterations in tyrosine hydroxylase described above (J. Kizer and D. Jacobowitz, *personal communication*). Apparently the changes in tyrosine hydroxylase levels observed after endocrine manipulations are occurring in dopaminergic neurons. It is interesting to note in this regard that dopamine turnover in the median eminence of normal rats is quite brisk and norepinephrine turnover slow (J. Zivin and J. Kizer, *personal communication*). The changes in tyrosine hydroxylase are most marked at the level of the median eminence. Whether endocrine-induced alterations in the activity of tyrosine hydroxylase are attributable to variations in the firing rate of dopaminergic nerves or to metabolic effects of hormones on these nerves remains to be determined.

CONCLUSION

Much of the information presented in this chapter has admittedly been of a preliminary nature. It is hoped that this information will provide a foundation on which future studies can be built. By combining anatomical, physiological, and biochemical approaches it will be possible to learn more about cells of the hypothalamic nuclei—cells which comprise the final common pathway in the brain's regulation of the anterior pituitary.

REFERENCES

Baba, Y., Matsuo, H., and Schally, A. V. (1971): Structure of the porcine LH- and FSH-releasing hormone. II. Confirmation of the proposed structure by conventional sequential analyses. *Biochem. Biophys. Res. Commun.,* 44:459–467.

Björklund, A., Falck, B., Hromek, F., Owman, C., and West, K. A. (1970): Identification and terminal distribution of the tubero-hypophyseal monoamine fibre system in the rat by means of stereotopic and microspectrofluorimetric techniques. *Brain Res.,* 17:1–23.

Bøler, J., Enzmann, F., Folkers, K., Bowers, C. Y., and Schally, A. V. (1969): The identity of chemical and hormonal properties of the thyrotropin releasing hormone and pyroglutamyl-histidyl-proline amide. *Biochem. Biophys. Res. Commun.,* 37:705–710.

Brazeau, P., Vale, W., Burgus, R., Ling, N., Butcher, M., Rivier, J., and Guillemin, R. (1973): Hypothalamic polypeptide that inhibits the secretion of immunoreactive pituitary growth hormone. *Science,* 179:77–79.

Brownstein, M., Saavedra, J. M., and Palkovits, M. (1974*a*): Norepinephrine and dopamine in the limbic system of the rat. *Brain Res.,* 79:431–436.

Brownstein, M., Saavedra, J. M., Palkovits, M., and Axelrod, J. (1974*b*): Histamine content of hypothalamic nuclei of the rat. *Brain Res.,* 77:151–156.

Brownstein, M., Palkovits, M., Saavedra, J. M., Bassiri, R. M., and Utiger, R. D. (1974*c*): Thyrotropin-releasing hormone in specific nuclei of the brain. *Science,* 185:267–269.

Brownstein, M., Arimura, A., Sato, H., Schally, A. V., and J. S. Kizer (1975*b*): The regional distribution of somatostatin in the rat brain. *Endocrinology (in press).*

Brownstein, M., Kobayashi, R., Palkovits, M., and Saavedra, J. M. (1975*a*): Choline acetyltransferase levels in diencephalic nuclei of the rat. *J. Neurochemistry,* 24:35–38.

Burgus, R., Dunn, T. F., Desiderio, D., and Guillemin, R. (1969): Structure moléculaire du facteur hypothalamique hypophysiotrope TRF d'origine ovine: Mise en évidence par spectrométrie de masse de la sequence. *C. R. Acad. Sci.* [D] (Paris), 269:1870–1893.

Carlini, E. A., and Green, J. P. (1963): The subcellular distribution of histamine, slow-reacting substance and 5-hydroxytryptamine in the brain of the rat. *Br. J. Pharmacol.,* 20:264–277.

Carlsson, A., Falck, B., and Hillarp, N-A. (1962a): Cellular localization of brain monoamines. *Acta Physiol. Scand. [Suppl.],* 196:1–28.

Carlsson, A., Falck, B., Hillarp, N-A., and Torp, A. (1962b): Histochemical localization of the cellular level of hypothalamic noradrenaline. *Acta Physiol. Scand.,* 54:385–386.

Crighton, D. B., Schneider, H. P. G., and McCann, S. M. (1970): Localization of LH-releasing factor in the hypothalamus and neurohypophysis as determined by an in vitro method. *Endocrinology,* 87:323 329.

Dahlstrom, A., and Fuxe, K. (1964): Evidence for the existence of monoamine-containing neurons in the central nervous system. I. Demonstration of monoamines in the cell bodies of brain stem neurones. *Acta Physiol. Scand. [Suppl.],* 323:1–55.

Fuxe, K. (1964): Cellular localization of monoamine in the median eminence and the infundibular stem of some mammals. *Z. Zellforsch.,* 61:710–724.

Fuxe, K. (1965): Evidence for the existence of monoamine neurons in the central nervous system. IV. Distribution of monoamine nerve terminals in the central nervous system. *Acta Physiol. Scand. [Suppl.],* 247:36–85.

Fuxe, K., and Hökfelt, T. (1966): Further evidence for the existence of tuberoinfundibular dopamine neurons. *Acta Physiol. Scand.,* 66:245–246.

Fuxe, K., and Hökfelt, T. (1969): Catecholamines in the hypothalamus and the pituitary gland. In: *Frontiers in Neuroendocrinology 1969,* edited by W. F. Ganong and L. Martini, pp. 47–96. Oxford University Press, New York.

Fuxe, K., and Hökfelt, T. (1970): Central monoaminergic system and hypothalamic function. In: *The Hypothalamus,* edited by L. Martini, N. Motta, and F. Fraschini, pp. 123–138. Academic Press, New York.

Garbarg, M., Baudry, M., Benda, P., and Schwartz, J. C. (1975): Simultaneous presence of histamine-N-methyltransferase and catechol-O-methyltransferase in neuronal and glial cells in culture. *Brain Res.,* 83:538–541.

Goldberg, A., and McCaman, R. E. (1973): The determination of picomole amounts of acetylcholine in mammalian brain. *J. Neurochem.,* 20:1–8.

Halász, B. (1969): The endocrine effects of isolation of the hypothalamus from the rest of the brain. In: *Frontiers in Neuroendocrinology 1969,* edited by W. F. Ganong and L. Martini, pp. 307–342. Oxford University Press, New York.

Hanin, I., and Schuberth, J. (1974): Labelling of acetylcholine in the brain of mice fed on a diet containing deuterium labelled choline: Studies utilizing gas chromatography-mass spectroscopy. *J. Neurochemistry,* 23:819 824.

Hökfelt, T., Fuxe, K., Goldstein, M., and Johansson, O. (1973): Evidence for adrenergic neurons in the rat brain. *Acta Physiol. Scand.,* 89:286–288.

Jackson, I. M., and Reichlin, S. (1974): Thyrotropin releasing hormone (TRH) distribution in the brain, blood, and urine of the rat. *Life Sci.,* 14:2259–2266.

Jacobowitz, D., and Palkovits, M. (1974): Topographic atlas of catecholamine and acetylcholinesterase-containing neurons in the rat brain. I. Forebrain (telencephalon, diencephalon). *J. Comp. Neurol.,* 157:13–28.

Kataoka, K., and De Robertis, E. (1967): Histamine in isolated small nerve endings and synaptic vesicles of rat brain cortex. *J. Pharmacol. Exp. Ther.,* 156:114–125.

Kizer, J. S., Palkovits, M., Zivin, J., Brownstein, M., Saavedra, J. M., and Kopin, I. J. (1974): The effect of endocrinological manipulations on tyrosine hydroxylase and dopamine-β-hydroxylase activities in individual hypothalamic nuclei of the adult male rat. *Endocrinology,* 85:799–812.

Kizer, J. S., Arimura, A., Schally, A. V., and Brownstein, M. J. (1975): Absence of luteinizing hormone releasing hormone (LH-RH) from catecholaminergic neurons. *Endocrinology (in press).*

Kobayashi, R. M., Palkovits, M., Kopin, I. J., and Jacobowitz, D. (1974): Biochemical mapping of noradrenergic nerves arising from the rat locus coeruleus. *Brain Res.,* 77:269–279.

Kobayashi, R. M., Brownstein, M., Saavedra, J. M., and Palkovits, M. (1975): Choline acetyltransferase content in discrete regions of the rat brain stem. *J. Neurochem.* (*in press*).

Koelle, G. B. (1954): The histochemical localization of cholinesterases in the central nervous system of the rat. *J. Comp. Neurol.,* 100:211–235.

Koelle, G. B. (1966): Cytological distributions and physiological functions of cholinesterases. In: *Handbuch der Experimentellen Pharmakologie,* Vol. 15, edited by O. Eichler and A. Farah, pp. 187–298. Springer, Berlin.

Koslow, S. H., and Schlumpf, M. (1974): Quantitation of adrenaline in rat brain nuclei and areas by mass fragmentography. *Nature (Lond.),* 251:530–531.

Koslow, S. H., Racagni, G., and Costa, E. (1974): Mass fragmentographic measurement of norepinephrine, dopamine, serotonin, and acetylcholine in seven discrete nuclei of the rat tel-diencephalon. *Neuropharmacology,* 13:1123–1130.

Krulich, L., Illner, P., Fawcett, C. P., Quijada, M., and McCann, S. M. (1971): Dual hypothalamic regulation of growth hormone secretion. In: *Growth and Growth Hormone,* pp. 306–316. International Congress Series No. 244. Excerpta Medica, Amsterdam.

Krulich, L., Quijada, M., Hefco, E., and Sundberg, D. K. (1974): Localization of thyrotropin-releasing factor (TRF) in the hypothalamus of the rat. *Endocrinology,* 95:9–17.

Kuhar, M. J., Taylor, K. M., and Snyder, S. H. (1971): The subcellular localization of histamine and histamine methyltransferase in rat brain. *J. Neurochem.,* 18:1515–1527.

Lidbrink, P., Jonsson, G., and Fuxe, K. (1974): Selective reserpine-resistant accumulation of catecholamines in central dopaminergic neurons after DOPA administration. *Brain Res.,* 67:439–456.

Loizou, L. A. (1972): The postnatal ontogeny of monoamine-containing neurons in the central nervous system of the albino rat. *Brain Res.,* 40:395–418.

Matsuo, H., Baba, Y., Nair, R. M. G., Arimura, A., and Schally, A. V. (1971): Structure of the porcine LH- and FSH-releasing hormone. I. The proposed amino acid sequence. *Biochem. Biophys. Res. Commun.,* 43:1334–1339.

Oliver, C., Eskay, R. L., Ben-Jonathan, N., and Porter, J. C. (1974): Distribution and concentration of TRH in the rat brain. *Endocrinology,* 95:540–553.

Palkovits, M. (1973): Isolated removal of hypothalamic or other brain nuclei of the rat. *Brain Res.,* 59:449–450.

Palkovits, M. (1975): Microdissection of discrete hypothalamic nuclei. In: *Topographical Neuroendocrinology,* edited by W. Stumpf and L. Grant. Karger, Basel (*in press*).

Palkovits, M., and Fisher, J. (1968): *Karyometric Investigations.* Akadémiai Kiadó, Budapest.

Palkovits, M., Brownstein, M., Saavedra, J. M., and Axelrod, J. (1974a): Norepinephrine and dopamine content of hypothalamic nuclei. *Brain Res.,* 77:137–149.

Palkovits, M., Brownstein, M., and Saavedra, J. M. (1974b): Serotonin content of the brain stem nuclei in the rat. *Brain Res.,* 80:237–249.

Palkovits, M., Saavedra, J. M., Kobayashi, R. M., and Brownstein, M. (1974c): Choline acetyltransferase content of limbic nuclei of the rat. *Brain Res.,* 79:443–450.

Palkovits, M., Arimura, A., Brownstein, M., and Saavedra, J. M. (1974d): Luteinizing hormone releasing hormone (LH-RH) content of the hypothalamic nuclei in rat. *Endocrinology,* 95:554–558.

Palkovits, M., Kobayashi, R., Kizer, J. S., Jacobowitz, D. M., and Kopin, I. J. (1975): Effect of stress on catecholamines and tyrosine hydroxylase activity of individual hypothalamic nuclei. *Neuroendocrinology* (*in press*).

Rivier, J., Brazeau, P., Vale, W., Ling, N., Burgus, R., Gilon, G., Yardley, J., and Guillemin, R. (1973): Synthèse totalé par phase solide d'un tétradécapeptide ayant les propriétés chemique et biologique de la somatostatine. *C. R. Acad. Sci.* [D] (*Paris*), 276:666–669.

Saavedra, J. M., Palkovits, M., Brownstein, M., and Axelrod, J. (1974a): Serotonin distribution in the nuclei of the rat hypothalamus and preoptic region. *Brain Res.*, 77:157–165.

Saavedra, J. M., Brownstein, M., and Palkovits, M. (1974*b*): Serotonin distribution in the limbic system of the rat. *Brain Res.*, 79:437–441.

Saavedra, J. M., Brownstein, M., Palkovits, M., Kizer, J. S., and Axelrod, J. (1974*c*): Tyrosine hydroxylase and dopamine-β-hydroxylase: Distribution in individual rat hypothalamic nuclei. *J. Neurochem.*, 23:869–871.

Saavedra, J. M., Palkovits, M., Brownstein, M., and Axelrod, J. (1974*d*): Localization of phenylethanolamine N-methyl-transferase in rat brain nuclei. *Nature (Lond.)*, 248:695–696.

Schwartz, J. C., Julien, C., Feger, I., and Garbarg, M. (1974): Histaminergic pathway in rat brain: Evidence by hypothalamic lesions. *Fed. Proc.*, 33:285.

Shute, C. C. D., and Lewis, P. R. (1961): The use of cholinesterase techniques combined with operative procedures to follow nervous pathways in the brain. *Bibl. Anat.*, 2:34–49.

Shute, C. C. D., and Lewis, P. R. (1967): The ascending cholinergic reticular system: Neocortical, olfactory and subcortical projections. *Brain*, 90:497–520.

Vale, W., Brazeau, P., Grant, G., Nussey, A., Burgus, R., Rivier, J., Ling, N., and Guillemin, R. (1972): Premières observations sur le mode d'action de la somatostatine un facteur hypothalamique qui inhibe la sécrétion de l'hormone de croisance. *C. R. Acad. Sci. [D] (Paris)*, 275:2913–2916.

Vale, W., Rivier, C., Palkovits, M., Saavedra, J. M., and Brownstein, M. (1974): Ubiquitous brain distribution of inhibitors of adenohypophysial secretion. *Endocrinology*, 94:A128.

Weiner, R. I., Shryne, J. E., Gorski, R. A., and Sawyer, C. H. (1972): Changes in the catecholamine content of the rat hypothalamus following deafferentation. *Endocrinology*, 90:867–873.

Wheaton, J. E., Krulich, L., and McCann, S. M. (1975): Localization of luteinizing hormone-releasing hormone in the preoptic area and hypothalamus of the rat using radioimmunoassay. *Endocrinology (in press)*.

Winokur, A., and Utiger, R. D. (1974): Thyrotropin releasing hormone: Regional distribution in rat brain. *Science*, 185:265–267.

Zimmerman, E. A., Robinson, A. G., Husain, M. K., Acosta, M., Frantz, A. G., and Sawyer, W. H. (1974): Neurohypophyseal peptides in the bovine hypothalamus: The relationship of neurophysin I to oxytocin, and neurophysin II to vasopressin in supraoptic and paraventricular regions. *Endocrinology*, 95:931–936.

Frontiers in Neuroendocrinology, Vol. 4,
edited by L. Martini and W. F. Ganong.
Raven Press, New York © 1976.

Chapter 2

Localization of Hypothalamic Hormones by Immunocytochemical Techniques

Earl A. Zimmerman

Department of Neurology and The International Institute for the Study of Human Reproduction,
Columbia University, New York, New York 10032

Although the hypothalamus has been considered the source of peptide hormones that influence the pituitary gland and other target tissues outside the brain, the specific cells of synthesis and secretion have not been completely characterized. In neuroendocrinology, and neurobiology in general, it is important to know the biochemical function of a specific cell or cell system. Because of the extreme complexity of its cellular structures compared to other endocrine organs, the hypothalamus has remained a black box. By assaying even a very small piece of hypothalamus obtained by microdissection (Palkovits, 1973; see also Chapter 1) or the content of granules separated by centrifugation (Taber and Karovolas, 1975), one cannot determine which cells and granules contain luteinizing hormone-releasing hormone (LRH). Despite the large numbers and types of cells in the hypothalamus, however, it is virtually certain that particular ones in certain regions synthesize and secrete specific neurohormones.

The classic histological work on the magnocellular neurosecretory system using selective Gomori stains (aldehyde fuchsin and chrome-alum-hematoxylin) demonstrated that a neurosecretory material was formed in the perikarya of supraoptic and paraventricular neurons and transported in their axons to the posterior pituitary gland (Scharrer and Scharrer, 1954; Bargmann, 1966, 1968). The concept that these specialized nerve cells can form oxytocin and vasopressin in the hypothalamus and secrete them into the general circulation at their terminals developed with these and subsequent studies (Sloper, 1966; Ginsburg, 1968). Gomori material, characteristic of the magnocellular system, was absent or scanty in the zona externa of the median eminence around capillaries of the hypophyseal portal system and absent from parvicellular neurons of the tuberoinfundibular system, which is thought to carry releasing hormones to the portal bed (Szentágothai et al., 1968; Kobayashi et al., 1970). Immunocytochemical studies now provide more direct *in situ* evidence, which supports the neurosecretory theory and the concept that oxytocin and vasopressin are secreted by the magnocellular

system and hypophysiotropins by the parvicellular system. The immunocytochemical approach is only a few years old and the data are incomplete, but
a few surprises have already been uncovered. Vasopressin appears to be
secreted into portal blood in the median eminence as well as into systemic
blood in the posterior pituitary (Zimmerman et al., 1973a). Hypothalamic
hormones may be secreted into the cerebrospinal fluid (CSF) of the third
ventricle and transported by tanycytes of the ependyma to the portal bed
(Zimmerman et al., 1975a). Discovery of LRH (Kordon, 1975) and
somatostatin (Pelletier et al., 1975) in the organum vasculosum of the
lamina terminalis (OVLT) suggests that this structure also plays a role in
neuroendocrine function.

IMMUNOCYTOCHEMICAL METHODS

A number of important technical advances have now permitted a beginning in the localization of hypothalamic hormones *in situ*. First was the
characterization of specific brain antigens and the generation of corresponding antisera. The localization of the larger, more stable carrier proteins of
vasopressin and oxytocin, the neurophysins, in the magnocellular system by
immunofluorescence (Livett et al., 1971) was an important first step that
encouraged subsequent attempts to localize the smaller peptides, vasopressin,
oxytocin, LRH, and somatostatin as antisera became available. Secondly,
immunoenzyme techniques, particularly the immunoperoxidase methods
(Avareameas, 1970; Nakane, 1971; Sternberger, 1974), were developed
for both light and electron microscopic immunocytochemical studies. Extensive work with fixatives, penetration, and the peroxidase-antiperoxidase
(PAP) technique that evolved during the many elegant studies of tropic
hormones in the anterior pituitary (Moriarty, 1973) provided the methods
and principles now being applied for the localization of hypothalamic hormones and other molecules such as tyrosine hydroxylase (Pickel et al.,
1975).

Despite the first exciting successes in brain localization, problems associated with the immunocytochemical approach remain to be resolved. Both
false-positive and false-negative results are sometimes obtained. Antiserum
to a small peptide generated to an immunogen in which the hormone was
conjugated to a larger protein may contain antibodies that cross react with a
sequence peculiar to the conjugate in brain tissue that is not the hormone.
Antibodies to bovine serum albumin (BSA) in a whole antiserum generated
by an immunogen prepared by conjugation of LRH to BSA cross react with
substances in the magnocelluar system that do not contain LRH (Kozlowski
et al., 1975). False-negative results can be produced by using fixatives that
may be ideal for cytological detail but which may destroy the immunoreactive
site (Silverman and Zimmerman, 1975). Therefore despite the most meticu-
lous controls (including absorption with purified hormone), immunocyto-

chemical data should be interpreted along with information obtained by bioassay and radioimmunoassay, and when possible by studying more than one antigen in the same cell. The neurophysins are additional antigens that can be localized along with oxytocin and vasopressin. Similarly, the immuno-histochemical localizing of dopamine-β-hydroxylase (DBH) and phenyl-ethanolamine-N-methyltransferase (PNMT) have enhanced the validity of histochemical data on norepinephrine (Hartman et al., 1972; Hökfelt et al., 1973) and epinephrine (Hökfelt et al., 1974a).

LOCALIZATION OF NEUROPHYSINS

Historical Review

Van Dyke and co-workers (1941) described a protein with a molecular weight of approximately 30,000 which had oxytocic, pressor, and antidiuretic effects. It was soon shown that the octapeptide hormones oxytocin and vaso-pressin (Du Vigneaud, 1956) were loosely bound to this carrier protein moiety (Acher and Du Vigneaud, 1958), which was then renamed neuro-physin. Further research revealed that most mammalian species probably have two major neurophysins although there is evidence for a third in some animals (Robinson and Frantz, 1973). Neurophysins have a molecular weight of about 10,000 (Walter et al., 1971; Capra and Walter, 1975). One neurophysin appears to be associated with oxytocin and another with vaso-pressin (Dean et al., 1968; Zimmerman et al., 1974a; 1975b). Since radio-immunoassays for oxytocin and vasopressin were not generally available, it was hoped that a specific radioimmunoassay for oxytocin-neurophysin and vasopressin-neurophysin would be useful for studying neurohypophyseal function in peripheral blood. In 1968 Fawcett, Powell, and Sachs provided some encouragement by demonstrating that radiolabeled neurophysin was present in peripheral plasma. This observation was soon confirmed by radio-immunoassay (Cheng and Friesen, 1972; Legros and Franchimont, 1972). Robinson et al. (1971a) succeeded in the radioimmunoassay of bovine neuro-physin I (NPI) and neurophysin II (NPII). There was a tendency for the NPI and NPII to be secreted independently in response to physiological stimuli for the secretion of oxytocin and vasopressin, respectively (Robinson et al., 1971b). An intragranular association of NPI with oxytocin and NPII with vasopressin had been previously suggested by Dean et al. (1968).

More recently radioimmunoassay produced physiological evidence for hormone-specific neurophysins in humans (Robinson, 1975). Nicotine in-halation releases a neurophysin (nicotine-stimulated neurophysin; NSN) along with vasopressin (Robinson, 1975). Another neurophysin is stimulated by estrogen administration (estrogen-stimulated neurophysin; ESN), which is elevated in plasma during pregnancy and at the time of ovulation (Legros and Franchimont, 1972; Robinson, 1975). These assays for specific human neurophysin provide similar results in plasma samples of rhesus monkeys (Robinson et al., 1974). Bovine NPI and NPII may be analogous to human and monkey ESN and NSN, respectively. Whether ESN is actually released with oxytocin remains to be determined, although it is likely as indicated by the immunocytochemical data provided below. It was shown by radioimmunoassay and bioassay that there is a relationship of NPI to oxytocin and of NPII to vasopressin in the bovine hypothalamus (Zimmerman et al., 1974a). In addition, NPI and NPII have been localized in oxytocin- and vasopressin-containing cells, respectively, in the ox (Vandesande et al., 1975a). A relationship of a particular neurophysin with oxytocin and another with vasopressin was also noted in the pig (Pickup et al., 1973). Further evidence for an oxytocin-neurophysin and a vasopressin-neurophysin was found in homozygous Brattleboro rats with diabetes insipidus (DI rats), which lack a neurophysin as well as vasopressin (Burford et al., 1971; Sunde and Sokol, 1975).

Intracellular Distribution of Neurophysins

A large number of immunocytochemical studies on the general distribution of neurophysins have been performed since 1970 using cross-species antisera with both immunofluorescence and immunoperoxidase techniques (Watkins, 1975a,b; Zimmerman et al., 1975b). These studies were possible because neurophysins of different species share many common amino acid sequences in a large portion of the body of the molecule (Capra and Walter, 1975). Neurophysin appears to be an ancestral protein. Antihuman and antibovine antisera cross react with material in the magnocellular system of many animals: lamprey, goldfish, chicken, mouse, rat, guinea pig, monkey, and man (Zimmerman et al., 1975b). In the mammalian hypothalamus neurophysin is found in the perikarya of virtually all the neurons in the supraoptic nucleus (SON) and in approximately 75% of magnocellular neurons in the paraventricular nucleus (PVN), although we could never stain all the cells in the PVN (Fig. 2–1a,c). Neurophysin is also found in magnocellular neurons scattered along the paraventricular tract (Fig. 2–1a,b; Zimmerman et al., 1973b) between the SON and the PVN in the rat, monkey, and man. It is also found in the retrochiasmatic portion of the SON in the lateral anterior tuberal floor, as seen in the mouse and rat (Zimmerman et al., 1975b). In most preparations there is normally a wide variation in the cytoplasmic content of immunoreactive material. In cells that appear partially filled, the neurophysin is concentrated in the perinuclear zone. This probably represents concentration of the neurophysin in the endoplasmic reticulum and Golgi apparatus, which packages it into granules (Clementi and Ceccarelli, 1970) along with vasopressin or the precursor of both (Sachs and Takabatake, 1964). By immunoelectron microscopy, it has been shown that neurophysin is located in the large granules of the magnocellular peri-

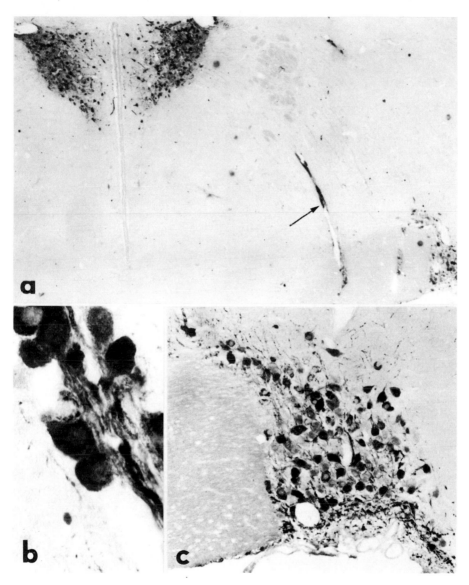

FIG. 2–1. Light microscopic study of the magnocellular system in the anterior hypothalamus of the albino rat using antiserum to bovine neurophysin I. Immunoperoxidase technique. *a:* At low power in the coronal plane, neurophysin is seen in large cell bodies of the paired paraventricular nuclei (at *upper left*), supra-optic nucleus (at *lower right*), and in cells (*arrow*) along the paraventricular tract. *b:* Higher magnification at *arrow* in *a.* ✕760. *c:* Higher power of supraoptic nucleus in *a,* showing neurophysin in all the cells. ✕200. (*a:* from Zimmerman et al., 1975b. *b:* from E. Zimmerman, *unpublished data.*)

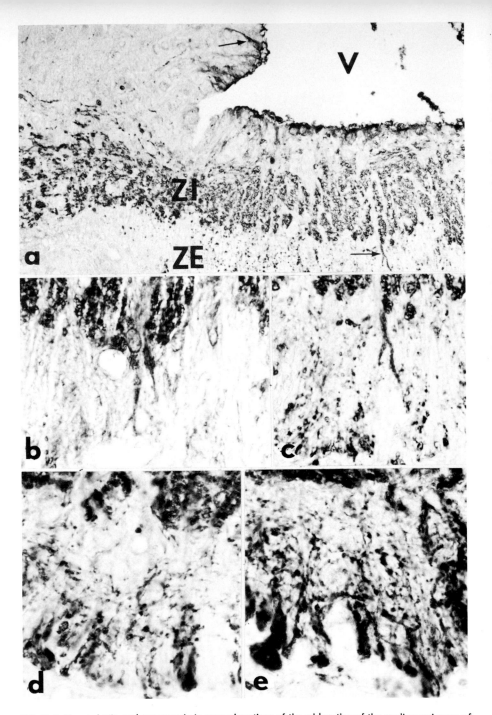

FIG. 2–2. Neurophysin and vasopressin in coronal sections of the midportion of the median eminence of albino rats reacts with antiserum to human neurophysin (*a* and *c*), antiserum to all rat neurophysins (*e*), and to vasopressin (*b* and *d*). Immunoperoxidase technique. *a:* Neurophysin is seen in axons of the hypothalamohypophyseal tract in zona interna (ZI). Some fibers appear to leave the tract (*lower arrow*) to project to zona externa (ZE) in normal rat. Some tanycytes contain neurophysin (*upper arrow*). V, third ventricle. Cresyl violet counterstain, ×270. *b:* Vasopressin fiber leaving the tract to end in the zona externa. Adjacent section to (*a* and *c*), ×690. *c:* Higher magnification of *a* at *lower arrow* showing neurophysin fiber to zona externa. ×690. *d:* Two weeks after bilateral adrenalectomy there is a marked increase in the vasopressin in the zona externa. ×690. *e:* Neurophysin in section adjacent to *d*. The antisera to human and rat neurophysins produce identical immunoperoxidase staining in the rat. ×690. (*a, b,* and *c:* from Zimmerman et al., 1975c. *d* and *e:* from E. Zimmerman, L. Recht, and M. Stillman, *unpublished micrographs.*)

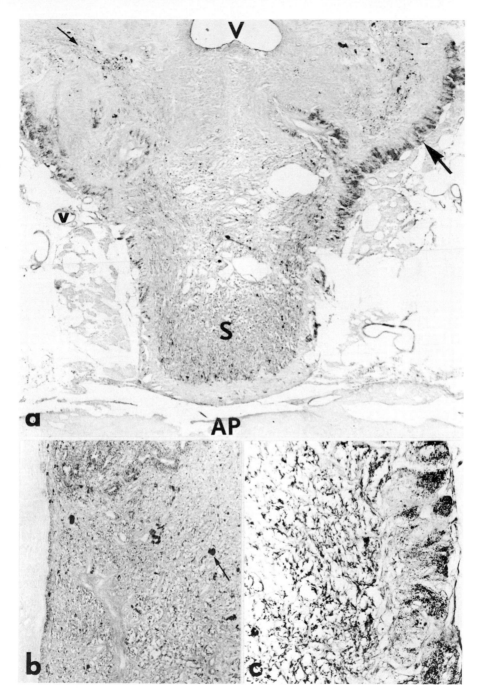

FIG. 2–3. Distribution of neurophysin in a rhesus monkey using antibovine neurophysin I. Immunoperoxidase method. *a*: Coronal section through the median eminence and pituitary stalk (S). Neurophysin is seen in fibers of the hypothalamohypophyseal tract as it passes ventromedially (*small arrow*) and in the zona externa (*large arrow*). v, portal vein. V, third ventricle. AP, anterior pituitary. ×43. *b*: Neurophysin in the posterior pituitary. *Arrow points to stained Herring body. Intermediate lobe (at left edge) does not react.* ×203. *c*: Higher magnification at larger arrow in *a* shows neurophysin in fibers of the tract in zona interna (*left*) and concentrated around portal capillaries in zona externa (*right*). ×504. (*a* and *c*: from Zimmerman et al., 1973a. *b*: from E. Zimmerman, K. Hsu, and M. Tannenbaum, *unpublished data.*)

karya (Pelletier et al., 1974*a*). As the neurons fill with neurophysin-containing granules, reaction products appear to extend into their dendrites and beaded axonal processes, which can be followed long distances through the fiber layer in the zona interna of the median eminence (Fig. 2–2), along the pituitary stalk, and into their endings on systemic capillaries in the posterior lobe (Fig. 2–3b). The neurophysin in these fibers and their swellings (Herring bodies) is also located in large granules (Pelletier et al., 1974*a*; Silverman et al., 1975). These findings confirm earlier studies using Gomori stains and transmission electron microscopy (Sloper, 1966). More sensitive and specific than previous techniques, however, the immunocytochemical studies have shown that the fields of the SON and PVN are more extensive than previously emphasized. Cells of this system are scattered anteriorly as far as the lamina terminalis, dorsally as far as the ventral anterior thalamus, laterally well beyond the fornix, and caudally to the midmedian eminence (Zimmerman et al., 1975*b*). Although concentrated in the SON and the PVN, neurophysin-positive cell bodies form a continuous trail between these two nuclei (Fig. 2–1a,b). It is impossible to make a sharp anatomical separation of this system into two distinct nuclei.

Neurophysin Around Hypophyseal Portal Capillaries

The immunocytochemical approach produced some unexpected findings. The first was the discovery of large concentrations of neurophysin in the zona externa of the median eminence of sheep (Parry and Livett, 1973; Kozlowski et al., 1975) and monkeys (Fig. 2–3a,c; Zimmerman et al., 1973*a*), and more recently in cats and dogs (Watkins, 1975*a*), guinea pigs (Silverman and Zimmerman, 1975), and rats (Zimmerman et al., 1975*a*). It had been shown in the rat that the scanty Gomori-positive material normally present in the zona externa increases markedly after adrenalectomy (Rinne, 1972; Wittowski and Bock, 1972), and this increase was thought to be due to an increase in corticotropin-releasing hormone (CRH). More recently increased amounts in the zona externa were found after adrenalectomy by immunoperoxidase techniques (Vandesande et al., 1974; Watkins et al., 1974). Whether a neurophysin is associated with CRH, as suggested by Watkins et al. (1974), remains to be established. At least some of the neurophysin in the zona externa is accompanied by vasopressin (Zimmerman et al., 1975*a*), which increases markedly after adrenalectomy as shown by the immunoperoxidase technique (Fig. 2–2; Seif et al., 1975).

It has been debated for years whether the magnocellular system projects to the portal bed (Knigge and Scott, 1970) and whether vasopressin normally plays a role in the release of ACTH (Martini, 1966; Yates et al., 1971). The immunohistochemical demonstration of neurophysin in the zona externa led us to measure neurophysin and vasopressin in blood collected from individual portal veins of monkeys (Zimmerman et al., 1973*a*). Large amounts of ESN, NSN, and vasopressin were detected (Table 2–1). The amount of vasopressin actually measured (mean 13,500 pg/ml) during the stress of surgery is more than enough to release ACTH and growth hormone (GH) and is similar to the amount previously estimated to reach the anterior pituitary (Goldman and Lindner, 1962). Since our study was reported, we have obtained further evidence that our radioimmunoassay for vasopressin was not detecting CRH. Extracts of equivalent amounts of the hypothalamus and posterior pituitary from normal and homozygous rats of the Brattleboro strain (DI rats) were assayed for vasopressin in the same assay used previously in the study of monkey portal blood (Zimmerman et al., 1973a). No vasopressin was detected in the homogenates of DI rats, whereas large

TABLE 2–1. *Radioimmunoassays of neurophysin and vasopressin in monkeys*

Monkey	ES-NP (ng/ml)		NS-NP (ng/ml)		VP (pg/ml)	
	SB	PB	SB	PB	SB	PB
557	1.4	124	4.4	100	—	—
561	3.0	25	2.0	10	35	11,000
564	4.6	240	2.1	88	50	16,000
448	2.2	28	2.0	48	40	14,500

ES-NP, estrogen-stimulated neurophysin. NS-NP, nicotine-stimulated neurophysin. VP, vasopressin. SB, systemic venous blood. PB, hypophyseal portal blood. The blood samples were obtained simultaneously.

amounts were found in the normal animals. It is known that DI rats secrete CRH, although the ACTH response to stress is not completely normal (Yates et al., 1971).

Immunoelectron microscopic studies have now shown that axon terminals near portal capillaries contain intragranular neurophysin and vasopressin (Fig. 2–4a; Goldsmith and Zimmerman, 1975; Silverman and Zimmerman, 1975). The precise source of these terminals remains to be defined. Axons from the magnocellular system appear to leave the hypothalamohypophyseal tract in the zona interna to run in palisade fashion to the zona externa (Fig. 2–2). It is not known if they originate in both the SON and PVN, and whether they run directly to zona externa or as collaterals of fibers going on to the posterior lobe. Vandesande et al. (1974) suggested that neurophysin-containing fibers in the zona externa come from parvicellular neurons in the suprachiasmatic nucleus in the rat. However, they could not trace these suprachiasmatic fibers to the median eminence. In both rats and mice we also have not been able to trace the fine fibers of the suprachiasmatic nucleus to the median eminence by this technique. In addition, in the guinea pig (Silverman and Zimmerman, 1975), monkey (Zimmerman et al., 1973a), and sheep (Kozlowski et al., 1975), where neurophysin normally abounds in the zona externa, it has not been found in the suprachiasmatic nucleus.

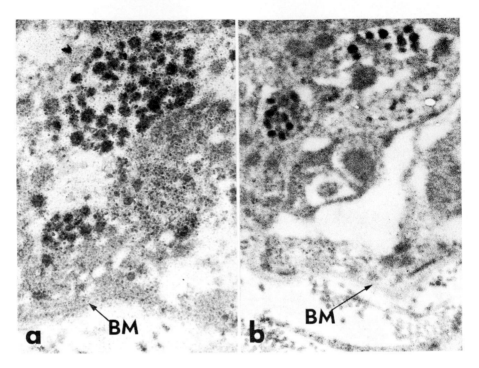

FIG. 2–4. Electron microscopic immunocytochemical staining of the zona externa of a rat median eminence using peroxidase antiperoxidase (PAP) technique. a: Antiserum to lysine vasopressin localizes the octapeptide in larger neurosecretory granules (1,300 to 1,700Å). ×23,000. b: Application of antiserum to LRH localizes the decapeptide to smaller granules (750 to 900 Å) in axon terminals different from those containing vasopressin. BM, basement membrane. ×23,000. a: from P. Goldsmith and E. Zimmerman, *unpublished data.* b: from P. Goldsmith and W. Ganong, *unpublished data.*

Two different-sized granules in different axon terminals on portal capillaries were found to contain vasopressin and neurophysin in the guinea pig. Terminals containing larger granules (1,300 to 1,500 Å) were rare, and endings containing smaller granules (900 to 1,000 Å) were common (Silverman and Zimmerman, 1975). It is possible but not proved that the axon terminals containing the smaller granules originate in magnocellular cells in the PVN (Silverman and Zimmerman, 1975).

CSF and Ependymal Neurophysin

Another unexpected finding was the presence of neurophysin in the tanycytes of the lower third ventricle at the level of the median eminence of some monkeys (Robinson and Zimmerman, 1973) and rats (Fig. 2–2a; Zimmerman et al., 1975a). The major function of these specialized ependymal cells in the median eminence is thought to be the transport of substances from the CSF to the portal blood (Knigge and Scott, 1970; Knowles, 1972; Ben-Jonathan et al., 1974; Knigge, 1974). Neurophysin concentrations were higher in cisternal and lumbar CSF than in peripheral blood of man and monkey, and radiolabeled neurophysin did not appear to be transferred from peripheral blood to CSF in dogs (Robinson and Zimmerman, 1973). Experiments of Vorheer and associates (1968) had suggested that vasopressin was secreted into CSF. On the basis of these data and the close proximity of neurophysin and vasopressin fibers to the third ventricle as seen by light microscopic immunocytochemistry (Zimmerman et al., 1975a), it was postulated that these peptides were secreted into CSF by axons of magnocellular neurons. By scanning and transmission electron microscopy, axons containing large electron-dense granules typical of magnocellular fibers are seen among the many different axon terminals that project into the third ventricle (Scott et al., 1974a). Immunoelectronmicroscopy has provided more direct evidence that axon terminals containing vasopressin and neurophysin enter the floor of the third ventricle in the median eminence of the rat (Goldsmith and Zimmerman, 1975). Axon terminals may enter the third ventricle at more anterior sites as well (Scott et al., 1974a). As seen by light microscopy and the immunoperoxidase technique, vasopressin- and neurophysin-containing fibers of the suprachiasmatic nucleus of the rat run dorsally and rostrally in the subependymal glial plate of the anterior third ventricle (E. Zimmerman, L. Recht, M. Stillman, and R. Defendini, in preparation).

The physiological role of neurohypophyseal peptides in CSF is not fully understood. How much if any vasopressin reaches the portal capillary system via tanycytes is not known. Although immunoreactive neurophysin has been found in tanycytes by light microscopy, vasopressin has not been demonstrated with certainty in tanycytes by these methods, and neither neurophysin nor vasopressin has been demonstrated in tanycytes by electron microscopy (LeClerc and Pelletier, 1974; Pelletier et al., 1974a; Goldsmith and Zimmerman, 1975; Silverman and Zimmerman, 1975). These substances may be difficult to demonstrate in tanycytes by immunocytochemistry owing to problems in fixation.

The CSF route may also be important in the transport of vasopressin to areas of the brain other than the hypothalamus where the hormone may be important in learning (Van Wimersma Greidanus et al., 1975a). It was shown that the normal route by which vasopressin reaches the midbrain limbic circuit, where it may act on memory, is a ventricular pathway. Injections of antiserum to vasopressin and not to oxytocin into the cerebral ventricles of the rat interfere with learning (Van Wimersma Greidanus et al., 1975b).

Localization of Specific Neurophysins, Vasopressin, and Oxytocin

Brattleboro Rats with Diabetes Insipidus

By application of antihuman ESN or an anti-rat neurophysin that cross reacts with all rat neurophysins in the immunoperoxidase technique, it was found that the neurophysin present in DI rats was located in cell bodies concentrated in the dorsal half of the SON and in the PVN, mainly in the lateral wings of the nucleus (Fig. 2–5a; Zimmerman et al., 1975c). In normal rats, including those of the Long-Evans strain, all cells of the SON and approximately 75% of the magnocellular neurons in the PVN contained neurophysin. The neurophysin previously shown to be absent in extracts of the posterior pituitary of vasopressin-deficient DI rats (Burford et al., 1971; Sunde and Sokol, 1975) appears to be missing from the cells of the more ventral SON and more medial PVN. These cells appear to be the neurons that produce vasopressin and its associated neurophysin in the normal rat.

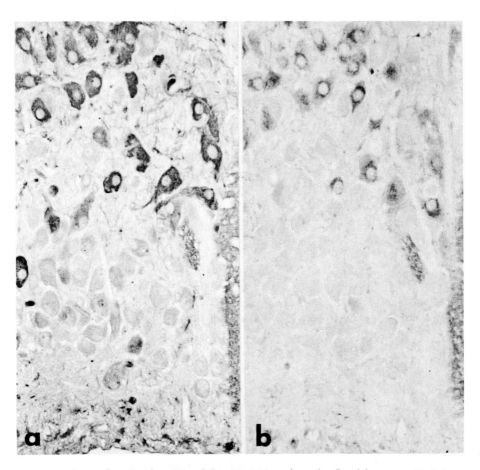

FIG. 2–5. Adjacent 5μ coronal sections of the supraoptic nucleus of a Brattleboro rat with diabetes insipidus (homozygote). *a*: Immunoperoxidase stain using an antiserum to all rat neurophysins. Neurophysin (dark staining) is located in dorsal cells and missing from ventral cells made visible by cresyl violet counter-stain. All supraoptic cells contain neurophysin in normal rat (Fig. 2-1c). *b*: Oxytocin localized in dorsal cells by the same technique using antiserum to oxytocin. ×260. (From E. Zimmerman and H. Sokol, *unpublished data.*)

The more dorsal cells of the SON and more lateral magnocellular neurons of the PVN would then be producing oxytocin and its neurophysin. By applying antioxytocin in the immunoperoxidase method, it has now been shown that the neurophysin-positive cells of DI rats contain oxytocin (Fig. 2–5b), and the oxytocin-containing cells occupy the same positions in the heterozygous Brattleboro rats and in normal rats of this and other strains (Zimmerman et al., 1975c). Rabbit antiserum to oxytocin was prepared using synthetic oxytocin conjugated to thyroglobulin as the immunogen. Antithyroglobulin was removed from the antiserum by absorption before use.

Normal Rats

Burlet et al. (1973) and Sahar et al. (1975; *personal communication*) found that almost all the cells in SON contained immunoreactive vasopressin. Elde (1974) and Zimmerman et al., (1975b,c) found that nearly all SON cells in the rat were vasopressin-positive by the immunoperoxidase technique. The distribution of vasopressin in the magnocellular neurons of the PVN is less certain. Zimmerman et al. (1974b,c) found that the majority of neurons contained the hormone, including cells in the lateral wings; all the other investigators cited above found a smaller number. There appears to be a relative separation of cells forming oxytocin and vasopressin and their associated neurophysins in the two nuclei. This separation was suggested by studies of DI rats with Gomori stains (Sokol and Valtin, 1967). Recent immunocytochemical studies of the bovine hypothalamus demonstrated a complete separation of cells containing oxytocin and NPI and vasopressin and NPII (De Mey et al., 1974; Vandesande et al., 1975a). Some overlap in hormone-neurophysin formation, however, appears to be possible in the rat, particularly in the dorsal SON and perhaps in the PVN as well (Zimmerman et al., 1975c). We also found suggestive evidence that the two hormones appear in the same cell in humans, but we still view this finding with caution. The possibility of some cross reactivity of our antivasopressin with oxytocin, however, appeared to be ruled out by absorption controls in the immunoperoxidase technique (Silverman and Zimmerman, 1975).

Human Hypothalamus

Four peptides were studied in the human hypothalamus (Zimmerman et al., 1975b; R. Defendini, E. Zimmerman, A. Robinson, *in preparation*). Utilizing light microscopy and the immunoperoxidase technique, ESN, NSN, oxytocin, and vasopressin were localized in adjacent serial paraffin sections (Fig. 2–6). Vasopressin and NSN were found in nearly all cells of the SON and in the majority of the magnocellular perikarya in the PVN. Oxytocin and ESN were distributed together, mainly in the medial portion of the dorsolateral part of the SON, and were concentrated in the dorsal cap of the

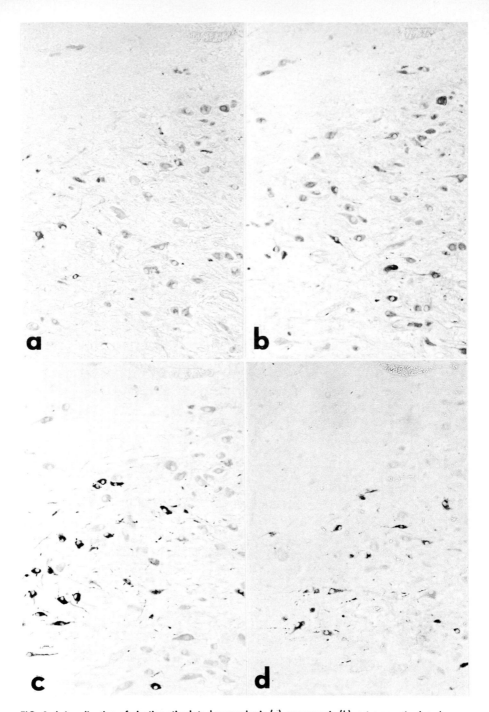

FIG. 2–6. Localization of nicotine-stimulated neurophysin (*a*), vasopressin (*b*), estrogen-stimulated neuro-physin (*c*), and oxytocin (*d*) in adjacent 5 μ sagittal sections of a human supraoptic nucleus by immuno-peroxidase method. Nicotine-stimulated neurophysin and vasopressin are found in virtually all the perikarya. Estrogen-stimulated neurophysin and oxytocin are concentrated in a smaller population of cells. ×100. (*a, b, c*: from Zimmerman et al., 1975b. *d*: from R. Defendini, E. Zimmerman, A. Robinson, *unpublished data.*)

PVN. In man as in the rat, both hormones and both neurophysins were found in large neurons scattered between the SON and PVN, although not necessarily in the same cells. In the magnocellular nuclei there were some cells that contained both hormones and both neurophysins, and other cells which appeared to contain only vasopressin and NSN.

These rat and human data may challenge the absolute one-cell-one-hormone theory and suggest that the independent control of vasopressin and oxytocin secretion is determined, at least in part, by subcellular mechanisms. Studies are in progress to establish this possibility more firmly. Evidence for the formation of more than one hormone in a particular cell has, however, been noted in the anterior pituitary, where the following pairs of hormones have been reported in the same cell: FSH and LH (Phifer et al., 1973), GH and prolactin (Zimmerman et al., 1974c), and MSH and ACTH (Moriarty, 1973).

Since NSN and vasopressin are secreted together into the systemic circulation (Robinson, 1975), it was no surprise to find them in the same cell. This confirmation was significantly supplemented by finding oxytocin in cells containing ESN. Although both oxytocin and ESN rise during pregnancy (Kumaresan et al., 1972; Robinson, 1975), direct physiological data that oxytocin is secreted along with ESN awaits simultaneous studies of the two peptides in plasma. It is expected, however, that oxytocin may be influenced by ovarian events. Roberts and Share (1969) demonstrated that estradiol administration for a week significantly increases the amount of oxytocin released after vaginal distention in sheep. The marked rise in ESN after estradiol administration and during the midcycle surge of LH in man (Robinson, 1975) and monkey (Robinson et al., 1974) may be accompanied by oxytocin. Since ESN is also present in high concentrations in monkey portal blood (Table 2–1), it is not unlikely that significant amounts of oxytocin also reach the anterior pituitary.

Vasopressin could normally play a role in the release of ACTH from the anterior pituitary, possibly assisting the action of CRH (Yates et al., 1971). Although a role for oxytocin in adenohypophyseal function has not been established (Doepfner, 1968; Reichlin and Mitnick, 1973), its administration did release FSH in man (Franchimont, 1971). Since it has been shown that oxytocin can compete with the enzymatic destruction of LRH *in vitro* (Griffith et al., 1974), a possible midcycle peak of oxytocin accompanying ESN would make more LRH available for the LH surge. Another role for oxytocin in the anterior pituitary may be to inhibit the release of melanocyte-stimulating hormone by the tripeptide fragment of the hormone formed enzymatically (Walter et al., 1973).

Suprachiasmatic Nucleus

It was recently shown that the suprachiasmatic nucleus (SCN) of the rat (Vandesande et al., 1974; Zimmerman et al., 1975b) and mouse (Zimmerman et al., 1975*b*) contains neurophysin and vasopressin (Zimmerman et al., 1975*b*). This first demonstration of neurophysin or vasopressin in parvicellular neurons strongly suggests a neurosecretory role for this nucleus (Fig. 2–7). These cells did not appear to contain oxytocin in the normal rat (Vandesande et al., 1975*b*).

On the basis of ultrastructural studies of the hypothalamus of the rat, Clementi and Ceccarelli (1970) suggested that the arcuate neurons were the only cells other than magnocellular neurons which might have neurosecretory function. They found that cells of the SCN contained some vesicles not interpreted as neurosecretory. In similar studies Suburo and Pellegrino de Iraldi (1969) found small granulated vesicles or granules, often near the Golgi apparatus, and small axons with varicosities containing mixed vesicles, which they thought compatible with neurosecretion. Clattenberg and co-workers (1972) found evidence for neurosecretion in the suprachiasmatic nucleus of the rabbit after coitus by demonstrating the appearance of larger (1,542 Å) vesicles.

Where are the terminations of suprachiasmatic axons? This question is particularly important in the light of reports that the SCN generates adrenal rhythms (Moore and Eichler, 1972). The studies of Szentágothai et al. (1968) and Vandesande et al. (1974) suggest that axons of the SCN project caudally to the portal system in the median eminence. Frontal cuts immedi-

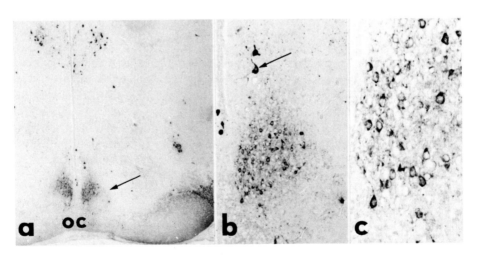

FIG. 2–7. Coronal section of albino rat anterior hypothalamus reacted with antihuman neurophysin. Immunoperoxidase stain. *a*: Low-power micrograph showing neurophysin in the paired suprachiasmatic nucleus (SCN) over the optic chiasm (OC). Arrow points to right portion of the SCN. Neurophysin is also seen in the paired anterior portions of the paraventricular nucleus (*upper left*) and in the supraoptic nucleus (*lower right*). *b*: High-power micrograph of area at arrow in *a* showing neurophysin concentrated in the dorsal cells of the SCN, which are about one-third the size of magnocellular neurons (*arrow*). Fine fibers pass dorsally from the apex of the SCN. ×180. *c*: Higher magnification of *b*. A stained fiber, presumably an axon, can be followed from a cell body (at *lower left*). ×260. (From E. Zimmerman, M. Stillman, L. Recht, and R. Defendini, *unpublished data.*)

ately caudal but not rostral to the SCN abolish the diurnal rhythm in corti-costerone secretion (Moore and Eichler, 1972). Since Vandesande et al. (1974) found an increase in neurophysin staining in the SCN and zona externa after adrenalectomy, it would be appealing to consider that vaso-pressin or CRH associated with a neurophysin (Watkins et al., 1974) medi-ates the influence of this system on ACTH in the rat. It is unlikely, however, that CRH is the mediator in the neurophysin-positive cells since these cells in the SCN are neurophysin- and vasopressin-negative in our unpublished studies of DI rats, which are known to have CRH (Yates et al., 1971).

The very fine axons of the SCN neurons are very difficult to follow by any staining method, and they could not be traced caudally for any distance by the immunoperoxidase technique for vasopressin and neurophysin. They could be seen passing directly dorsally (Fig. 2–7) and rostrally to run up under the ependyma in the lateral wall and floor of the third ventricle (E. Zimmerman, L. Recht, M. Stillman, and R. Defendini, *in preparation*). Unlike Vandesande et al. (1974), we noticed no changes in neurophysin or vasopressin in the SCN 1 to 3 weeks after adrenalectomy.

If axons of the SCN pass caudally to hypothalamic regions other than the zona externa, as discussed recently by Moore and Klein (1974) in reference to a possible polysynaptic pathway from SCN to the pineal, one wonders if vasopressin fibers of SCN might end on CRH-secreting neurons. In this situation vasopressin would be acting as a neurotransmitter to release CRH. A central action of vasopressin on CRH release was postulated by Hedge and associates (1966), who found that vasopressin was more effective in releasing ACTH when it was injected into the ventral hypothalamus than when injected into the anterior pituitary. Further studies are needed to de-termine if vasopressin-containing fibers from the SCN serve to mediate the diurnal rhythm in ACTH in rodents, and if the direct retinal pathways to the ventral portions of the SCN (Moore and Lenn, 1972; Moore, 1973; Campbell and Ramaley, 1974) terminate on vasopressin and neurophysin neurons.

LOCALIZATION OF LRH

Zona Externa

LRH, a decapeptide, has been the subject of a number of immunocyto-chemical studies during the last 2 yr by both fluorescence and peroxidase labeling methods (Kordon and Ramirez, 1975; Kozlowski et al., 1975). The most consistent finding in a variety of mammals has been the concentration of LRH in the zona externa of the median eminence (Barry et al., 1973; Baker et al., 1974; King et al., 1974; Kordon et al., 1974; Hökfelt et al., 1975; Kozlowski et al., 1975; Sétaló et al., 1975). As shown by Baker et al. (1974) in coronal sections of the midmedian eminence in many species,

LRH tends to be concentrated in the lateral portions of the contact zone (Fig. 2–8) compared to vasopressin, which is present in all portions (Zimmerman et al., 1975*b*). In coronal sections of the guinea pig, LRH is located along the entire sweep of the contact zone (Baker et al., 1974). In the rat LRH is also found in the anterior median eminence and can be traced to the retrochiasmatic area (Kordon et al., 1974). There is also a large concentration of LRH in the caudal median eminence in the guinea pig (Leonardelli et al., 1973) and rat (Kordon et al., 1974). By both light and electron microscopy LRH-containing fibers are also seen in the zona interna and even more dorsally in the median eminence in the subependymal lining of the floor of the third ventricle (Kordon et al., 1974; Goldsmith and Ganong, 1975; Kordon and Ramirez, 1975).

Most investigators have interpreted the light microscopic findings in the zona externa to mean that LRH is contained in axon terminals on portal capillaries because of their course and beaded appearance as well as the lack of staining in the cell bodies of tanycytes, which also project to the portal capillaries (Kobayashi and Matsui, 1969). The lateral concentration of LRH in the zona externa appears to correspond to the region occupied by terminals of the tuberoinfundibular tract from the arcuate nucleus as shown by silver stains (Szentágothai et al., 1968; King et al., 1974), and to the area of terminals of arcuate dopaminergic fibers (Hökfelt et al., 1975).

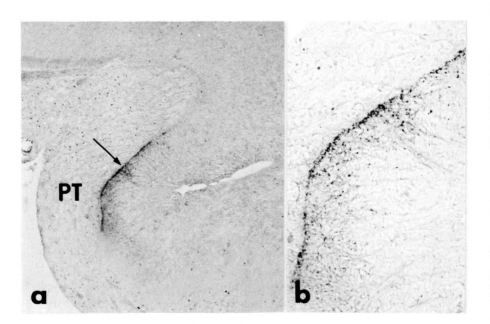

FIG. 2-8. Concentration of LRH in the lateral zona externa (arrow) along the pars tuberalis (PT) of a sheep median eminence. Coronal section. Immunoperoxidase technique. *a:* ×65. *b:* ×280. (From Kozlowski et al., 1975.)

Two immunoelectron microscopic studies have now confirmed that LRH is contained in granules within axon terminals near portal capillaries in the rat (Goldsmith and Ganong, 1974; 1975; Pelletier et al., 1974b). The presence of LRH in small (750 to 950 Å) granules (Pelletier et al., 1974b) in these axon terminals lends strong support to the concept that LRH is a neurosecretory product. Vasopressin and neurophysin were found in large granules in different terminals on portal capillaries in the same rat preparations (Fig. 2–4; Goldsmith and Zimmerman, 1975). It was previously found by centrifugation that 1,000 Å granules contained LRH, and 1,200 to 1,800 Å granules from the median eminence were rich in vasopressin, oxytocin, and CRH (Kobayashi et al., 1970). By immunoelectron microscopy somatostatin has been localized in granules of about 1,000 Å diameter in terminals in rat zona externa (Pelletier et al., 1974c).

Arcuate Nucleus

Immunocytochemical data support the concept that LRH is a secretory product of the hypothalamus. The largest regional hypothalamic concentration of LRH by radioimmunoassay (Palkovits et al., 1974a; Wheaton et al., 1975) and by bioassay (McCann et al., 1975; Wheaton et al., 1975) is located in the median eminence, where LRH is concentrated in axon terminals. The next highest concentration is in the arcuate nucleus (Palkovits et al., 1974a; Wheaton et al., 1975), which contains the cell bodies that contribute the largest number of fibers to the tuberoinfundibular tract (Haymaker, 1969) and is the presumed site of LRH formation (Szentágothai et al., 1968; Zambrano, 1969; Raisman, 1972; Zimmerman et al., 1974b). If the neurosecretory theory applies to LRH in parvicellular perikarya in the arcuate nucleus as it does to vasopressin in magnocellular neurons, then the LRH-containing granules seen in the zona externa should be traceable to their cell bodies of origin. The most pressing problem in the immunocytochemical localization of LRH is the inability of most studies to identify LRH in perikarya (Kordon et al., 1974; Kordon, 1975; Kordon and Ramirez, 1975). A major reason for failure may simply be a low concentration of LRH in the cell body compared to the terminal, or loss of LRH or its immunoreactivity from the tissues by the procedures so that only the highest concentrations can be seen. Goldsmith and Ganong (1975) found that 98% of the immunoreactive LRH was lost from their hypothalamic tissues during the dehydrating and embedding procedures for electron microscopy. Differences in tissue processing may be the reason why vasopressin has been localized in magnocellular perikarya using immunoperoxidase techniques with light microscopy but not with electron microscopy (Le Clerc and Pelletier, 1974). Kordon (1975) suggested that there may be too little LRH stored in perikarya to be detected, or that LRH may be in the form of a prohormone that does not react with the antiserum.

The extensive work of Barry and co-workers focused on the problem of visualization of perikaryal LRH (Barry and Dubois, 1974; Barry et al., 1974). Since significant amounts of LRH may be stored only at the terminals, Barry's group used a number of procedures to stop axonal flow, *viz.,* colchicine and intraventricular methanol (Barry et al., 1974). By these and other methods primarily in guinea pigs, they showed LRH by immunofluorescence in the cell bodies of arcuate neurons and noted a number of reactive cells in the preoptic region. They described a preopticoinfundibular pathway containing LRH. That such a pathway exists was supported in earlier localization studies by bioassay of extracts of hypothalamic regions. These studies showed significant amounts of LRH in the preoptic-suprachiasmatic region and decreased LRH in the median eminence after lesions had been produced in the suprachiasmatic region (Schneider et al., 1969). Electrical stimulation of the preoptic region induced ovulation (Terasawa and Sawyer, 1969), and knife cuts caudal to it abolished ovulation in the rat (Szentágothai et al., 1968). The LRH-containing cells described by Barry et al. (1974) were scattered. Some were located around the anterior commissure and others in the parolfactory cortex. Positive fibers were seen passing to "extrahypothalamic" regions as well. Hökfelt and associates (1974b) reported LRH-containing fibers in the amygdala. More recent regional studies by bioassay and radioimmunoassay have shown that most of the LRH in the preoptic area is located in the area of the OVLT (Wheaton, 1975; Wheaton et al., 1975). Most of the cell bodies described by Barry and co-workers in the preoptic area lie outside this structure, although some may project to it (Barry et al., 1974).

In our own studies there was LRH staining in about 10% of arcuate perikarya (Fig. 2–9a,c) in both male and female adult mice (Zimmerman et al., 1974b). The positive cells were located primarily in the dorsomedial parts of the nucleus. As seen by light microscopy, this staining was peculiar in that it was often located at the periphery of the cell and in some cases even appeared to lie outside the cell body. In some cells, however, it seemed to be entirely intracytoplasmic. Rarely the staining could be followed for a short distance, presumably in an axon process. Since our previous report (Zimmerman et al., 1974b), we have reproduced our findings in the murine arcuate nucleus by using three different anti-LRH antisera in several different strains and with dilutions as high as 1:4,000 (A. Silverman, G. Kozlowski, and E. Zimmerman, *unpublished observations*). (Two of these antisera were provided by G. Niswender and another by S. Sorrentino, Jr.) All the antisera had been prepared using BSA conjugates, and anti-BSA was removed by absorption before use. Arcuate perikarya comprised the only neuronal group we could identify, and this may be the only nucleus (except for the lateral portion of the ventromedial nucleus) that contains LRH (Palkovits et al., 1974a; Wheaton et al., 1975).

Another significant problem in LRH localization by immunocytochemistry is the differences in staining peculiar to different species. For example, in

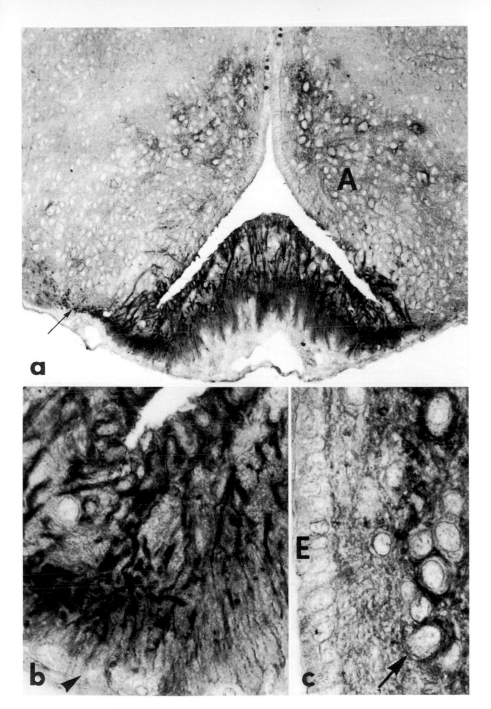

FIG. 2–9. Demonstration of LRH in the middle portion of the mouse median eminence by immunoperoxidase method. Coronal section. *a:* LRH concentrated in dorsomedial cells of the arcuate nucleus (A), lateral zona externa (*arrow*), and tanycytes. ✕200. *b:* Higher magnification of the left side of the median eminence in *a* shows LRH-reaction products in the cytoplasm of the entire length of numerous tanycytes from the floor and lower walls of the third ventricle to their endings in the zona externa (*arrow head*). ✕600. *c:* Arcuate perikarya near the ependymal lining (E) along the right side of the ventricle in *a*. Fine reaction products to LRH are seen within the entire cytoplasm of some cells (*arrow*) at the periphery of others. ✕600. (From Zimmerman et al., 1974a.)

the mouse we see what appears to be some axonal staining in the lateral zona externa, as well as tanycyte and arcuate reactivity. The same procedure on the rat produces staining in the lateral zona externa as described by Baker et al. (1974), some staining in tanycytes, and none in arcuate nucleus (Zimmerman et al., 1974a). Kozlowski and Zimmerman (*unpublished observations*) were unable to stain LRH in the rhesus monkey, but Kordon (1975) found it in the zona externa of the baboon. Antisera to LRH in the radioimmunoassay, however, detect high concentrations of LRH in rhesus monkey portal blood (Carmel et al., 1975) and extracts of rat hypothalamus (Araki et al., 1975). These species differences in immunostaining are totally without explanation but may reflect some physical chemical differences in the may the same molecule is held in the tissues.

Tanycytes

Although the immunostaining system showed an LRH concentration in the lateral zona externa in the mouse (Fig. 2–9a), as it does in rat and sheep (Kozlowski et al., 1975), marked staining was found throughout the length of many tanycytes in the median eminence of the mouse (Fig. 2–9b). The immunostaining was intracytoplasmic, dense, and granular—not the usual "fuzzy" reaction products found in a "nonspecific" background. The staining was so strong that the procedure appeared to be one of the best stains available for studying tanycyte morphology. Using anti-BSA and absorption with BSA, controls revealed that the reaction was not due to the presence of anti-BSA, although anti-BSA did react with material in the proximal portions of some tanycytes and in CSF, presumably albumin (Zimmerman et al., 1974b).

The presence of LRH in tanycytes would lend support to the ventricular route hypothesis as a pathway for releasing factors to the portal bed (Ben-Jonathan et al., 1974; Knigge, 1974). LRH could be secreted into the CSF of the third ventricle and carried to the tanycytes in the floor and lower walls of the median eminence and then transported to portal blood (Scott et al., 1974b). The significant amounts of LRH recently reported in the CSF obtained from the third ventricle of rats (Joseph et al., 1975), if confirmed, would also support a CSF-tanycyte pathway to portal blood. It is not known whether tanycytes can take up LRH from their terminals in the contact zone and transport it in the reverse direction to CSF or store it and resecrete it (Oota et al., 1974; Zimmerman et al., 1974b). The marked changes in the ultrastructure of tanycytes during the menstrual cycle or after estrogen treatment in the monkey, however, does suggest that they have some role in reproduction (Kumar and Knowles, 1967).

Organum Vasculosum of the Lamina Terminalis

Immunoreactive LRH was found around the OVLT of the mouse (Fig. 2–10a,b; Zimmerman et al., 1974b), guinea pig (Barry et al., 1974, and rat

(Fig. 2–10c; Kordon, 1975). Whether the LRH was in axon or tanycyte terminals could not be established in the mouse, but the studies of Barry et al. (1974) and Kordon (1975) suggested it was located in axon terminals.

The OVLT is a circumventricular organ located just anterior to the optic chiasm in the midline in the floor (Fig. 2–10a,b) and the very anterior end of the third ventricle in the lamina terminalis (Weindl and Joynt, 1972; Weindl, 1973). Also called the supraoptic crest, this structure has axon and tanycyte terminals on fenestrated capillaries as in the median eminence (Röhlich and Wenger, 1969). The earlier studies of the hypophyseal vascular system revealed that the OVLT shares a peculiar permeability to vital dyes with the more caudal hypophyseal portal system (Wislocki and King, 1936). LRH might then be secreted into the fenestrated capillaries of the OVLT as it is in the median eminence. That OVLT plays a role in reproduction was suggested previously by Leveque (1972).

The OVLT is the subject of considerable interest at present as both immunohistochemical and regional assay approaches have localized LRH in or near this structure, which lies in the middle of the preoptic area. Although Palkovits et al. (1974a) did not report LRH anterior to the arcuate nucleus in the rat, it was described in earlier (Crighton et al., 1970) and more recent (Araki et al., 1975) regional studies. McCann and co-workers (Wheaton, 1975; Wheaton et al., 1975) have now repeated their earlier studies using frozen serial sections in three planes and new bioassays for LRH and FRH and a radioimmunoassay for LRH. Nearly all the LRH in the preoptic area was located in extracts of the region of the OVLT. Smaller amounts were found in the very basal midline of the hypothalamus from the region behind the OVLT to the arcuate nucleus and median eminence.

Recently, R. Weiner, working in Kordon's laboratory (personal communication) found evidence that the LRH in the OVLT is independent from that in the mediobasal hypothalamus. In the rat, after deafferentation of the mediobasal hypothalamus by Halasz-type knife cuts (Halasz, 1969), there was about a 75% decrease in the LRH content in the island and a reduction in immunoperoxidase staining in LRH-containing fibers in the median eminence, whereas there was no change in LRH in the OVLT by either method. These observations suggest that the LRH which appears to be in axon terminals in the OVLT is formed in cell bodies outside the arcuate or ventromedial nucleus, perhaps in parikarya in the preoptic area (Barry et al., 1974). Additional evidence for an LRH system anterior to and independent from the midhypothalamus was also recently reported in relation to ovarian function in the rat (Araki et al., 1975). Variations in the content of LRH were different in the two regions during the estrous cycle and after castration. The studies of Wheaton et al. (1975) would indicate that most of the LRH measured in the anterior region by Araki et al. (1975) was located in the OVLT.

These new findings raise important questions about the mechanism by which the preoptic area and projections from the amygdala and other brain

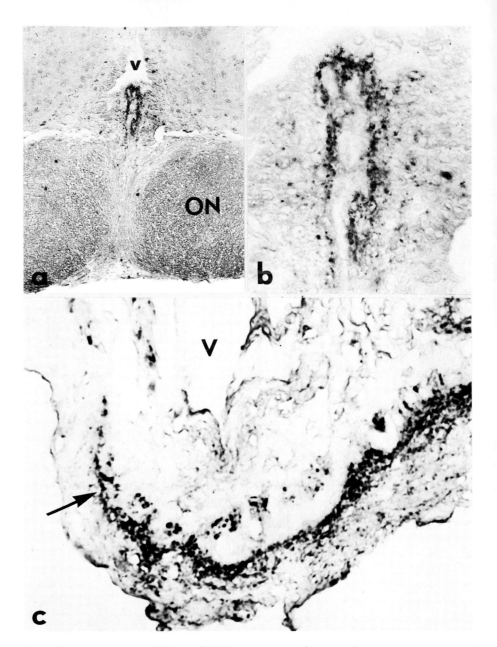

FIG. 2–10. Demonstration of LRH in the OVLT by immunoperoxidase procedures. *a:* Low-power view of LRH in a coronal section of mouse OVLT which lies between and above the optic nerves (ON) and rostral to the chiasm. V, anterior tip of the third ventricle. *b:* Higher magnification of *a,* demonstrating LRH around the vascular structure of the OVLT. ×350. *c:* Sagittal section of rat hypothalamus demonstrating LRH-containing terminals in the OVLT (*arrow*). V, third ventricle. ×600. (*a* and *b:* from Zimmerman et al., 1974a. *c:* from Kordon and Ramirez, 1975.)

regions (Raisman and Field, 1971) that converge on this area regulate ovulation (Everett, 1965). If all "preoptic" LRH is located in the OVLT, does this structure represent the final common pathway for the secretion of LRH by this region? If the venous drainage of the OVLT reaches the anterior pituitary gland, the specialized capillary system in the preoptic region would represent an "anterior accessory hypophyseal portal system." There is no evidence at present, however, that the venous drainage of the OVLT communicates with the hypophyseal portal system. Duvernoy et al. (1969), in a careful study of 30 human brains in which they injected India ink and gelatin solution into the cerebral vasculature at autopsy, determined that the veins of the OVLT drain into the systemic circulation via the anterior cerebral veins. They also reviewed the work of Mergner on the OVLT of the monkey and concluded that this organ does not have a venous connection with the portal system in man or monkey. Their histological studies did suggest neurosecretion into the capillary bed of the OVLT in primates. These studies raise the possibility that LRH is secreted into the systemic circulation at a very specific site in the preoptic area. The physiological importance of this pathway is not immediately evident since there is no known role for LRH in the systemic circulation. Studies of the OVLT are needed in the rat since there may be species differences in its drainage and the preoptic area appears to be important in the ovulatory surge in the rat (Halász, 1969) and not in the monkey (Krey et al., 1975).

The preoptic area may also control the ovulatory surge in the rat by pathways to the arcuate-median eminence region that do not contain LRH or by a ventricular route carrying LRH from the anterior to the middle third ventricle. It is not known, however, if the axon terminals in the anterior third ventricle (Scott et al., 1974a) contain LRH. In addition, the transport capacity of the numerous tanycytes in the OVLT to or from CSF has not been studied (Weindl, 1973). Theoretical portal or CSF pathways that might transport LRH from the OVLT would not fully explain the findings of Tejasen and Everett (1967) concerning the preopticotuberal pathway. It seems unlikely that the specific point-to-point relationship between the preoptic area and the hypophysiotropic region, demonstrated in rats by unilateral stimulation of the preoptic area and unilateral frontal cuts near the suprachiasmatic region which abolished ovulation, would involve the OVLT, which appears to be a common midline structure. Future studies of the preoptic area and ovulation, however, must consider the OVLT.

Pineal Gland

Large amounts of LRH and TRH have been reported in the pineal gland (White et al., 1974). Using bioassay and radioimmunoassay, four to 10 times more LRH was found in extracts of porcine, ovine, and bovine pineal than in hypothalamus extracts. Kozlowski and Zimmerman (1974) reported

LRH in the mouse and sheep pineal using an immunoperoxidase technique, although the staining proved inconsistent in subsequent studies. LRH was not found in extracts of sheep and monkey pineal glands by radioimmunoassay (Araki et al., 1975). Further studies are needed to establish the presence and importance of LRH in the pineal gland.

LOCALIZATION OF SOMATOSTATIN

At present there are only four immunocytochemical studies of the most recently characterized hypothalamic hormone, somatostatin (Burgus et al., 1973). Using an antiserum generated by a conjugate of this tetradecapeptide to human α-globulin in an immunofluorescence technique, Hökfelt et al. (1974b) found somatostatin close to portal capillaries in the caudal zona externa and upper stalk of the guinea pig. Staining was also seen around portal capillary loops deeper in the median eminence. A similar distribution was found in the rat median eminence by light microscopy and an immunoperoxidase technique (Pelletier et al., 1975), except that somatostatin staining was more intense in the lateral parts of the zona externa. This is reminiscent of the differences in the distribution of LRH in these two species (Baker et al., 1974). Although Pelletier et al. (1975) did not report somatostatin in other regions of the hypothalamus, Hökfelt et al. (1974b) noted a dot-fiber pattern, probably axonal, primarily in the ventromedial nucleus. Some somatostatin-containing fibers were also seen in the periventricular nucleus, basal lateral hypothalamus, and amygdala. Hökfelt et al. (1974b) reported a similar distribution for somatostatin- and LRH-positive fibers except that LRH was also found in the more anterior portions of the zona externa but not in the ventromedial nucleus.

Like thyrotropin-releasing hormone (TRH; Brownstein et al., 1974a), somatostatin is concentrated in the zona externa and is widely distributed in the brain, as seen in regional studies in the rat (Brownstein et al., 1975). Somatostatin was concentrated in the hypothalamus and was highest in the median eminence. There was some somatostatin in all hypothalamic nuclei but relatively more in the arcuate, ventral premammillary, and ventromedial nuclei. In the rest of the brain the amygdala was one of the areas relatively rich in somatostatin (Brownstein et al., 1975). Hökfelt et al. (1974b) discussed the possibility that the somatostatin present in nerve fibers in the ventromedial nucleus may serve to inhibit cells that secrete GH-releasing factor (Martin, 1974; see also Chapter 5).

Using immunoelectron microscopic techniques, Pelletier and associates (1974b) localized somatostatin within 900 to 1,100-Å granules in 30% of the nerve endings on portal capillaries in the zona externa of the rat. Some positive fibers were also present in zona interna close to negative fibers of the hypothalamohypophyseal tract. Somatostatin has not been localized in perikarya in the brain but has been found in the cytoplasm of pancreatic cells, which are probably α-cells (Luft et al., 1974). Somatostatin may be produced in these cells to inhibit glucagon secretion.

Pelletier et al. (1975) found somatostatin in three circumventricular organs other than the median eminence in the rat: the OVLT, subcommissural organ, and pineal gland. Immunostaining in the OVLT and pineal gland was close to capillaries, and in the subcommissural organ was in the ependyma. Somatostatin as well as LRH may be secreted into the capillaries of the OVLT.

LOCALIZATION OF TRH

TRH, like somatostatin, is generally distributed in the brain, with a large concentration in the hypothalamus (Brownstein et al., 1974a; Jackson and Reichlin, 1974; Winokur and Utiger, 1974). There are no reported immunochemistry studies in which TRH was localized intracellularly. One reason for this failure is the possibility that TRH may not be formed on ribosomes and packaged and transported in granules. It may be formed instead by enzymatic action in the cytoplasm (Reichlin and Mitnick, 1973). In addition, the tripeptide TRH may be more easily lost during tissue processing than the larger peptide hormones or neurophysin proteins.

INTERACTIONS OF HORMONE-SECRETING NEURONS WITH STEROID HORMONES, TRANSMITTERS, AND OTHER REGULATORS

Once the hormone-forming cells are identified, the signals which regulate neurosecretion can be better understood. Interactions between specific neurosecretory cells, steroid receptors, brain pathways containing specific neurotransmitters, and homeostatic signals such as osmolality will be the subject of many future studies. Some of these correlations can be suggested from existing data.

Steroid Hormones

Estrogen-stimulated neurophysin offers one hypothalamic parameter to help unravel the mechanisms involved in the positive feedback effect of estradiol on the monkey hypothalamus (Knobil, 1974). As in the rat (Stumpf, 1970; Pfaff and Keiner, 1973), preliminary autoradiographic studies of the monkey hypothalamus (Gerlach et al., 1974) show that some magnocellular neurons incorporate estrogen. It remains to be proved, possibly by simultaneous autoradiographic and immunocytochemical studies, whether the same cells which contain ESN have estradiol receptors. Estrogen-sensitive neurons ending on ESN-forming cells may also be involved in the ovarian regulation of ESN. There is a good correlation between the avid incorporation of estrogen (Stumpf, 1970; Pfaff and Keiner, 1973) and the probable formation of LRH in the arcuate nucleus (Palkovits et al., 1974a; Zimmerman et al., 1974b).

Adrenal steroids appear to have significant and complicated effects on neurophysin (Vandesande et al., 1974; Watkins et al., 1974), vasopressin (Seif et al., 1975), and CRH (Yates et al., 1971). It is not known if the adrenal steroids incorporated by the hypothalamus (McEwen and Pfaff, 1973; Gerlach et al., 1974) act differently on the cell bodies or terminals of vasopressin- and neurophysin-containing neurons in the zona externa. Investigations of the increased immunostaining of these peptides in the zona externa after adrenalectomy will have to consider the inhibitory role of norepinephrine (Cross, 1973) present in fibers innervating this region (Bjorklund et al., 1973). In addition, inhibitory actions of glucocorticoids on tyrosine hydroxylase in the median eminence may regulate the catecholamine terminals in the zona externa (Kizer et al., 1974).

Biogenic Amines

The distribution of catecholamines in the hypothalamus is detailed in Chapter 1. A few correlations with hormone-producing cells should be mentioned. Both norepinephrine (Abrahams and Pickford, 1956) and epinephrine (Olsson, 1970) can inhibit the secretion of vasopressin and oxytocin (Ginsburg, 1968) when given by several routes. Evidence that these catecholamines, particularly norepinephrine, could act on the cells of the SON and PVN was shown by histofluorescence studies. Catecholamine-containing terminals were found on these cells (Fuxe, 1965) which appeared to be axosomatic (Fuxe and Hökfelt, 1969). These findings have been confirmed by immunofluorescence studies using anti-DBH as a marker for norepinephrine (Hartman et al., 1972; Hökfelt et al., 1973) and anti-PNMT for epinephrine (Hökfelt et al., 1974a). It is of interest that more norepinephrine (Palkovits et al., 1974b), DBH (Saavedra et al., 1974a), and PNMT (Saavedra et al., 1974b) were contained in the PVN than the SON. Since both oxytocin and vasopressin are formed in both nuclei, a differential control of the two hormones may be regulated in part by difference in catecholamine innervation. The concentration of norepinephrine terminals on ventral vasopressin cells of the SON and parvicellular neurons of the PVN (Fuxe, 1965), which contain neither octapeptide, suggests that this transmitter may normally inhibit vasopressin more than oxytocin.

Norepinephrine is in the outer rim of the SCN, whereas serotonin is more central (Saavedra et al., 1974c).

It is interesting that the neurophysin- and vasopressin-containing cells tend to cap and encircle the major portion of the nucleus (Fig. 2–7). Fuxe (1965) demonstrated that serotonin-containing fibers end in the ventral part of the SCN. These data suggest that norepinephrine may regulate vasopressin in the SCN as in the SON. Serotonin may have a different function in the three vasopressin-forming nuclei in the rat. Brownstein and associates (1974b) have also shown that these three nuclei contain significant concentrations of histamine, a putative transmitter which may stimulate vasopressin secretion (Bennett et al., 1973).

Combined immunohistochemical studies using antisera to the hormones and to synthesizing enzymes of putative transmitters should further clarify the structural relationships between the glandular and neural functions of the brain. Labeling specific cells after electrophysiological studies by unit recording techniques (Cross, 1973) will also advance our understanding of neurosecretory mechanisms. It may be possible to determine if units in the PVN which respond to suckling (Cross, 1973) contain oxytocin, and if osmosensitive cells near or in the SON (Hayward and Vincent, 1970) produce vasopressin.

SUMMARY AND CONCLUSIONS

Immunocytochemistry is a new approach to neurosecretion. Information concerning the specific sites of synthesis and the pathways that transport and secrete a number of hypothalamic hormones has been obtained by these methods during the last few years.

It is now known that vasopressin and oxytocin and their associated neurophysins are located in the perikarya of magnocellular neurons of both the SON and PVN. Although there is a regional separation of the cells containing each of the hormones, there is some evidence that oxytocin cells may also form vasopressin.

Vasopressin and neurophysin are found in parvicellular neurons in the SCN of the rat and mouse. Although the significance of this new finding is not known, the location of these cells might suggest a role for vasopressin in mediating the diurnal variation of ACTH. In addition to the classic terminals in the posterior pituitary gland, there is now ample evidence that vasopressin and neurophysin are also contained in axon terminals on the portal capillary bed in the median eminence. Vasopressin may normally participate in ACTH and GH release from the anterior pituitary gland. The high concentrations of ESN in hypophyseal portal blood and the localization of oxytocin in ESN cells suggest that significant amounts of this hormone also reach the anterior pituitary.

LRH and somatostatin are found in granules within axon terminals near portal capillaries in the median eminence. These appear to be terminals of small neurons, which supports the earlier theory that the parvicellular system secretes hormones into the hypophyseal portal blood. The exact sites and mechanism of formation and transport of the hormones to these terminals remain uncertain. Unlike the octapeptides, LRH and somatostatin have not been adequately localized in cell bodies and their axons. Failure to localize perikaryal hormone may be due to problems in the techniques currently used, which may result in a loss of most of the hormone antigen from the tissues.

Both LRH and somatostatin are found by light microscopy in the OVLT of rodents. The nature of the staining suggests that they may be secreted into this vascular organ. Available evidence concerning venous drainage of the OVLT in primates suggests that these hormones are secreted into the systemic circulation at this site in the preoptic region. Since recent regional assay studies reveal that most of the LRH in the preoptic area of the rat is in the OVLT, further studies will be concerned with the possibility of a communication of the OVLT with the hypophyseal portal system by veins or by a CSF route.

A new interest in the CSF and a ventricular route for neuroendocrine communication has been stimulated by a variety of scattered reports of secretory peptides in a number of circumventricular organs; LRH and somatostatin are found in the pineal gland and the OVLT, somatostatin in the subcommissural organ, LRH and neurophysin in median eminence tanycytes, and vasopressin and neurophysin in axon terminals projecting into the floor of the third ventricle from the median eminence. Confirmation of these reports and further studies of these hormones in CSF may add importance to the proposed tanycyte route to portal blood and suggest a route by which hypophysiotropic hormones may reach extrahypothalamic sites of action.

ACKNOWLEDGMENTS

The author's work was supported by a Teacher-Investigator Award from the NINDS (USPHS, NS 11008) and by a Ford Foundation grant to the International Institute for The Study of Human Reproduction, Columbia University.

The contributions of many fellow scientists made this chapter possible: R. Defendini, P. C. Goldsmith, K. C. Hsu, C. Kordon, C. P. Kozlowski, A. G. Robinson, A. J. Silverman, H. W. Sokol, and M. Tannenbaum. The chapter was made more current by investigators quoted in the text who kindly reported work in progress and manuscripts in press. Special appreciation is expressed to my assistant S. Rosario; to R. Defendini, D. Toran-Allerand, and A. Lamme for excellent photographic assistance; and to M. Ferin and B. Scharrer for helpful criticism of the manuscript. P. Czernichow prepared the rabbit antiserum to oxytocin. M. K. Husain performed the vasopressin assays on the Brattleboro strain rats.

REFERENCES

Abrahams, V. C., and Pickford, M. (1956): Observations on a central antagonism between adrenaline and acetyl choline. *J. Physiol. (Lond.)*, 131:712–718.

Acher, R. R., and Du Vigneaud, V. (1958): Purification of oxytocin and vasopressin by way of a protein complex. *J. Biol. Chem.*, 233:116–119.

Araki, S., Ferin, M., Zimmerman, E. A., and Vande Wiele, R. L. (1975): Ovarian modulation of immunoreactive gonadotropin releasing hormone (Gn-RH) in the rat brain: Evidence for a differential effect on the anterior and mid-hypothalamus. *Endocrinology*, 96:644–650.

Avareameas, S. (1970): Immunoenzyme techniques: Enzymes as markers for localization of antigens and antibodies. *Int. Rev. Cytol.*, 27:349–385.

Baker, B. L., Dermody, W. C., and Reel, J. R. (1974): Localization of luteinizing hormone-releasing hormone in the mammalian hypothalamus. *Am. J. Anat.*, 139:129–134.

Bargmann, W. (1966): Neurosecretion. *Int. Rev. Cytol.*, 19:183–201.

Bargmann, W. (1968): Neurohypophysis: structure and function. In: *Handbook of Experimental Pharmacology, Vol. 23: Neurohypophyseal Hormones and Similar Polypeptides*, edited by B. Berde, pp. 1–39. Springer-Verlag, New York.

Barry, J., and Dubois, M. P. (1974): Étude en immunofluorescence de la différenciation prénatale des cellules hypothalamiques élaboratrices de LH-RH de la maturation de la voie neurosécrétice préoptico-infundibulaire chez le cobaye. *Brain Res.*, 67:103–113.

Barry, J., Dubois, M. P., and Poulain, P. (1973): LRF producing cells of the mammalian hypothalamus. *Z. Zellforsch.*, 146:351–366.

Barry, J., Dubois, M. P., and Carette, B. (1974): Immunofluorescence study of the preoptico-infundibular LRF neurosecretory pathway in the normal, castrated or testosterone-treated male guinea pig. *Endocrinology*, 95:1416–1423.

Ben-Jonathan, N., Mical, R. S., and Porter, J. C. (1974): Transport of LRF from CSF to hypophysial portal and systemic blood and the release of LH. *Endocrinology*, 95:18–25.

Bennett, C. T., Pert, A., Gall, K. J., and Blair, J. R. (1973): Histamine release of vasopressin: Functional role of histamine in the cat supraoptic nucleus. *Fed. Proc.*, 32:221 (abstract A53).

Björklund, A., Moore, R. Y., Nobin, A., and Stenevi, U. (1973): The organization of the tubero-hypophyseal and reticulo-infundibular catecholamine neuron systems in the rat brain. *Brain Res.*, 51:171–191.

Brownstein, M. J., Palkovits, M., Saavedra, J. M., Bassiri, R., and Utiger, R. D. (1974a): Thyrotropin-releasing hormone in specific nuclei of rat brain. *Science*, 185:267–269.

Brownstein, M. J., Saavedra, J. M., Palkovits, M., and Axelrod, J. (1974b): Histamine content of hypothalamic nuclei of the rat. *Brain Res.*, 77:151–156.

Brownstein, M., Arimura, A., Sato, H., Schally, A. V., and Kizer, J. S. (1975): The regional distribution of somatostatin in the rat brain. *Endocrinology*, 96:1456–1461.

Burford, G. D., Jones, C. W., and Pickering, B. T. (1971): Tentative identification of a vasopressin-neurophysin and an oxytocin-neurophysin in the rat. *Biochem. J.*, 124:809–813.

Burgus, R., Ling, N., Butcher, M., and Guillemin, R. (1973): Primary structure of somatostatin, a hypothalamic peptide that inhibits the secretion of pituitary growth hormone. *Proc. Natl. Acad. Sci., U.S.A.*, 70:684–688.

Burlet, A., Marchetti, J., Duhielle, J. (1973): Etude par immunofluorescence de la réparatition de la vasopressine au niveau du système hypothalamo-neurohypophysaire du rat. *C. R. Soc. Biol. [D] (Paris)*, 167:924–928.

Campbell, C. B. G., and Ramaley, J. (1974): Retinohypothalamic projections: Correlation with onset and the adrenal rhythm in infant rats. *Endocrinology*, 94:1201–1204.

Capra, J. D., and Walter, R. (1975): Primary structure and evolution of neurophysins. *Ann. N.Y. Acad. Sci.*, 248:92–111.

Carmel, P. W., Araki, S., and Ferin, M. (1975): Prolonged stalk blood collection in rhesus monkeys: Pulsatile release of gonadotropin-releasing hormone (GN-RH). *Endocrinology*, 96:Abs. 107.

Cheng, K. W., and Friesen, H. G. (1972): The isolation and characterization of human neurophysin. *J. Clin. Endocrinol. Metab.*, 34:165–176.

Clattenberg, R. E., Singh, R. P., and Montemurro, D. G. (1972): Post coital ultrastructural changes in neurons of the suprachiasmatic nucleus in the rabbit. *Z. Zellforsch.*, 125:448–459.

Clementi, F., and Ceccarelli, B. (1970): Fine structure of rat hypothalamic nuclei. In:

The Hypothalamus, edited by L. Martini, M. Motta, and F. Fraschini, pp. 17–44. Academic Press, New York.

Crighton, D. G., Schneider, H. P. G., and McCann, S. M. (1970): Localization of LH-releasing factor in the hypothalamus and neurohypophysis as determined by in vitro assay. *Endocrinology,* 87:323–329.

Cross, B. A. (1973): Unit responses in the hypothalamus. In: *Frontiers in Neuroendocrinology 1973,* edited by W. F. Ganong and L. Martini, pp. 133–171. Oxford University Press, New York.

Dean, C. R., Hope, D. B., and Kazic, T. (1968): Evidence for the storage of oxytocin with neurophysin-I and vasopressin with neurophysin-II in separate neurosecretory granules. *Br. J. Pharmacol.,* 24:192–193.

DeMey, J., Vandesande, F., and Dierickx, K. (1974): Identification of neurophysin producing cells. II. Identification of neurophysin II and the neurophysin II producing neurons in the bovine hypothalamus. *Cell Tissue Res.,* 153:531–543.

Doepfner, W. (1968): The influence of neurohypophysial peptides on adenohypophysial function. In: *Handbook of Experimental Pharmacology, Vol. 23: Neurohypophysial Hormones and Similar Polypeptides,* edited by B. Berde, pp. 625–654. Springer-Verlag, New York.

Duvernoy, H., Koritké, J. G., and Monnier, G. (1969): Sur la vascularisation de la lame terminale humaine. *Z. Zellforsch.,* 102:49–77.

Du Vigneaud, V. (1956): Hormones of the posterior pituitary gland: Oxytocin and vasopressin. In: *The Harvey Lectures 1954–55,* pp. 1–26. Academic Press, New York.

Elde, R. P. (1974): The production and characterization of anti-vasopressin antibodies and their use in the immunoenzyme histochemical localization of vasopressins in the hypothalamo-neurohypophysial neurosecretory system of several mammals. Ph.D. Thesis, University of Minnesota.

Everett, J. W. (1965): Ovulation in rats from pre-optic stimulation through platinum electrodes: Importance of duration and spread of stimulus. *Endocrinology,* 76:1195–1201.

Fawcett, C. P., Powell, A. E., and Sachs, H. (1968): Biosynthesis and release of neurophysin. *Endocrinology,* 83:1299–1310.

Franchimont, P. (1971): The regulation of follicle stimulating hormone and luteinizing hormone secretions in humans. In: *Frontiers in Neuroendocrinology 1971,* edited by L. Martini and W. F. Ganong, pp. 331–358. Oxford University Press, New York.

Fuxe, K. (1965): Evidence of the existence of monoamine terminals in the central nervous system. *Acta Physiol. Scand.* [*Suppl. 247*], 64:37–85.

Fuxe, K., and Hökfelt, T. (1969): Catecholamines in the hypothalamus and the pituitary gland. In: *Frontiers in Neuroendocrinology 1969,* edited by W. F. Ganong and L. Martini, pp. 47–96. Oxford University Press, London.

Gerlach, J. L., McEwen, B. S., Pfaff, D. W., Ferin, M., and Carmel, P. W. (1974): Rhesus monkey brain binds radioactivity from ^{3}H-estradiol and ^{3}H-corticosterone, demonstrated by nuclear isolation and radioautography. *Endocrinology,* 94:A370.

Ginsburg, M. (1968): Production, release, transportation and elimination of neurohypophyseal hormones. In: *Handbook of Experimental Pharmacology, Vol. 23: Neurohypophyseal Hormones and Similar Polypeptides,* edited by B. Berde, pp. 286–371. Springer-Verlag. New York.

Goldman, H., and Lindner, L. (1962): Antidiuretic hormone concentration in blood perfusing the adenohypophysis. *Experientia,* 18:279.

Goldsmith, P. C., and Ganong, W. F. (1974): Ultrastructural localization of luteinizing hormone-releasing hormone in the rat hypothalamus. Program, Abstracts of the 4th Annual Meeting of the Society of Neuroscience (abstract A250).

Goldsmith, P. C., and Ganong, W. F. (1975): Ultrastructural localization of luteinizing hormone-releasing hormone in the median eminence of the rat. *Brain Res. (in press).*

Goldsmith, P. C., and Zimmerman, E. A. (1975): Ultrastructural localization of neurophysin and vasopressin in rat median eminence. *Endocrinology,* 96:A239.

Griffith, E. C., Hooper, K. C., Jeffcoate, S. L., and Holland, D. T. (1974): The presence of peptidases in the rat hypothalamus inactivating LHRH. *Acta Endocrinol. (Kbh.),* 75:435–441.

Halász, B. (1969): The endocrine effects of isolation of the hypothalamus from the rest of the brain. In: *Frontiers in Neuroendocrinology 1969,* edited by W. F. Ganong and L. Martini, pp. 307–342. Oxford University Press, New York.

Hartman, B. K., Zide, O., and Udenfriend, S. (1972): The use of dopamine-β-hydroxylase as a marker for the central noradrenergic system in the rat brain. *Proc. Natl. Acad. Sci. U.S.A.,* 6:2722–2721.

Haymaker, W. (1969): The hypothalamo-pituitary neural pathways and the circulatory system of the pituitary. In: *The Hypothalamus,* edited by W. Haymaker, E. Anderson, and W. J. H. Nauta, pp. 219–250. Charles C Thomas, Springfield, Ill.

Hayward, J. N., and Vincent, J. D. (1970): Osmosensitive single neurones in the hypothalamus of unanesthetized monkeys. *J. Physiol. (Lond.),* 210:947–972.

Hedge, G. A., Yates, M. B., Marcus, R., and Yates, F. E. (1966): Site of action of vasopressin causing corticotropin release. *Endocrinology,* 79:328–340.

Hökfelt, T., Fuxe, K., and Goldstein, M. (1973): Immunohistochemical studies on monoamine-containing cell systems. *Brain Res.,* 62:461–469.

Hökfelt, T., Fuxe, K., Goldstein, M., and Johansson, O. (1974a): Immunohistochemical evidence for the existence of adrenalin neurons in the rat brain. *Brain Res.,* 66:235–251.

Hökfelt, T., Efendic, S., Johansson, O., Luft, R., and Arumura, A. (1974b): Immunohistochemical localization of somatostatin (growth hormone release-inhibiting factor) in the guinea pig brain. *Brain Res.,* 80:165–169.

Hökfelt, T., Fuxe, K., Goldstein, M., Johansson, O., Fraser, H., and Jeffcoate, S. L. (1975): Immunofluorescence mapping of central monoamine and releasing hormone (LRH) systems. In: *Anatomical Neuroendocrinology,* edited by W. E. Stumpf and L. D. Grant. Karger, Basel *(in press).*

Jackson, I. M. D., and Reichlin, S. (1974): Thyrotropin-releasing hormone (TRH): Distribution in hypothalamic and extrahypothalamic brain tissues of mammalian and sub-mammalian chordates. *Endocrinology,* 95:854–862.

Joseph, S. A., Sorrentino, S., Jr., and Sundberg, D. K. (1975): Releasing hormones, LRF, and TRF, in the cerebrospinal fluid of the third ventricle. In: *Brain Endocrine Interaction. II. The Ventricular System, 2nd International Symposium, Tokyo, 1974,* edited by K. M. Knigge, D. E. Scott, H. Kobayashi, and S. Ishli, Karger, Basel, pp. 306–312.

King, J. C., Parsons, J. A., Erlandsen, S. L., and Williams, T. H. (1974): Luteinizing hormone-releasing hormone (LH-RH) pathway of the rat hypothalamus revealed by the unlabeled antibody peroxidase-antiperoxidase method. *Cell Tissue Res.,* 153:211–217.

Kizer, J. S., Palkovits, M., Zivin, Jr., Brownstein, M., Saavedra, J. M., and Kopin, I. J. (1974): The effect of endocrinological manipulations on tyrosine hydroxylase and dopamine-β-hydroxylase in individual hypothalamic nuclei of the adult male rat. *Endocrinology,* 95:799–812.

Knigge, K. M. (1974): Role of the ventricular system in neuroendocrine processes: initial studies on the role of catecholamines in transport of thyrotropin releasing factor. In: *Frontiers in Neurology and Neuroscience Research,* edited by P. Seeman and G. M. Brown, pp. 40–47. University of Toronto Press, Toronto.

Knigge, K. M., and Scott, D. E. (1970): Structure and function of the median eminence. *Am. J. Anat.,* 129:223–228.

Knobil, E. (1974): On the control of gonadotropin secretion in the rhesus monkey. *Recent Prog. Horm. Res.,* 30:1–46.

Knowles, F. (1972): Ependyma of the third ventricle in relation to pituitary function. *Prog. Brain Res.,* 38:255–270.

Kobayashi, H., and Matsui, T. (1969): Fine structure of the median eminence and its functional significance. In: *Frontiers of Neuroendocrinology 1969,* edited by W. F. Ganong and L. Martini, pp. 1–46. Oxford University Press, New York.

Kobayashi, H., Matsui, T., and Ishii, S. (1970): Functional electron microscopy of the hypothalamic median eminence. *Int. Rev. Cytol.,* 29:281–381.

Kordon, C. (1975): New data on hormone-transmitter interaction in gonadotropic regulation. *Manuscript submitted.*

Kordon, C., and Ramirez, V. D. (1975): Recent developments in neurotransmitter-hormone interactions. In: *Anatomical Neuroendocrinology,* edited by W. E. Stumpf and L. D. Grant. Karger, Basel (*in press*).

Kordon, C., Kerdelhué, B., Pattou, E., and Jutisz, M. (1974): Immunocytochemical localization of LHRH in axons and nerve terminals of the rat median eminence. *Proc. Soc. Exp. Biol. Med.,* 147:122–127.

Kozlowski, G. P., and Zimmerman, E. A. (1974): Localization of gonadotropin-releasing hormone (Gn-RH) in sheep and mouse brain. *Anat. Rec.,* 178:396.

Kozlowski, G. P., Nett, T. M., and Zimmerman, E. A. (1975): Immunocytochemical localization of Gn-RH and neurophysin. In: *Anatomical Neuroendocrinology,* edited by W. E. Stumpf and L. D. Grant. Karger, Basel (*in press*).

Krey, L. C., Butler, W. R., and Knobil, E. (1975): Surgical disconnection of the medial basal hypothalamus and pituitary function in the rhesus monkey. I. Gonadotropin secretion. *Endocrinology* (*in press*).

Kumar, T. C. A., and Knowles, F. G. W. (1967): A system linking the third ventricle with the pars tuberali sof the rhesus monkey. *Nature (Lond.),* 215:54–55.

Kumaresan, P., Anandarangam, B., and Vasicka, A. (1972): Studies of human oxytocin with radioimmunoassay. Excerpta Medica International Congress Series No. 256, Abstract 516. Excerpta Medica, Amsterdam.

LeClerc, R., and Pelletier, G. (1974): Electron microscope localization of vasopressin in the hypothalamus and neurohypophysis of the normal and Brattleboro rat. *Am. J. Anat.,* 140:583–588.

Legros, J. J., and Franchimont, P. (1972): Human neurophysin blood levels under normal, experimental, and pathological conditions. *Clin. Endocrinol.,* 1:99–113.

Leonardelli, J., Barry, J., and Dubois, M-P. (1973): Mise en évidence par immunofluorescence d'un constituant immunologiquement apparenté au LH-RF dans l'hypothalamus et l'éminence mediane chez les Mammifères. *C. R. Acad. Sci. [D] (Paris),* 276:2043–2046.

Leveque, T. F. (1972): The medial prechiasmatic area in the rat and LH secretion. In: *Brain-Endocrine Interaction. Median Eminence: Structure and Function,* edited by K. M. Knigge, D. E. Scott, and A. Weindl, pp. 298–305. Karger, Basel.

Livett, B. G., Uttenthal, L. O., and Hope, D. B. (1971): Localization of neurophysin II in the hypothalamo-neurohypophyseal system of the pig by immunofluorescence histology. *Philos. Trans. R. Soc. Lond. [Biol. Sci.],* 261:371–378.

Luft, R., Efendic, S., Hökfelt, T., Johansson, O., and Arimura, A. (1974): Immunohistochemical evidence for the localization of somatostatin-like immunoreactivity in a cell population of the pancreatic islets. *Med. Biol.,* 52:428–430.

Martin J. B. (1974): Inhibitory effect of somatostatin (SRIF) on the release of growth hormone (GH) induced in the rat by electrical stimulation. *Endocrinology,* 94:497–502.

Martini, L. (1966): Neurohypophysis and anterior pituitary activity. In: *The Pituitary Gland,* Vol. 3, edited by G. W. Harris and B. T. Donovan, pp. 535–577. University of California Press, Berkeley.

McCann, S. M., Krulich, L., Quijada, M., Wheaton, J., and Moss, R. L. (1975): Gonadotropin-releasing factors: sites of production, secretion and action in the brain. In: *Anatomical Neuroendocrinology,* edited by W. E. Stumpf and L. D. Grant. Karger, Basel (*in press*).

McEwen, B. S., and Pfaff, D. W. (1973): Chemical and physiological approaches to neuroendocrine mechanisms: attempts at integration. In: *Frontiers in Neuroendocrinology 1973,* edited by W. F. Ganong and L. Martini, pp. 267–335. Oxford University Press, London.

Moore, R. Y. (1973): Retinohypothalamic projections in mammals: A comparative study. *Brain Res.,* 49:403–409.

Moore, R. Y., and Eichler, V. B. (1972): Loss of a circadian adrenal corticosterone rhythm following suprachiasmatic lesions in the rat. *Brain Res.,* 42:201–206.

Moore, R. Y., and Klein, D. C. (1974): Visual pathways and central control of a circadian rhythm in pineal serotonin-N-acetyltransferase activity. *Brain Res.,* 71:17–34.

Moore, R. Y., and Lenn, N. J. (1972): A retinohypothalamic projection in the rat. *J. Comp. Neurol.,* 146:1–14.

Moriarty, G. C. (1973): Adenohypophysis: Ultrastructural cytochemistry: A review. *J. Histochem. Cytochem.*, 21:855–894.

Nakane, P. K. (1971): Application of percxidase-labelled antibodies to the intracellular localization of hormones. In: *In Vitro Methods in Reproductive Cell Biology*, edited by A. Diczfalusy, pp. 190–204. Karolinska Symposia on Research Methods in Reproductive Endocrinology, No. 3. Bogtrykkeriet Forum, Copenhagen.

Olsson, K. (1970): Effects on water diuresis of infusions of transmitter substances into the third ventricle. *Acta Physiol. Scand.*, 79:133–135.

Oota, Y., Kobayashi, H., Nishioka, R. S., and Bern, H. A. (1974): Relationship between neurosecretory axon and ependymal terminals on capillary walls in the median eminence of several vertebrates. *Neuroendocrinology*, 16:127–136.

Palkovits, M. (1973): Isolated removal of hypothalamic or other brain nuclei of the rat. *Brain Res.*, 59:449–450.

Palkovits, M., Brownstein, M., Saavedra, J. M., and Axelrod, J. (1974a): Luteinizing hormone releasing hormone (LH-RH) content of the hypothalamic nuclei in rat. *Endocrinology*, 96:554–558.

Palkovits, M., Brownstein, M., Saavedra, J. M., and Axelrod, J. (1974b): Norepinephrine and dopamine content of hypothalamic nuclei of the rat. *Brain Res.*, 77:137–149.

Parry, H. B., and Livett, B. G. (1973): A new hypothalamic pathway to the median eminence containing neurophysin and its hypertrophy in sheep with natural scrapie. *Nature (Lond.)*, 242:63–65.

Pelletier, G., Le Clerc, R., LaBrie, F., and Puviani, R. (1974a): Electron microscopic immunohistochemical localization of neurophysin in the rat hypothalamus and pituitary. *Mol. Cell Endocrinol.*, 1:157–166.

Pelletier, G., Labrie, F., Puviani, R., Arimura, A., and Schally, A. V. (1974b): Electron microscope localization of luteinizing hormone-releasing hormone in the rat median eminence. *Endocrinology*, 95:314–315.

Pelletier, G., Labrie, F., Arimura, A., and Schally, A. V. (1974c): Electron microscopic immunohistochemical localization of growth hormone-release inhibiting hormone (somatostatin) in the rat median eminence. *Am. J. Anat.*, 140:445–450.

Pelletier, G., LeClerc, R., Dube, D., Labrie, F., Puviani, R., Arimura, A., and Schally, A. V. (1975): Localization of growth hormone-release inhibiting hormone (somatostatin) in the rat brain. *Am. J. Anat*, 142:397–400.

Pfaff, D. W., and Keiner, M. (1973): Atlas of estradio-concentrating cells in the central nervous system of the female rat. *J. Comp. Neurol.*, 151:121–158.

Phifer, R. F., Midgley, A. R., and Spicer, S. S. (1973): Immunohistologic evidence that follicle-stimulating and luteinizing hormones are present in the same cell types in the human pars distalis. *J. Clin. Endocrinol. Metab.*, 36:125–141.

Pickel, V. M., Joh, T. H., Field, P. M., Becker, C. G., and Reis, D. J. (1975): Cellular localization of tyrosine hydroxylase by immunohistochemistry. *J. Histochem. Cytochem.*, 23:1–12.

Pickup, J. C., Johnston, C. I., Nakamura, S., Uttenthal, L. O., and Hope, D. B. (1973): Subcellular organization of neurophysins, oxytocin, (8-lysine)-vasopressin and adenosine triphosphatase in porcine posterior pituitary lobes. *Biochem. J.*, 132:316–317.

Raisman, G. (1972): A second look at the parvicellular neurosecretory system. In: *Brain-Endocrine Interaction. Median Eminence: Structure and Function*, edited by K. M. Knigge, D. E. Scott, and A. Weindl, pp. 109–118. Karger, Basel.

Raisman, G., and Field, P. (1971): Sexual dimorphism in the preoptic area of the rat. *Science*, 173:731–733.

Reichlin, S., and Mitnick, M. (1973): Biosynthesis of hypothalamic hypophysiotropic factors. In: *Frontiers in Neuroendocrinology 1973*, edited by W. F. Ganong and L. Martini, pp. 61–88. Oxford University Press, New York.

Rinne, U. K. (1972): Effect of adrenalectomy on the ultrastructure and catecholamine fluorescence of nerve endings in the median eminence of the rat. In: *Brain-Endocrine Interaction. Median Eminence: Structure and Function*, edited by K. M. Knigge, D. E. Scott, and A. Weindl, pp. 164–170. Karger, Basel.

Roberts, J. S., and Share, L. (1969): Effects of progesterone and estrogen on blood levels of oxytocin during vaginal distention. *Endocrinology*, 84:1076–1081.

Robinson, A. G. (1975): Isolation, assay, and secretion of individual human neurophysins. *J. Clin. Invest.,* 55:360–367.

Robinson, A. G., and Frantz, A. G. (1973): Radioimmunoassay of posterior pituitary peptides: A review. *Metabolism (Clin. Exp.),* 22:1047–1057.

Robinson, A. G., and Zimmerman, E. A. (1973): Cerebrospinal fluid and ependymal neurophysin. *J. Clin. Invest.,* 52:1260–1267.

Robinson, A. G., Zimmerman, E. A., Engleman, E. G., and Frantz, A. G. (1971a): Radioimmunoassay of bovine neurophysin: Specificity of neurophysin I and neurophysin II. *Metabolism (Clin. Exp.),* 20:1138–1147.

Robinson, A. G., Zimmerman, E. A., and Frantz, A. G. (1971b): Physiologic investigation of posterior pituitary binding proteins neurophysin I and neurophysin II. *Metabolism (Clin. Exp.),* 20:1148–1155.

Robinson, A. G., Ferin, M., and Zimmerman, E. A. (1974) Neurophysin in monkey: Correlation with mid-cycle estrogen and LH. *Endocrinology,* 94:A213.

Röhlich, P., and Wenger, T. (1969): Elektronenmikroskopische untersuchungen am organon vasculosum laminae terminalis der ratte. *Z. Zellforsch.,* 102:483–506.

Saavedra, J. M., Brownstein, M., Palkovits, M., Kizer, S., and Axelrod, J. (1974a): Tyrosine hydroxylase and dopamine-β-hydroxylase: Distribution in the individual rat hypothalamic nuclei. *J. Neurochem.,* 23:869–871.

Saavedra, J. M., Palkovits, M., Brownstein, M., and Axelrod, J. (1974b): Localization of phenylethanolamine N-methyltransferase in rat brain nuclei. *Nature (Lond.),* 248:695–696.

Saavedra, J., Palkovits, M., Brownstein, M., and Axelrod, J. (1974c): Serotonin distribution in the nuclei of the rat hypothalamus and preoptic region. *Brain Res.,* 77:157–165.

Sachs, H., and Takabatake, Y. (1964): Evidence for a precursor in vasopressin biosynthesis. *Endocrinology,* 75:943–948.

Sahar, M., Castel, M., and Hochman, J. (1975): Biological applications of antibodies to vasopressin. Israel Society of Physiology, February 1975 (abstract).

Scharrer, E., and Scharrer, B. (1954): Hormones produced by neurosecretory cells. *Recent Prog. Horm. Res.,* 10:183–240.

Schneider, H. P. G., Crighton, D. B., and McCann, S. M. (1969): Suprachiasmatic LH-releasing factor. *Neuroendocrinology,* 5:271–380.

Scott, D. E., Kozlowski, G. P., and Sheridan, M. N. (1974a): Scanning electromicroscopy in the ultrastructural analysis of the mammalian cerebral ventricular system. *Int. Rev. Cytol.,* 37:349–388.

Scott, D. E., Dudley, G. K., Knigge, K. M., and Kozlowski, G. P. (1974b): In vitro analysis of the cellular localization of luteinizing hormone releasing factor (LRF) in the basal hypothalamus of the rat. *Cell Tissue Res.,* 149:371–378.

Seif, S. M., Huellmantel, A. B., Stillman, M., Recht, L., and Robinson, A. G. (1975): Neurophysin and vasopressin in the plasma and hypothalamus of adrenalectomized and normal rats. *Endocrinology,* 96:A-272.

Sétaló, G., Vigh, S., Schally, A. V., Arimura, A., and Flerkó, B. (1975): LH-RH containing neural elements in the rat hypothalamus. *Endocrinology,* 96:135–142.

Silverman, A. J., and Zimmerman, E. A. (1975): Ultrastructural immunocytochemical localization of neurophysin and vasopressin in the median eminence and posterior pituitary of the guinea pig. *Cell Tissue Res.,* 159:291–301.

Silverman, A. J., Knigge, K. M., and Zimmerman, E. A. (1975): Ultrastructural immunocytochemical localization of neurophysin in freeze-substituted neurohypophysis. *Am. J. Anat.,* 142:265–271.

Sloper, J. C. (1966): The experimental and cytopathological investigation of neurosecretion in the hypothalamus and pituitary. In: *The Pituitary Gland,* Vol. 3, edited by G. W. Harris and B. T. Donovan, pp. 131–239. University of California Press, Berkeley.

Sokol, H. W., and Valtin, H. (1967): Evidence for the synthesis of oxytocin and vasopressin in separate neurones. *Nature (Lond.),* 214:314–316.

Sternberger, L. A. (1974): *Immunocytochemistry.* Prentice-Hall, Englewood Cliffs, N.J.

Stumpf, W. E. (1970): Estrogen-neurons and estrogen-neuron systems in the periventricular brain. *Am. J. Anat.,* 129:207–218.

Suburo, A. M., and Pellgrino de Iraldi, A. (1969): An ultrastructural study of the rat's suprachiasmatic nucleus. *J. Anat.,* 105:439–446.

Sunde, D., and Sokol, H. W. (1975): Quantification of rat neurophysins by polyacrylamide gel electrophoresis: Applications to the rat with hereditary hypothalamic diabetes insipidus. *Ann. N.Y. Acad. Sci.,* 248:345–364.

Szentágothai, J., Flerkó, B., Mess, B., and Halász, B. (1968): *Hypothalamic Control of the Anterior Pituitary.* Akademiai Kiadó, Budapest.

Taber, C. A., and Karovolas, H. J. (1975): Subcellular localization of LH releasing activity in the rat hypothalamus. *Endocrinology,* 96:446–452.

Tejasen, T., and Everett, J. W. (1967): Surgical analysis of the preoptico-tuberal pathway controlling ovulatory release of gonadotropins in the rat. *Endocrinology,* 81:1387–1396.

Terasawa, E. I., and Sawyer, C. H. (1969): Changes in electrical activity in the rat hypothalamus related to electrochemical stimulation of adenohypophyseal function. *Endocrinology,* 85:143–149.

Vandesande, F., DeMey, J., and Dierickx, K. (1974): Identification of neurophysin producing cells. I. The origin of the neurophysin-like substance-containing nerve fibers of the external region of the median eminence of the rat. *Cell Tissue Res.,* 151:187–200.

Vandesande, F., Dierickx, K., and DeMey, J. (1975a): Identification of the vasopressin-neurophysin II and the oxytocin-neurophysin I producing neurons in the bovine hypothalamus. *Cell Tissue Res.,* 156:189–200.

Vandesande, F., Dierickx, K., and DeMey, J. (1975b): Identification of vasopressin-neurophysin producing neurons of the rat suprachiasmatic nuclei. *Cell Tissue Res.,* 156:337–342.

Van Dyke, H. B., Chow, B. F., Greep, R. O., and Rothen, A. (1941): The isolation of a protein from pars neuralis of the ox pituitary with constant oxytocic, pressor and diuresis-inhibiting effects. *J. Pharmacol. (Kyoto),* 74:190–209.

Van Wimersma Greidanus, Tj. B., Bohus, B., and De Wied, D. (1975a): The role of vasopressin in memory processes. *Prog. Brain Res. (in press).*

Van Wimersma Greidanus, Tj. B., Dogterom, J., and De Wied, D. (1975b): Intraventricular administration of anti-vasopressin serum inhibits memory consolidation in rats. *Life Sci.* (in press).

Vorherr, H., Bradbury, M. W. B., Hoghoughi, M., and Kleeman, C. R. (1968): Antidiuretic hormone in cerebrospinal fluid during endogenous and exogenous changes in its blood level. *Endocrinology,* 83:246–250.

Walter, R., Schlesinger, D. H., Schwartz, I. L., and Capra, J. D. (1971): Complete amino acid sequence of bovine neurophysin II. *Biochem. Biophys. Res. Commun.,* 44:293–298.

Walter, R., Griffiths, E. C., and Hooper, K. C. (1973): Production of MSH-release-inhibiting hormone by a particulate preparation of hypothalami: Mechanisms of oxytocin inactivation. *Brain Res.,* 60:449–457.

Watkins, W. B. (1975a): Neurosecretion in the external and internal zone of the median eminence of the cat and dog. *Cell Tissue Res. (in press).*

Watkins, W. B. (1975b): Immunohistochemical demonstration of neurophysin in the hypothalamoneurohypophysial system. *Int. Rev. Cytol.,* 41:241–284.

Watkins, W. B., Schwabedal, P., and Bock, R. (1974): Immunohistochemical demonstration of a CRF-associated neurophysin in the external zone of the rat median eminence. *Cell Tissue Res.,* 152:411–421.

Weindl, A. (1973): Neuroendocrine aspects of circumventricular organs. In: *Frontiers in Neuroendocrinology 1973,* edited by W. F. Ganong and L. Martini, pp. 3–33. Oxford University Press, New York.

Weindl, A., and Joynt, R. J. (1972): The median eminence as a circumventricular organ. In: *Brain Endocrine Interaction. Median Eminence: Structure and Function,* edited by K. M. Knigge, D. E. Scott, and A. Weindl, pp. 280–297. Karger, Basel.

Wheaton, J. E. (1975): Localization of LH-releasing hormone (LRH) in the preoptic area and hypothalamus of the rat brain. *Fed. Proc.,* 34:113.

Wheaton, J. E., Krulich, J., and McCann, S. M. (1975): Localization of luteinizing hormone-releasing hormone (LRH) in the preoptic area and hypothalamus of the rat using radioimmunoassay. *Endocrinology (in press).*

White, W. F., Hedlund, M. T., Weber, G. F., Rippel, R. H., Johnson, E. S., and Wilber, J. F. (1974:) The pineal gland: A supplemental source of hypothalamic releasing hormones. *Endocrinology,* 94:1422–1426.

Winokur, A., and Utiger, R. D. (1974): Thyrotropin-releasing hormone: Regional distribution in rat brain. *Science,* 185:265–267.

Wislocki, G. B., and King, L. S. (1936): The permeability of the hypophysis and hypothalamus to vital dyes with a study of the hypophyseal vascular supply. *Am. J. Anat.,* 58:421–472.

Wittowski, W., and Bock, R. (1972): Electron microscopical studies of the median eminence following interference with the feedback system anterior pituitary-adrenal cortex. In: *Brain Endocrine Interaction. Median Eminence Structure and Function,* edited by K. M. Knigge, D. E. Scott, and A. Weindl, pp. 171–180. Karger, Basel.

Yates, F. E., Russell, S. M., Dallman, M. F., Hedge, G. A., McCann, S. M., and Dhariwal, A. P. S. (1971): Potentiation by vasopressin of corticotropin release induced by corticotropin-releasing factor. *Endocrinology,* 88:3–15.

Zambrano, D. (1969): The arcuate complex of the female rat during the sexual cycle. *Z. Zellforsch.,* 93:560–570.

Zimmerman, E. A., Carmel, P. W., Husain, M. K., Ferin, M., Tannenbaum, M., Frantz, A. G., and Robinson, A. G. (1973a): Vasopressin and neurophysin: High concentrations in monkey hypophyseal portal blood. *Science,* 182:925–957.

Zimmerman, E. A., Hsu, K. C., Robinson, A. G., Carmel, P. W., Frantz, A. G., and Tannenbaum, M. (1973b): Studies on neurophysin secreting neurons with immunoperoxidase techniques employing antibody to bovine neurophysin. I. Light microscopic findings in monkey and bovine tissues. *Endocrinology,* 92:931–940.

Zimmerman, E. A., Robinson, A. G., Husain, M. K., Acosta, M., Frantz, A. G., and Sawyer, W. H. (1974a): Neurohypophyseal peptides in the bovine hypothalamus: The relationship of neurophysin I to oxytocin, and neurophysin II to vasopressin in supraoptic and paraventricular regions. *Endocrinology,* 95:931–936.

Zimmerman, E. A., Hsu, K. C., Ferin, M., and Kozlowski, G. P. (1974b): Localization of gonadotropin-releasing hormone (Gn-RH) in the hypothalamus of the mouse by immunoperoxidase technique. *Endocrinology,* 95:1–8.

Zimmerman, E. A., Defendini, R., and Frantz, A. G. (1974c): Prolactin and growth hormone in patients with pituitary adenomas: A correlative study in tumor and plasma by immunoperoxidase and radioimmunoassay. *J. Clin. Endocrinol. Metab.,* 38:577–585.

Zimmerman, E. A., Kozlowski, G. P., and Scott, D. E. (1975a): Axonal and ependymal pathways for the secretion of biologically active peptides into hypophysial portal blood. In: *Brain-Endocrine Interaction. II. The Ventricular System, 2nd International Symposium, Tokyo,* edited by K. M. Knigge, D. E. Scott, H. Kobayashi, and S. Ishii, pp. 123–134. Karger, Basel.

Zimmerman, E. A., Defendini, R., Sokol, H. W., and Robinson, A. G. (1975b): The distribution of neurophysin-secreting pathways in the mammalian brain: Light microscopic studies using the immunoperoxidase technique. *Ann. N.Y. Acad. Sci.,* 248:92–111.

Zimmerman, E. A., Defendini, R., Sokol, H. W., and Robinson, A. G. (1975c): The intracellular distribution of oxytocin, vasopressin and respective neurophysins in mammalian hypothalamus. *Endocrinology,* 96:A95.

Frontiers in Neuroendocrinology, Vol. 4,
edited by L. Martini and W. F. Ganong.
Raven Press, New York © 1976.

Chapter 3

Mode of Action of Hypothalamic Regulatory Hormones in the Adenohypophysis

Fernand Labrie, Georges Pelletier, Pierre Borgeat, Jacques Drouin, Louise Ferland, and Alain Belanger

Medical Research Council Group in Molecular Endocrinology, Centre Hospitalier de l'Université Laval, Québec, Québec, GIV 4G2, Canada

Although important information about the mechanism of action of hypothalamic regulatory hormones could be obtained using hypothalamic extracts at different stages of purification, elucidation of the structures of thyrotropin-releasing hormone (Bøler et al., 1969; Burgus et al., 1969), luteinizing hormone-releasing hormone (Matsuo et al., 1971; Burgus et al., 1971), and somatostatin (Brazeau et al., 1973; Schally et al., 1975) has only recently been accomplished. The relative ease of synthesis of these peptides and their analogues has opened new possibilities for studying their mechanisms of action and has already permitted many interesting structure-function studies.

EFFECT OF HYPOTHALAMIC REGULATORY HORMONES ON CYCLIC AMP ACCUMULATION IN THE ANTERIOR PITUITARY

The first suggestive evidence for a role of adenosine 3',5'-monophosphate (cyclic AMP) as mediator of the action of hypothalamic regulatory hormones in the anterior pituitary gland originated from the observations that cyclic AMP derivatives or theophylline, an inhibitor of cyclic nucleotide phosphodiesterase, stimulate the release of all six main anterior pituitary hormones (Labrie et al., 1975a). However, proof of the role of cyclic AMP had to be obtained by measuring changes of adenylate cyclase activity or cyclic AMP concentrations under the influence of pure or synthetic neurohormones.

Much recent evidence indicates that cyclic AMP is involved as mediator of the action of luteinizing hormone-releasing hormone (LRH) in the anterior pituitary gland. Addition of LRH leads to stimulation of cyclic AMP accumulation in rat anterior pituitary gland *in vitro* (Borgeat et al., 1972; Jutisz et al., 1972; Kaneko et al., 1973; Labrie et al., 1973; Makino, 1973; Borgeat et al., 1974a,b). The concentration of LRH required for half-maximal stimulation of cyclic AMP accumulation is 0.1 to 1.0 ng/ml or

1×10^{-10} to 1×10^{-9} M LRH (Borgeat et al., 1972). A close correlation is always observed between rates of LH and FSH release and changes of intracellular cyclic AMP concentrations, both as a function of time of incubation and concentration of the neurohormone.

When LRH analogues having a spectrum of biological activity ranging between 0.001% and 500% to 1,000% the activity of LRH itself were used, the same close parallelism between stimulation of cyclic AMP accumulation and both LH and FSH release was found under all experimental conditions (Borgeat et al., 1974a). That LRH exerts its action by activating adenylate cyclase and not by inhibiting cyclic nucleotide phosphodiesterase is indicated by the observation that a similar effect of the neurohormone is observed in the presence or absence of theophylline (Borgeat et al., 1972).

The possibility of developing a contraceptive method based on inhibitory LRH analogues has led to the synthesis of many such substances, some of which are potent inhibitors of LRH action both *in vivo* (Ferland et al., 1975a) and *in vitro* (Labrie et al., 1975b). The availability of LRH antagonists offered the possibility of investigating the correlation between their inhibitory effect on LRH-induced cyclic AMP accumulation and LH and FSH release.

Using rat anterior pituitary cells in monolayer culture, we had previously found (Labrie et al., 1975b) that the release of LH induced by 3×10^{-9} M LRH was 50% inhibited by adding [Des-His^2, D-Ala^6] LRH at 3×10^{-6} M, [Des-His^2, D-Ala^6, Des-Gly-NH$_2$^{10}] LRH ethylamide at 6×10^{-6} M, [Des-His^2, D-Leu^6] LRH at 4×10^{-6} M, [D-Phe^2] LRH at 6×10^{-6} M, [Des-His^2, Des-Gly-NH$_2$^{10}] LRH propylamide at 2×10^{-5} M, and [D-Phe^2, D-Ala^6] LRH at 10^{-7} M (M. Savary and F. Labrie, *unpublished observations*). Since none of these analogues has important inherent LH-releasing activity, they were first tested in the present studies at a molar ratio of 10,000 against 5×10^{-9} M LRH. All six LRH antagonists led to marked inhibition of LRH-induced cyclic AMP accumulation (62.0% to 38.0% inhibition), and LH (87.4% to 47.5%) and FSH (75.4% to 29.7%) release.

As an example, Fig. 3–1 shows the inhibitory effect of increasing concentrations of [D-Phe^2, D-Leu^6] LRH on cyclic AMP accumulation and LH and FSH release in rat anterior pituitary gland *in vitro*. The close correlation between inhibition of LRH-induced cyclic AMP accumulation and LH and FSH release adds strong support to the concept of an obligatory role of the adenylate cyclase system as mediator of LRH action in the anterior pituitary gland. Although the changes are of somewhat smaller magnitude, addition of thyrotropin-releasing hormone (TRH) to anterior pituitary tissue leads also to increased intracellular levels of cyclic AMP accompanied by increased thyrotropin (thyroid-stimulating hormone; TSH) release (Bowers, 1971; Labrie et al., 1975a,c).

Recently it was shown that somatostatin leads to rapid inhibition of cyclic AMP accumulation in the anterior pituitary gland *in vitro* (Kaneko et al.,

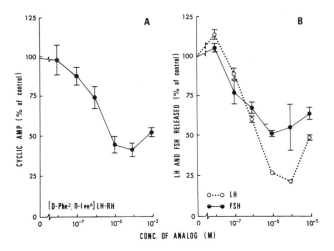

FIG. 3–1. Effect of increasing concentrations of [D-Phe², D-Leu⁶] LH-RH (LRH) on 3 × 10⁻⁹ M LRH-induced cyclic AMP accumulation (A) and LH and FSH release (B) in rat hemipituitaries *in vitro*.

1973; Borgeat et al., 1974*b*), this inhibitory effect being accompanied by marked inhibition of both GH and TSH release (Borgeat et al., 1974*b*). The effect of somatostatin on cyclic AMP accumulation in rat anterior pituitary tissue is illustrated on Fig. 3–2; maximal inhibition (approximately 35% of the control level) occurs 10 min after adding the peptide.

Since growth hormone (GH)- and TSH-secreting cells account for 50% to 70% of the total adenohypophyseal cell population in adult male rats, the 50% inhibition of cyclic AMP accumulation in total pituitary tissue suggests

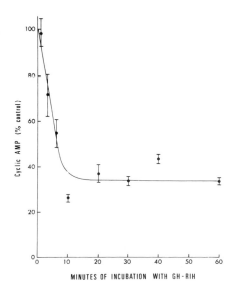

FIG. 3–2. Time course of the effect of somatostatin (GH-RIH) on cyclic AMP accumulation in anterior pituitary gland. Incubation and assay were performed as described by Borgeat et al. (1974*b*).

almost complete inhibition of cyclic AMP accumulation in the GH- and TSH-secreting cells. The inhibitory effect of somatostatin is observed under both basal and prostaglandin E_2- or theophylline-induced conditions, thus suggesting an inhibitory action of somatostatin on adenylate cyclase activity.

The data presented show clearly that two stimulatory hypothalamic hormones—TRH and LRH—lead to parallel stimulation of cyclic AMP accumulation and specific hormone release, and one inhibitory peptide, somatostatin, leads to parallel inhibition of cyclic AMP accumulation and GH and TSH release. Such findings suggest strongly that changes of adenylate cyclase activity are involved in the mechanism of action of these three peptides in the anterior pituitary gland.

TRH RECEPTOR—PROTEIN KINASE

Analogous to other cyclic AMP-mediated hormonal systems (Robison et al., 1968), the sequence of events in the action of TRH is presumably: (1) binding of TRH to specific receptor sites on the external surface of the plasma membrane of thyrotrophs or mammotrophs; and (2) activation of adenylate cyclase with elevation of intracellular levels of cyclic AMP leading to activation of protein kinase, phosphorylation of protein substrates, and altered rates of specific subcellular functions.

Since there are recent reviews detailing the characteristics of ^{3}H-TRH binding to isolated plasma membranes and intact cells (Labrie et al., 1975c) and the properties of protein kinase and phosphorylation of adenohypophyseal protein substrates (Labrie et al., 1975a), these aspects are not discussed here.

SIMILARITY OF FUNCTIONAL RECEPTORS FOR TRH AND SOMATOSTATIN IN DIFFERENT CELL TYPES

Functional TRH Receptors in TSH- and PRL-Secreting Cells

Since TRH stimulates both TSH and prolactin (PRL) secretion, it is of interest to investigate the degree of similarity of the receptors for TRH in the two cell types. Using plasma membranes isolated from bovine anterior pituitaries during lactation when PRL-secreting cells are much more numerous than thyrotrophs, we found that the affinity of the receptor for ^{3}H-TRH was approximately 3×10^{-8} M (Labrie et al., 1972). An almost identical K_D for TRH was found using membranes prepared from PRL/GH-secreting tumor cells (Hinkle and Tashjian, 1973), a TSH-secreting tumor (Grant et al., 1973), and anterior pituitary homogenates prepared from rats under a variety of physiological conditions (De Léan et al., 1974). In competition experiments various TRH analogues were found to displace ^{3}H-TRH with equal potency using receptors from PRL/GH-secreting GH$_3$ cells (Hinkle et al., 1974) and a TSH-secreting tumor (Grant et al., 1973). Working with five analogues having a wide range of biological activity, Rivier and Vale (1974) found almost identical potencies of these analogues on both TSH and PRL release. These data suggest strongly that the receptors for TRH in TSH- and PRL-secreting cells are very similar in both their affinity for the hormone and their ability to express a specific biological response (hormone release).

Functional Somatostatin Receptors in GH-, TSH-, and PRL-Secreting Cells

Somatostatin not only inhibits the basal release of GH but also the release induced by theophylline, prostaglandin E_2, N^6-monobutyryl cyclic AMP, and N^6,2'O-dibutyryl cyclic AMP (Vale et al., 1972; Bélanger et al., 1974; Borgeat et al., 1974b).

Although not affecting the basal release of TSH (Hall et al., 1973; Vale et al., 1974; Drouin et al., 1975), somatostatin markedly inhibits TRH-induced TSH release *in vitro* and *in vivo* (Vale et al., 1974; Drouin et al., 1975) in rats and *in vivo* in humans (Hall et al., 1973; Siler et al., 1974). Moreover, under certain experimental conditions, PRL release in cells in monolayer culture is also inhibited by somatostatin (Vale et al., 1974; Drouin et al., 1975), whereas partial suppression of basal plasma PRL levels has been reported in some acromegalic patients (Yen et al., 1974).

In addition to its action at the pituitary level, somatostatin has been found to inhibit insulin (Alberti et al., 1973; De Vane et al., 1974; Mortimer et al., 1974; Yen et al., 1974), glucagon (Gerich et al., 1974; Mortimer et al., 1974, and gastrin (Bloom et al., 1974) secretion. This large spectrum of actions of somatostatin raises the question of specificity of the receptor(s) for the tetradecapeptide in different responsive cell types. Taking advantage of the availability of synthetic analogues of somatostatin having a wide range of biological activity, we studied the relative potencies of somatostatin and its analogues on the release of GH, TSH, and PRL in rat anterior pituitary cells in monolayer culture.

Using somatostatin and two of its analogues with respective potencies of 1% and 0.1% that of the natural peptide on GH release, we found almost identical potencies of each peptide on the release of the three pituitary hormones (GH, TSH, and PRL); the ED_{50} was 3×10^{-10} M for somatostatin, 3×10^{-8} M for analogue I, and 2×10^{-7} M for analogue II. These findings indicate that the functional receptors for somatostatin are very similar in the three corresponding anterior pituitary cell types: somatotrophs, thyrotrophs, and mammotrophs.

We previously observed that somatostatin leads to parallel inhibition of spontaneous GH and PRL release as well as TRH-induced TSH release (Drouin et al., 1975), but the present data obtained with peptides having such a wide range of biological activity provide stronger evidence for a close similarity of the functional somatostatin receptors in the anterior pituitary gland.

CHARACTERISTICS OF THE INTERACTION BETWEEN TRH AND SOMATOSTATIN

Since it is possible that the secretion rate of both TSH and PRL may be dependent on the relative concentrations of TRH (stimulatory) and somatostatin (inhibitory) in the portal hypothalamohypophyseal blood, we studied the characteristics of the interaction of these two hypothalamic peptides on TSH and PRL secretion, using pituitary cells in culture. Somatostatin, at concentrations up to 10^{-7} M, does not affect the basal release of TSH from anterior pituitary cells in monolayer culture (Fig. 3–3A). However, the 12-fold increase of TSH release observed in the presence of 10^{-8} M TRH is reduced by approximately 65% by adding 10^{-8} M somatostatin, half-maximal inhibition being produced at 2.5×10^{-10} M somatostatin.

In agreement with these data, Fig. 3–3B shows that 10^{-8} M somatostatin inhibits TSH release induced by 10^{-8} to 10^{-7} M TRH to approximately 30% of the maximal response obtained in the absence of the tetradecapeptide. It can be seen in Fig. 3–3B that the concentration of TRH giving half-maximal stimulation (ED_{50}) of TSH release is only slightly increased from 1 to 3×10^{-9} M in the presence of somatostatin. We also studied the possible effect of somatostatin on the ED_{50} values for TRH-stimulated PRL release. As shown in Fig. 3–4, somatostatin (3×10^{-10} M and 10^{-8} M) led to a progressive inhibition of PRL release and inhibited the maximal response obtained with TRH. However, the TRH ED_{50} for PRL release was not affected by the presence of somatostatin.

The interaction between TRH and somatostatin in TSH-producing cells is noncompetitive, since the inhibition is only 30% reversed by a 10-molar excess of TRH (Fig. 3–3B). In addition, the TRH ED_{50} of stimulation of TSH release is not significantly increased by adding 10^{-8} M somatostatin.

That somatostatin does not compete with TRH at the TRH receptor site is clearly illustrated by the finding that somatostatin does not affect ^{3}H-TRH binding to isolated adenohypophyseal plasma membranes (Drouin et al., 1975). This and the data which show that somatostatin has no effect on the apparent K_m of stimulation of TSH (Fig. 3–3B) or PRL (Fig. 3–4) release by TRH indicate quite clearly that the two hypothalamic peptides act on different receptors in both TSH- and PRL-secreting cells.

We previously found that TRH stimulates (Labrie et al., 1975a) and somatostatin inhibits (Borgeat et al., 1974a; Labrie et al., 1975a) cyclic AMP accumulation in anterior pituitary tissue, whereas TRH receptors are associated to a major extent with plasma membranes (Labrie et al., 1972; Poirier et al., 1972), which are also the site of adenylate cyclase. It is thus likely that the first step in the action of these two peptides is binding to

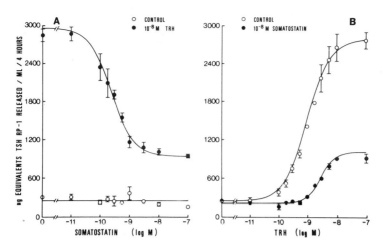

FIG. 3–3. A: Effect of increasing concentrations of somatostatin on TSH release in female rat anterior pituitary cells in monolayer culture in the absence (O— O) or presence (●—●) of 10^{-8} M TRH B: Effect of increasing concentrations of TRH on TSH release in the absence (O— O) or presence (●—●) of 10^{-8} M somatostatin.

specific receptors on the external surface of the plasma membrane with resultant activation (for TRH) or inhibition (for somatostatin) of adenylate cyclase activity.

The incomplete inhibition by somatostatin of the TRH-induced TSH release (Fig. 3–3) suggests that in thyrotrophs the receptors for somatostatin are less numerous than those for TRH, and/or that there are two classes of

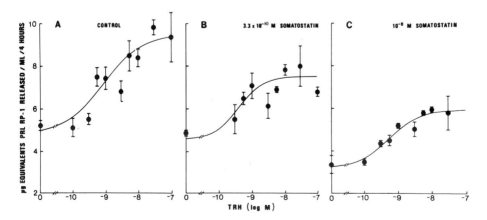

FIG. 3–4. Effect of increasing concentrations of TRH on the release of PRL in female rat anterior pituitary cells in culture in the absence (A) or presence (B and C) of 3.3 × 10^{-10} M or 10^{-8} M somatostatin.

functional receptors for somatostatin and/or TRH. Assuming the existence of different populations of receptors, a certain proportion of the somatostatin-receptor complexes would have the ability to reverse the action of the TRH-receptor complexes, thus explaining the 70% inhibition of the TRH response. The rest of the population of receptors for somatostatin could not efficiently compete with a unique population of TRH receptors, thus explaining the remaining TRH stimulatory effect in the presence of somatostatin. Another possibility would be the presence of two populations of TRH receptors. One would have a coupling mechanism less efficient than that of somatostatin, thereby explaining the 70% inhibition by the tetradecapeptide. The other would have a more efficient coupling mechanism than somatostatin, thus explaining the absence of total reversal of the TRH effect on TSH release by an excess of somatostatin. The absence of an inhibitory effect of somatostatin on basal TSH release could be due to the inability of the receptor-somatostatin complexes to inhibit the activity of the minimal number of adenylate cyclase molecules responsible for basal hormone release.

In PRL-secreting cells, somatostatin inhibits by 50% to 60% the basal release of PRL; the inhibition is also incomplete (approximately 50%) in the presence of TRH. Since the stimulation of PRL release by TRH is small, it is quite possible that the inhibition observed with somatostatin in the presence of TRH is secondary to inhibition of basal PRL release. As observed for thyrotrophs, these data indicate that the receptors for TRH in mammotrophs are more numerous than those for somatostatin or they are more efficient in coupling for expression of cellular function (PRL release).

Although there is a constant inhibition of PRL release by somatostatin *in vitro,* the situation is different *in vivo;* at least at the dose used, somatostatin has no effect on basal plasma PRL levels. This may be due to the already existing inhibitory tonic influence of the hypothalamus on PRL release *in vivo.*

It should be mentioned that somatostatin has been found to inhibit plasma PRL levels in some acromegalic patients (Yen et al., 1974). Under those pathological conditions the availability of somatostatin receptors might be quite different, and this might explain the observed discrepancy between normal and neoplastic PRL-secreting cells. The physiological significance of the inhibitory effect of somatostatin on basal PRL release *in vitro* cannot be properly assessed. Somatostatin does not affect basal or TRH-induced PRL release *in vivo* in the rat, or basal or TRH-induced levels of PRL in normal humans (Hall et al., 1973).

CHANGES IN PITUITARY SENSITIVITY TO LRH

There is good evidence for an essential role of estrogens as inducers of the preovulatory surge of LH. These data pertain to the induction of LH release and ovulation by the injection of estrogens early in the estrous cycle (Everett, 1948) and the abolition of the ovulatory surge of LH at proestrus by administration of an estrogen antiserum (Ferin et al., 1969). These findings do not differentiate between a positive estrogen action on LRH release at the hypothalamic level, an action on the sensitivity of the pituitary gonadotrops to LRH, or an action at both sites.

In order to investigate possible changes of pituitary sensitivity to LRH during the estrous cycle, the plasma LH response curve to LRH was studied in rats at different stages of the estrous cycle under conditions leading to blockage of endogenous LRH secretion (Surital or pentobarbital anesthesia). In order to eliminate interference by changes in endogenous LRH secretion during the course of the *in vivo* experiments, the animals were anesthetized with Surital 1 hr before subcutaneous injection of LRH and were kept deeply anesthetized up to the last blood collection. Surital anesthesia maintains constant plasma LH levels during the afternoon of proestrus and completely blocks ovulation. As shown in Fig. 3–5, the subcutaneous injection of increasing doses of LRH led to a much greater plasma LH response on the afternoon of proestrus than on diestrus I. In fact, the response to LRH is approximately seven-fold higher during proestrus than diestrus I (Ferland et al., 1975*b*).

The data obtained *in vivo* could be influenced by changes in endogenous LRH release in spite of pentobarbital or Surital anesthesia, changes in the transport or metabolism of exogenous LRH, changes of LH metabolism, or by a combination of these factors. We therefore studied the sensitivity to LRH *in vitro*, using pituitaries collected at the different stages of the estrous cycle. Figure 3–6A shows that during the first 45 min of incubation, the sensitivity of the pituitary to LRH is maximal during proestrus. It remains high on the morning of estrus and diminishes to minimal values during

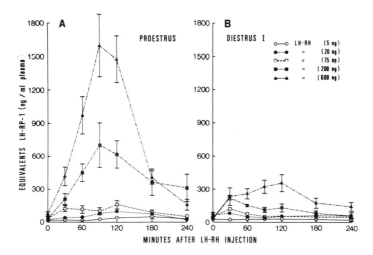

FIG. 3–5. Effect of increasing doses of LH-RH (LRH) on the plasma LH response in the rat on the afternoon of proestrus (A) and diestrus I (B). Experimental conditions were as described by Ferland et al. (1975b).

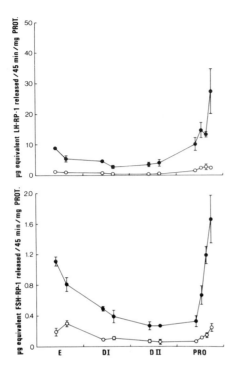

FIG. 3–6. Effect of 10^{-8} M LRH on LH and FSH release from rat anterior pituitary *in vitro* at different stages of the estrous cycle. Experimental conditions were as described by Ferland et al. (1975b). The incubation period was 0 to 45 min. E, estrus. DI, diestrus I. D II, diestrus II. PRO, proestrus. ○—○, control. ●—●, LRH 10^{-8} M.

diestrus. Thus the changes in the response to LRH *in vivo* are due to changes in pituitary sensitivity.

In the rat estrogen levels begin to rise on diestrus day II, a peak being reached on the morning of proestrus (Brown-Grant et al., 1970; Naftolin et al., 1972). It is thus possible that the estrogen surge is responsible for the increased pituitary sensitivity to LRH during the afternoon of proestrus. In agreement with this hypothesis, it has been found that treatment of rats with estradiol benzoate on diestrus day I increased the LRH response on the following day (Arimura and Schally, 1971).

In order to differentiate between an effect of steroids at the hypothalamic and pituitary levels, the response to LRH has been studied in pituitary cells in culture. Preincubation of cells for 36 hr in the presence of 3×10^{-9} M testosterone produces an approximately 10-fold increase in the apparent K_m of activation (ED_{50}) of LH release by LRH (Fig. 3–7). A possible explanation for this effect of the steroid could be a reduction of the number of binding sites for LRH on gonadotrops. The reverse has been found after 17β-estradiol treatment, the addition of this steroid leading to lowering of the ED_{50} for LRH. Such steroid-induced changes in the number of receptor sites for LRH may well explain the marked changes in pituitary sensitivity to LRH during the estrous cycle (Ferland et al., 1975b).

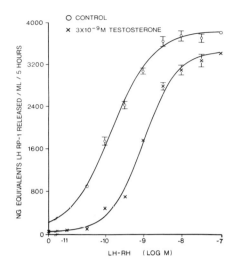

FIG. 3–7. Effect of 3×10^{-9} M testosterone on LH release induced by increasing concentrations of LH-RH (LRH) in pituitary cells in culture. After 3 days in culture, the cells were incubated for 5 hr with the indicated concentrations of LRH.

LRH ANALOGUES

The possibility of developing a contraceptive method based on inhibitory analogues of LRH has generated the current interest in synthesizing and carefully evaluating the activity of compounds of varying potency. The useful analogues antagonistic to LRH are those which: (1) have high affinity for the LRH receptor but interact in a way not leading to LH and FSH release; and (2) are resistant to *in vivo* degradation. The binding ability can best be evaluated by an *in vitro* system, and the second characteristic is best measured by *in vivo* studies. Structure-activity studies performed independently at these two levels (receptor affinity and peripheral degradation) should give the information required for the synthesis of improved compounds.

In our first study (Labrie et al., 1975*b*), 16 synthetic analogues of LRH were tested for their ability to inhibit the stimulation of LH release induced by 3×10^{-9} M LRH in anterior pituitary cells in monolayer culture. Half-maximal inhibition of LRH-induced LH release was obtained with [Des-His², D-Ala⁶] LRH at approximately 3×10^{-6} M, [Des-His², D-Ala⁶, Des-Gly-NH₂¹⁰] LRH ethylamide at 6×10^{-6} M, [Des-His², D-Leu⁶] LRH at 4×10^{-6} M (Fig. 3–8), [Des-His², Des-Gly-NH₂¹⁰] LRH trifluoroethylamide at 3×10^{-5} M, [Des-His²] LRH propylamide at 2×10^{-5} M, and [Leu² Leu³, D-Ala⁶, Des-Gly-NH₂¹⁰] LRH ethylamide at 1×10^{-5} M. [Des-His², Leu³, D-Ala⁶, Des-Gly-NH₂¹⁰] LRH ethylamide, [Pro¹, D-Ala⁶, Des-Gly-NH₂¹⁰] LRH ethylamide, and [D(Pyro) Glu, Des-His², Des-Gly-NH₂¹⁰] LRH ethylamide had no detectable antagonistic activity when tested up to a 3,000-fold molar ratio (analogue /LRH). Among the analogues tested, the most potent was

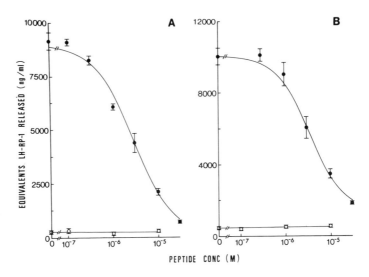

FIG. 3–8. Effect of increasing concentrations of [Des-His², D-Leu⁶] LH-RH (LRH) (A) or [D-Phe²] LH-RH (LRH) (B) on LH release in anterior pituitary cells in monolayer culture in the absence (○—○) or presence (●—●) of 3 × 10⁻⁹ M LRH.

[D-Phe², D-Leu⁶] LRH, 50% inhibition of LRH action being obtained at a molar ratio of 30:1.

Figure 3–9 shows that the subcutaneous injection of 30 μg [Des-His², D-Ala⁶] LRH, [Des-His², D-Leu⁶] LRH, or [D-Phe², D-Leu⁶] LRH in two equal doses 20 min before and at the same time as the injection of 100 ng LRH leads to an approximately 90% inhibition of the plasma LH response.

[Des-His²] LRH and [Gly²] LRH were the first analogues reported to be

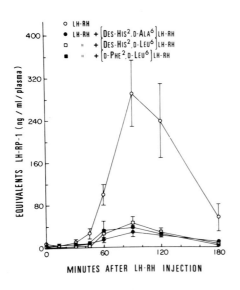

FIG. 3–9. Effect of [Des-His², D-Ala⁶] LH-RH (LRH), [Des-His², D-Leu⁶] LRH, and [D-Phe², D-Leu⁶] LRH on the plasma LH response to 100 ng LRH in the anesthetized female rat on the afternoon of proestrus. A total of 30 μg of the indicated analogues was injected subcutaneously in two equal doses 20 min before and at the time of LRH injection.

inhibitory to the action of LRH on LH release *in vitro* (Monahan et al., 1972; Vale et al., 1972). Much improved inhibitors are those which, in addition to a modification at position 2, include structural modifications of LRH shown to result in peptides more active than the natural hormone. Such modifications are those at the C-terminal end and those replacing the glycine residue at position 6 by a D-amino acid (Monahan et al., 1973; Vilchez-Martinez et al., 1974; Ferland et al., 1975a; Labrie et al., 1975b).

We previously observed that *in vivo* (Ferland et al., 1975a) and *in vitro* (Labrie et al., 1975b) the C-terminal ethylamide modification does not improve the inhibitory activity of the peptide. For example, [Des-His^2, D-Ala^6, des-Gly-NH$_2$^{10}] LRH ethylamide leads to a lower inhibition of cyclic AMP accumulation and LH and FSH release than [Des-His^2, D-Ala^6] LRH (M. Beaulieu, F. Labrie, D. Coy, E. Coy, and A. Schally, *unpublished observations*). This may be due, at least in part, to the low inherent stimulatory activity of the analogue at such a high concentration (Labrie et al., 1975b). However, in combination with the [Des-His^2] modification, the substitution of D-amino acids for glycine at position 6 of LRH (Monahan et al., 1973; Vilchez-Martinez et al., 1974; Ferland et al., 1975a; Labrie et al., 1975b) produces potent LRH inhibitors. An example of the effectiveness of such analogues is [Des-His^2, D-Ala^6] LRH and [Des-His^2, D-Leu^6] LRH.

A still better modification at position 2 appears to be replacement of the His residue by D-Phe (Rees et al., 1974; Ferland et al., 1975a; Labrie et al., 1975b). In fact, [D-Phe^2, D-Leu^6] LRH and [D-Phe^2, D-Phe^6] LRH can inhibit 50% of LRH action *in vitro* at molar ratios of approximately 100 and 30, respectively (M. Beaulieu, F. Labrie, D. Coy, E. Coy, and A. Schally, *unpublished observations*). These findings using hemipituitaries are in close agreement with data obtained using LRH-induced LH release in pituitary cells in monolayer culture (Labrie et al., 1975b).

ROLE OF PROSTAGLANDINS IN THE SECRETION AND ACTION OF HYPOTHALAMIC REGULATORY HORMONES

Do prostaglandins (PGs) play a mediator role in the action of hypothalamic hormones in the anterior pituitary gland? Such a role in the action of LH at the ovarian level was first suggested by Kuehl and associates (1970). *In vivo* evidence suggesting a role for PGs in certain actions of LH on the ovary has been provided by the findings of elevated levels of PGF and PGE in ovarian follicles following coitus or LH injection in rabbits (LeMaire et al., 1973; Armstrong et al., 1974) and prevention of ovulation by treatment with indomethacin (Yang et al., 1973) or injection of serum anti-PGF$_{2\alpha}$ (Armstrong et al., 1974). PGs have also been found to exert effects on many other endocrine tissues including the adrenal (De Wied et al., 1969; Flack et al., 1969) and thyroid (Burke et al., 1971).

In monkey granulosa cells in culture, PGE$_1$ stimulates (Channing, 1972) whereas $PGF_{2\alpha}$ inhibits (Chatterjee, 1972) progesterone secretion. Thus the effects of PGs can be stimulatory or inhibitory. Since the hypothalamus exerts both stimulatory and inhibitory influences on adenohypophyseal hormone secretion, PGs might theoretically appear as good candidates for controlling pituitary hormone secretion.

Prostaglandins and Adenohypophyseal Cyclic AMP

The stimulatory effect of PGE_1 and PGE_2 on cyclic AMP accumulation in anterior pituitary tissue is well substantiated (Zor et al., 1969, 1970; MacLeod and Lehmeyer, 1970; Makino, 1973; Ratner et al., 1974; Borgeat et al., 1975). At increasing concentrations ranging from 10^{-7} to 10^{-4} M, the various PGs exhibit markedly different potencies in inducing cyclic AMP accumulation in rat anterior pituitary tissue after 120 min of incubation (Fig. 3–10). The order of potency is: prostaglandin $E_1 \simeq E_2 > A_1 \simeq A_2 > F_{1\alpha} \simeq F_{2\alpha}$.

At 1×10^{-7} M the stimulatory effect of PGE_2 is already significant at 2 min and becomes maximal at 30 min (Borgeat et al., 1975). This maximal effect is followed by a progressive decrease to basal levels at 120 min. On addition of higher concentrations of PGE_2, cyclic AMP levels remain higher than controls at least up to 180 min (Borgeat et al., 1975). When studied at short time intervals (15 and 30 min), PGA_1 stimulates cyclic AMP accumulation only at high concentrations (10^{-4} M) and $PGF_{1\alpha}$ has only a mini-

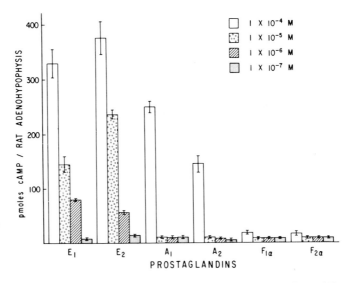

FIG. 3–10. Effect of increasing concentrations of prostaglandins E_1, E_2, A_1, A_2, $F_{1\alpha}$, and $F_{2\alpha}$ on cyclic AMP accumulation in rat anterior pituitary gland *in vitro*. Cyclic AMP was measured after 120 min of exposure to the indicated prostaglandin concentrations.

mal effect (Borgeat et al., 1975). PGs of the E type are thus the most potent activators of cyclic AMP accumulation in anterior pituitary tissue. PGE_1 and PGE_2 are in fact more potent than PGA_1 and PGA_2, and slight stimulation by $PGF_{1\alpha}$ is observed only at high concentrations (10^{-4} M).

Prostaglandins and GH Secretion

Data obtained from many *in vitro* studies using ox pituitary slices (Schofield, 1970; Cooper et al., 1972) and rat hemipituitaries (MacLeod and Lehmeyer, 1970; Hertelendy, 1971; Hertelendy et al., 1971, 1972; Kato et al., 1973; Bélanger et al., 1974; Ratner et al., 1974; Borgeat et al., 1975) leave no doubt about the stimulatory effect of PGs of the E series on GH release. As shown in Fig. 3–11, the order of potency of various PGs in stimulating GH release from rat anterior pituitary cells in culture closely parallels the potency previously observed on cyclic AMP accumulation (Fig. 3–10). In fact, half-maximal stimulation of GH release by PGE_1 and PGE_2 is observed at 5×10^{-7} M, 8 to 10×10^{-6} M for PGA_1 and PGA_2, and approximately 3×10^{-4} M for $PGF_{1\alpha}$ and $PGF_{2\alpha}$. As shown in Fig. 3–12, the *in vitro* stimulatory effect of PGE_1 and PGE_2 on GH release is confirmed *in vivo*. In fact, both PGE_1 and PGE_2 injected into the right superior vena cava in conscious rats lead to rapid and markedly elevated plasma GH levels, the effect of PGE_2 being approximately twice that of PGE_1. At doses up to 250 μg, PGA_1 and PGA_2 had no effect on plasma GH levels (data not shown). These data obtained in unanesthetized animals agree with the stimulatory effect of PGE_1 on plasma GH levels found in rats anesthetized

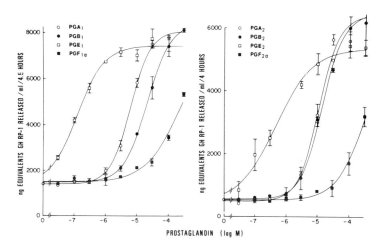

FIG. 3–11. Effect of increasing concentrations of prostaglandins E_1, A_1, B_1, $F_{1\alpha}$, E_2, A_2, B_2, and $F_{2\alpha}$ on GH release in anterior pituitary cells in culture. After 3 days in culture, the cells were incubated for 4 or 4.5 hr with the indicated prostaglandin concentrations.

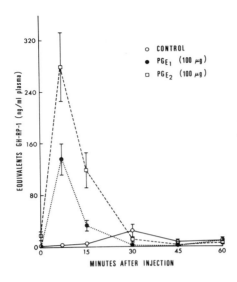

FIG. 3–12. Effect of intravenous injection of 100 μg PGE₁ or PGE₂ on plasma GH levels in the conscious male rat. Serial blood sampling after prostaglandin injection was achieved through a cannula inserted into the right superior vena cava 3 days previously.

with pentobarbital (Hertelendy et al., 1972) or urethane (Kato et al., 1973).

Intravenous infusion of PGE_1 at the rate of 50 to 140 ng/kg/min led to a marked rise of plasma GH levels in humans (Ito et al., 1971), whereas PGA_1 was found not to be effective (Wilson et al., 1971). A single dose of $PGF_{1\alpha}$ (20 μg/kg) was also reported to raise plasma GH levels in conscious sheep (Hertelendy et al., 1972).

Using a partially purified fraction of GH-releasing hormone (GRH), we recently found a rapid and concomitant stimulation of cyclic AMP accumulation and GH release in rat anterior pituitary tissue (Borgeat et al., 1973); comparable data have been obtained using a crude hypothalamic extract (Steiner et al., 1970). This close parallelism between changes of cyclic AMP levels and GH release induced by PGs and purified GRH may well indicate a role of PGs and cyclic AMP in the control of GH secretion. However, definitive proof of the role of PGs in the control of the activity of the somatotrops will be obtained only by direct measurement of the synthesis or mobilization of PGs under the influence of the corresponding neurohormones.

Prostaglandins and ACTH Secretion

In rats pretreated with a small dose of dexamethasone (25 μg/100 g body weight) and anesthetized with pentobarbital, the injection of PGE_1 (1.0 μg), $PGF_{1\alpha}$ (0.5 μg), or $PGF_{2\alpha}$ (0.5 μg) into the median eminence increased ACTH secretion (estimated by plasma corticosterone levels). Intravenous injections and injections into the lateral hypothalamus or pituitary had no effect (Hedge, 1972). In animals treated with pentobarbital only, ACTH secretion is very sensitive to the injection of PGE_1, a maximal response of plasma corticosterone being obtained at a dose of 1 μg. PGF$_{1\alpha}$ is much less potent by this route (Hedge, 1972). These data confirm those of Peng et al. (1970) who found that under similar conditions, PGE$_1$ produced maximal adrenal ascorbic acid depletion at a dose of 2 μg intravenously. PGA$_1$ or PGF$_{2\alpha}$ were not effective at even higher doses (5 μg/rat). De Wied et al. (1969) also found that in pentobarbital-chlorpromazine-pretreated rats a dose of 10 μg PGE$_1$ or PGE$_2$ (but not PGF$_{1\alpha}$ or PGF$_{2\alpha}$) stimulated plasma corticosterone levels. The possibility of a direct stimulatory effect of PGs at the adrenal level was ruled out because the response was abolished by hypophysectomy.

Since morphine, a drug believed to act mainly at the level of the CNS, inhibited the stimulatory response of ACTH secretion to PGs injected into the median eminence or intravenously (De Wied et al., 1969; Peng et al., 1970; Hedge, 1972), it is quite likely that PGs act at the hypothalamic level to stimulate the release of corticotropin-releasing hormone (CRH), which secondarily increases ACTH secretion. This proposed hypothalamic site of action of PGs is in agreement with the conclusions reached by De Wied et al. (1969). These investigators found that PGE$_1$ had a stimulatory effect on ACTH secretion in several systems commonly used for CRH assays, but that the response was abolished in rats with median eminence lesions; furthermore, they found that the addition of PGs had no effect on rat pituitaries incubated *in vitro*. The lower activity of PGF$_{1\alpha}$ and PGF$_{2\alpha}$ relative to PGE$_1$ when injected intravenously was attributed to a more rapid inactivation of PGs of the F than E types by plasma (Hedge, 1972). However, Vale et al. (1971) reported a stimulatory effect of PGE$_2$ on ACTH release *in vitro*.

The reported experiments indicate quite clearly that PGs can stimulate ACTH secretion *in vivo* by an action at the hypothalamic level leading to release of CRH(s). According to the data of Hedge (1972) and De Wied et al. (1969), PGE$_1$, PGE$_2$, PGF$_{1\alpha}$, and PGF$_{2\alpha}$ are all effective stimulators of CRH release.

As far as the action of PGs at the pituitary level is concerned, most of the *in vivo* evidence suggests a minor role at this site. However, the increase in ACTH release observed by Hedge (1972) after intrapituitary injection of a small dose (0.5 μg) of PGE$_1$ and the data of Vale et al. (1971) obtained *in vitro* indicate that further studies are needed.

Prostaglandins and LH and FSH Secretion

Studies Using Inhibitors of PG Synthetase

Indomethacin, an inhibitor of PG biosynthesis (Vane, 1971), prevents ovulation in rats when given early in the afternoon of proestrus (Tsafiri et al., 1972, 1973) or in the afternoon of the expected surge of LH in immature rats treated with pregnant mare's serum gonadotropin (PMS)

(Armstrong and Grinwich, 1972; Orczyk and Behrman, 1972; Armstrong and Zamecnik, 1975). However, there have been contradictory opinions about whether the action of the drug was on LH secretion (Behrman et al., 1972; Orcyk and Behrman, 1972) or directly on the ovary (Armstrong and Grinwich, 1972; Tsafiri et al., 1972, 1973; Armstrong and Zamecnik, 1975).

Indirect evidence suggested an action of PGs at the hypothalamic-pituitary level. It was found that ovulation blocked by indomethacin could be reversed by administering exogenous LH or a mixture of PGE_1 and $PGF_{2\alpha}$ (Orczyk and Behrman, 1972), and that ovulation blocked by aspirin in PMS-treated immature rats could be induced by LH or LRH (Behrman et al., 1972). These studies led to the suggestion (Behrman et al., 1972; Orczyk and Behrman, 1972) that PGs exert an effect at the pituitary level to stimulate LH release and at the hypothalamic level to induce LRH secretion. Treatment with either aspirin or indomethacin was accompanied by a reduction of hypothalamic and pituitary levels of PGFs.

Although acute (3 hr) and chronic (2 days) treatment with indomethacin blocked ovulation in all PMS-treated immature rats, LH administration could only reverse the acute effect of the drug (Orczyk and Behrman, 1972). Moreover, the number of ova was reduced from ten to five, thus indicating that the drug was acting at least partially at the ovarian level. The ability of exogenous LH to reverse the indomethacin-induced block of ovulation could also depend on the dose of LH used. In fact, a dose higher than that occurring during the spontaneous LH peak was more likely to counteract the effect of the PG synthetase inhibitor at the ovarian level.

That the main site of action of indomethacin was at the ovarian level was clearly shown by the finding that indomethacin administered during proestrus at a dosage found to inhibit ovulation failed to prevent the preovulatory elevation of serum LH following PMS injection in immature animals (Armstrong and Zamecnik, 1975). In agreement with this suggestion, the increase of ovarian PGF concentration that normally coincides with the LH peak was blocked by indomethacin. Similar conclusions about a main site of action of indomethacin being at the ovarian level were reached by Tsafiri et al. (1972, 1973), who found that indomethacin in high doses (10 mg) injected before the proestrous LH surge blocks ovulation without preventing the LH peak.

In agreement with the chronic experiments of Orczyk and Behrman (1972), Tsafiri et al. (1972) and Armstrong and Grinwich (1972) found that the indomethacin-induced block of ovulation could not be overcome by administering LH at a dose sufficient to induce ovulation in pentobarbital-anesthetized rats. Another argument which favors the theory that indomethacin acts on follicular rupture is that although indomethacin blocked follicular rupture it did not prevent maturation of follicle-entrapped oocytes, an effect attributed to LH. On the other hand, no oocyte maturation was observed in pentobarbital-anesthetized rats regardless of whether they were treated with indomethacin (Tsafiri et al., 1972).

The above experiments using indomethacin *in vivo* clearly indicate that the blockade of ovulation induced by the drug is secondary to an action at the ovarian level. However, these data do not rule out a role of PGs on LRH secretion and/or LH release. It is possible that indomethacin uptake is more efficient in the ovary than the hypothalamus and pituitary (Hucker et al., 1966) or that the inhibition of PG biosynthesis by indomethacin at the hypothalamic and pituitary levels was only partial and insufficient to prevent both LRH and LH release. In fact, as shown later, we find clear evidence for a stimulatory effect of PGs on LRH release. It is of interest that although LRH administration could not induce ovulation in indomethacin-treated rats, fluid retention disappeared after administration of the neurohormone (Behrman et al., 1972). Since uterine fluid release is considered to be a manifestation of progesterone secretion necessary for cervical relaxation, it is likely that LH release occurred and that progesterone secretion induced uterine fluid release in indomethacin-treated animals.

Effect of Intravenous PGs on Gonadotropin Release

As shown in Fig. 3–13, 250 μg PGE$_1$ or PGE$_2$ administered intravenously raised plasma LH levels in thiamylal-anesthetized animals. The study was performed during the afternoon of proestrus, a time of maximal pituitary sensitivity to LRH. It can also be seen that PGE$_2$ is approximately twice as potent as PGE$_1$. These data are in agreement with those of Tsafiri et al. (1973), who reported that subcutaneous injection of a higher dose (750 μg)

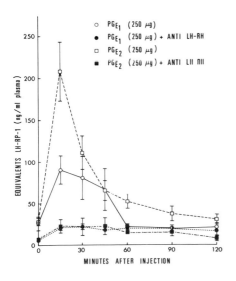

FIG. 3–13. Effect of intravenous injection of 250 μg PGE$_1$ or PGE$_2$ in the presence or absence of 0,5 ml anti-LH-RH (anti-LRH) serum. Female rats were anesthetized with sodium thiamylal on the afternoon of proestrus, and a cannula was inserted into the right superior vena cava before the indicated injections and serial blood sampling for measurement of plasma LH levels.

of PGE_2 increased plasma LH levels in pentobarbital-blocked proestrous rats. In steroid-primed ovariectomized rats, Harms et al. (1974) found that at doses up to 50 $\mu g/100$ g PGE_2 (but not PGE_1, $PGF_{1\alpha}$, or $PGF_{2\alpha}$) raised plasma LH levels in ether-anesthetized animals. Sato et al. (1974a) reported that injection of a relatively high dose (670 μg) of PGE_1, PGE_2, and $PGF_{2\alpha}$ increased serum LH levels measured 10 to 60 min later in estrogen/progesterone-primed ovariectomized rats. The minimal doses required were 0.2 μg PGE_2, 20 μg PGE_1, and 200 μg $PGF_{2\alpha}$.

Using male rats Ratner et al. (1974) reported stimulation of LH release after the intravenous injection of 20 μg PGE_1, and Sato et al. (1974b) found a stimulatory effect of PGE_2 on plasma FSH levels. Although etherization by itself stimulates LH release in the rat, most *in vivo* studies on the effect of PGs on gonadotropin release have been performed under ether anesthesia.

Labhsetwar (1973) reported that $PGF_{2\alpha}$ injected on pregnancy day 3 in hamsters increased plasma LH levels. Evidence for a stimulatory effect of $PGF_{2\alpha}$ on LH release has also been obtained in sheep. In fact, when 5 or 25 mg $PGF_{2\alpha}$ was given subcutaneously at midcycle, there was a small increase in plasma LH concentration (McCracken et al., 1973). Moreover, between days 5 and 10 of the estrous cycle in the ewe, the intracarotid infusion of $PGF_{2\alpha}$ at a rate of 6 $\mu g/hr$ or more was accompanied by a rise of plasma LH (Carlson et al., 1973). When estrous or ovariectomized ewes were used, $PGF_{2\alpha}$ did not affect plasma LH levels.

Effect of Intraventricular PGs on Gonadotropin Release

The findings of a stimulatory effect of intravenously injected PGE_1 or PGE_2 on LH release do not differentiate between an effect of PGs at the hypothalamic level on LRH release and a pituitary site of action on LH secretion. These approaches have been used to further elucidate the site of action of PGs by injecting PGEs intraventricularly and into the pituitary and then investigating the effect of anti-LRH serum on PG-induced LH release.

As shown in Fig. 3–14, 50 μg PGE_2 infused into the lateral ventricle of unanesthetized ovariectomized rats raised plasma LH levels. A significant effect was found 20 min after the beginning of the 30-min infusion, and a plateau was observed betwen 20 and 60 min, with a return to basal levels at 90 min. These data are in agreement with those of Harms et al. (1974), who found increased plasma LH levels after injecting 5 μg PGE_2 but not PGE_1 into the third ventricle of ether-anesthetized, ovariectomized rats. However, PGE_1 was found to have about 50% of the LH-releasing activity of PGE_2 when steroid-primed animals were used (Harms et al., 1974). When injected at a dose of 5 μg into the third ventricle of ovariectomized rats under ether anesthesia, PGE_1 (but not PGE_2, $PGF_{1\alpha}$, and $PGF_{2\alpha}$) led to increased plasma levels of LH and FSH (Harms et al., 1973).

Spies and Norman (1973) found that infusion of 10 or 30 μg PGE_1 into

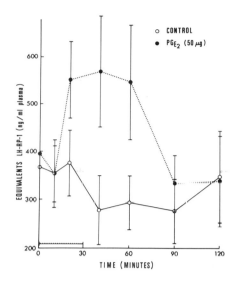

FIG. 3–14. Effect on plasma LH levels of a 0- to 30-min infusion of 50 μg PGE2 into the lateral ventricle of conscious ovariectomized rats.

the third ventricle of pentobarbital-anesthetized animals on the afternoon of proestrus induced ovulation in a large number of animals, whereas PGE2 and PGF2α were relatively ineffective. A role of PGs in the control of hypothalamic release of LRH is also suggested by the experiments of Labhsetwar and Zolovick (1973) who reported that injection of aspirin into the anterior hypothalamic area induced a PGF2α-reversible inhibition of ovulation in the PMS/progesterone-treated immature rat. Similar injections of either aspirin or PGF2α had no effect when administered into the pituitary.

It thus appears clear that intraventricular injection of PGs of the E and possibly of the F types leads to increased LH release in unanesthetized and ether- or pentobarbital-anesthetized rats. Although these data suggest a stimulatory effect of PGs on LRH secretion, material injected into the third or lateral ventricle may well reach the anterior pituitary gland and exert its action directly on LH release. Pelletier et al. (1975, *unpublished data*) have in fact found that after injecting ³H-TRH, ³H-LRH, or peroxidase into the lateral ventricle radioactivity and enzymatic activity diffuse through the median eminence and reach the primary plexus of the hypothalamopituitary portal system very quickly. It is thus possible that highly lipophilic compounds such as PGs diffuse quite freely between cells and nerve terminals of the median eminence. However, the amount of substances injected into the third ventricle that reach the adenohypophysis is very small (Ondo et al., 1972).

Effect of Intrapituitary Injection of PGs on Gonadotropin Release

Harms et al. (1974) found that although intrapituitary infusion of 5 μg PGE2 did not affect plasma LH levels in ovariectomized rats it did raise plasma LH levels in ovariectomized animals primed with estrogens; the same dose of PGE_1 was without effect. Sato et al. (1975), using a much higher dose (100 μg), found that both PGE_1 and PGE_2 (but not $PGF_{2\alpha}$) raised plasma LH levels in ovariectomized rats. An action of PGs at the pituitary level is also suggested by the fact that the response of plasma LH to LRH is slightly decreased after a 3-day treatment of female castrated animals with indomethacin (Sato et al., 1975). However, Spies and Norman (1973) found that the intrapituitary injection of 10 μg PGE_1 had little effect on the induction of ovulation.

Data obtained with the technique of intrapituitary injection or infusion of PGs can only be taken as suggestive evidence for a role of PGs at the pituitary level. Two limitations are apparent in this system: (1) backflow of PGs to the median eminence could occur with a resultant release of LRH; and (2) negative results could be due to limited diffusion of the injected compound.

Effect of Anti-LRH Serum on PG-Induced LH Release

The use of anti-LRH serum offers an approach that should permit differentiation between a hypothalamic and pituitary site of action in the induction of LH release after intravenous or intraventricular injection of PGs. As shown in Fig. 3–13, intravenous injection of LRH antiserum leads to a marked inhibition of PGE_2- or PGE_1-induced LH release. These data indicate that the stimulatory action of PGE_1 and PGE_2 on LH release after intravenous injection is mainly due to increased LRH secretion.

Since PGE_2 and PGE_1 raise plasma LH levels in unanesthetized as well as pentobarbital- or thiamylal-treated animals, it is likely that in the median eminence PGs act at a site close to the nerve endings containing LRH. In fact, it is likely that the centers controlling LH release (McCann and Porter, 1969) are inhibited by the anesthetics and are thus unresponsive to stimuli. The entry into the brain of peripherally administered PGs is very limited (Holmes and Horton, 1968), but the hypothalamus does not show a barrier to many small molecules (G. Pelletier, *unpublished observations*). Thus it seems likely that PGs injected peripherally act on the median eminence to induce the release of LRH from nerve endings. A role for PGs in the control of vasopressin secretion has also been suggested (Villhardt and Hedquist, 1970).

Effect of PGs on Gonadotropin Release In Vitro

Although many *in vitro* studies have been performed on the effect of PGs on LH and FSH release, the data are still conflicting. Using PGA_1, PGE_1, PGB_1, or $PGF_{1\alpha}$ in concentrations up to 200 μg/ml, Zor et al. (1969) found no significant stimulatory effect on LH release in rat anterior pituitaries *in vitro.* Using a similar system responding to the addition of PGE_1 or PGE_2 by a marked stimulation of GH release (Borgeat et al., 1975), we were unable to find a significant effect on either LH or FSH release for up to 3 hr of incubation. Chobsieng et al. (1975) did not find a stimulatory effect of PGE_2 on LH release from rat hemipituitaries during a 4-hr incubation.

The same negative results were obtained when the effect of increasing concentrations of different PGs was studied on hormone release in rat anterior pituitary cells in monolayer culture (Drouin and Labrie, 1975). PGE_1 and PGE_2 stimulated GH release at an apparent K_m value of 5×10^{-7} M, whereas the release of both LH and FSH was unaffected up to 10^{-5} M. A slight stimulation of both LH and FSII release was observed at very high concentrations of PGA_1 and PGA_2 (10^{-4} M). The physiological significance of the effect of such high concentrations of PGs is doubtful. In agreement with these data, Zor and associates (Z. Naor, Y. Koch, S. Bauminger, and U. Zor, *unpublished observations*) found that indomethacin, at a dose which reduced pituitary PG concentration, did not prevent the stimulation of cyclic AMP accumulation by LRH *in vitro* or LRH-induced LH release.

On the other hand, Sato et al. (1975) found a stimulatory effect of PGE_1, PGE_2, and $PGF_{2\alpha}$ on LH release from male rat anterior pituitaries *in vitro*. Makino (1973) and Ratner et al. (1974) also reported that PGE_1 stimulated LH release *in vitro;* and Dowd et al. (1973), using a perfusion system, reported a stimulatory effect of PGE_1 and PGE_2 on LH release.

Thus *in vitro* experiments do not provide definitive information on the role of PGs in LH release. However, it is clear that under many conditions where PGE_1 and PGE_2 lead to marked stimulation of GH release, there is no detectable effect of PGs on LH and FSH release.

Prostaglandins and TSH Secretion

Vale et al. (1971) found that TSH release from rat hemipituitaries *in vitro* is increased by PGE_1, whereas the TRH-induced release of TSH is inhibited by the PG antagonist 7-oxa-13-prostynoic acid. However, Tal et al. (1974) reported that PGs do not increase TSH release *in vitro*.

In an *in vivo* study Brown and Hedge (1974) found that none of the PGs they tested (A_1, E_1, B_1, and $F_{1\alpha}$) stimulated TSH secretion when injected intravenously into the anterior pituitary or the basal hypothalamus. PGE_1 injected intravenously was even found to be a potent inhibitor of TRH-induced TSH release. Prostaglandins E_1, A_1, B_1, and $F_{1\alpha}$ were all found to potentiate the action of TRH on TSH release when both PG and TRH were injected into the pituitary gland (Brown and Hedge, 1974). A role of PGs in the control of TSH secretion is also indicated by the finding of a decreased plasma TSH response to TRH in thyroidectomized rats on thyroid replacement therapy when treated for 48 hr with indomethacin (Thompson and Hedge, *personal communication*).

Since PGs injected intravenously or into the basal hypothalamus could directly influence the rate of TSH release or the release of TRH and somatostatin (two peptides having opposite effects on TSH release), data obtained in this way are difficult to interpret. However, injection of PGs into the pituitary gland and some *in vitro* studies suggest a role of PGs in the control of TSH secretion. A particularly interesting finding is the potentiation of the TRH-induced TSH release by PGs injected directly into the pituitary (Brown and Hedge, 1974).

Prostaglandins and Prolactin Secretion

When injected at a dose of 5 μg into the third ventricle of ovariectomized or ovariectomized/estrogen-treated rats under ether anesthesia, PGE_1 (but not PGE_2, $PGF_{1\alpha}$, or $PGF_{2\alpha}$) led to increased plasma PRL levels within 15 to 30 min (Harms et al., 1973; Ojeda et al., 1974a). PGE_1 and PGE_2 had no effect when injected directly into the anterior pituitary, suggesting that the stimulatory effect of PGE_1 was at the hypothalamic level. Sato et al. (1974b) also found that after intravenous injection PGE_1, PGE_2, and $PGF_{2\alpha}$ increased plasma PRL levels in castrated female rats pretreated with estrogens and progesterone. Vermouth and Deis (1972) reported that the intraperitoneal injection of $PGF_{2\alpha}$ on day 18 of pregnancy raised plasma PRL levels in rats.

These *in vivo* studies indicate that PGE_1 after intraventricular injection and PGE_1, PGE_2, and $PGF_{2\alpha}$ after intravenous injection raise plasma PRL levels in the rat. Since PGs do not seem to stimulate PRL secretion at the pituitary level (Labrie et al., 1973), it appears that the stimulatory effect of PGs is exerted on the release of the hypothalamic hormones controlling PRL secretion. Since PRL secretion is controlled by both positive and negative influences from the hypothalamus, the global stimulatory effect of PGE_1 could be due to stimulation of PRH secretion, inhibition of prolactin-inhibiting hormone(s) (PIH) release, or a combination of these. However, the net influence of the hypothalamus on PRL secretion is inhibitory (McCann and Porter, 1969; Schally et al., 1974). This inhibitory influence may be exerted by catecholamines (Ojeda et al., 1974b; MacLeod and Lehmeyer, 1974) and/or a PRL release-inhibiting substance different from catecholamines (Dupont and Redding, 1975). It thus appears that the reported stimulatory effect of PGs on PRL release could be more easily exerted by inhibiting the release of PIH, although stimulation of PRH release is also possible.

SUMMARY

Strong evidence has now been obtained for a role of cyclic AMP as mediator of the action of TRH, LRH, and somatostatin in the anterior pituitary gland. It has in fact been found that LRH and its agonistic analogues having a wide range of biological activity lead to simultaneous changes in cyclic AMP levels and LH and FSH release as a function of both concentration of the peptides and time of incubation. Moreover, when LRH antagonists are used, a close parallelism is found between their inhibitory effect on gonadotropin release and adenohypophyseal cyclic AMP levels. Somatostatin leads to rapid inhibition of cyclic AMP accumulation in anterior pituitary gland *in vitro,* this inhibitory effect being accompanied by parallel inhibition of pituitary hormone secretion.

Studies with somatostatin analogues indicate that the functional receptors for the tetradecapeptide are very similar in three anterior pituitary cell types: somatotrophs, thyrotrophs, and mammotrophs. There is also good evidence for similar properties of the functional receptor for TRH in both thyrotrophs and mammotrophs. The inhibition by somatostatin of the TRH-induced TSH and PRL release is of a noncompetitive type and occurs at a step subsequent to binding to receptors. The decreasing order of efficiency of somatostatin to inhibit GH, TSH, and PRL release could be secondary to the presence of different numbers of efficient receptors for the tetradecapeptide in the three corresponding cell types.

As ascertained by *in vitro* studies using pituitaries collected at different stages of the rat estrous cycle, the increased plasma LH response to LRH observed *in vivo* during proestrus is due to changes at the pituitary level. Studies with anterior pituitary cells in culture show that testosterone increases while estradiol decreases the apparent K_m of activation (ED_{50}) of LH release by LRH. Such effects could be secondary to steroid-induced changes of the level of LRH receptors in gonadotrophs.

Structural modifications of LRH at positions 2 and 6 lead to potent antagonists of LRH action both *in vivo* and *in vitro.* Prostaglandins exhibit markedly different potencies to induce cyclic AMP accumulation in anterior pituitary tissue, the order of potency being prostaglandin $E_1 \simeq E_2 > A_1 \simeq A_2 > F_{1\alpha} \simeq F_{2\alpha}$. The order of potency of various PGs to induce GH release in cells in culture closely parallels their effect on cyclic AMP accumulation, whereas no significant effect of PGs is measured on LH, FSH, or PRL secretion *in vitro.* When administered *in vivo,* PGE_1 and PGE_2 lead to marked increases of plasma GH and LH levels. Since the PG-induced stimulation of plasma LH concentration is completely abolished by pretreatment of the animals with anti-LRH antibodies, it is concluded that the increased plasma LH levels observed *in vivo* after PG administration are secondary to increased LRH release.

REFERENCES

Alberti, K. G. M. M., Christensen, S. E., Iversen, J., Seyer-Hansen, K., Christensen, N. J., Prange-Hansen, A., Lundbaek, K., and Orskov, H. (1973): Inhibition of insulin secretion by somatostatin. *Lancet,* 2:1299–1301.

Arimura, A., and Schally, A. V. (1971): Augmentation of pituitary responsiveness to

LH-releasing hormone (LH-RH) by estrogen. *Proc. Soc. Exp. Biol. Med.,* 136:290–293.

Armstrong, D. T., and Grinwich, D. L. (1972): Blockade of spontaneous and LH-induced ovulation in rats by indomethacin, an inhibitor of prostaglandin biosynthesis. *Prostaglandins,* 1:21–28.

Armstrong, D. T., and Zamenick, J. (1975): Pre-ovulatory elevation of rat ovarian prostaglandins F and its blockade by indomethacin. *Mol. Cell. Endocrinol.,* 2:125–131.

Armstrong, D. T., Grinwich, D. L., Moon, U. S., and Zamenick, J. (1974): Inhibition of ovulation in rabbits by intrafollicular injection of indomethacin and prostaglandin F antiserum. *Life Sci.,* 14:129–140.

Behrman, H. R., Orczyk, G. P., and Greep, R. O. (1972): Effect of synthetic gonadotropin-releasing hormone (GH-RH) on ovulation blockade by aspirin and indomethacin. *Prostaglandins,* 1:245–249.

Bélanger, A., Labrie, F., Borgeat, P., Savary, M., Côté, J., and Drouin, J. (1974): Inhibition of growth hormone and thyrotropin release by growth hormone-release inhibiting hormone. *Mol. Cell. Endocrinol.,* 1:329–339.

Bloom, S. R., Mortimer, C. H., Thorner, M. O., Besser, G. M., Hall, R., Gomez-Pan, A., Roy, V. M., Russel, R. C. G., Coy, D. H., Kastin, A. J., and Schally, A. V. (1974): Inhibition of gastrin and gastric-acid secretion by growth-hormone release-inhibiting hormone. *Lancet,* 2:1106.

Bøler, J., Enzman, F., Folkers, K., Bowers, C. Y., and Schally, A. V. (1969): The identity of chemical and hormonal properties of the thyrotropin releasing hormone and pyroglutamyl-histidyl-proline amide. *Biochem. Biophys. Res. Commun.,* 37:705–710.

Borgeat, P., Chavancy, G., Dupont, A., Labrie, F., Arimura, A., and Schally, A. V. (1972): Stimulation of adenosine 3′,5′-cyclic monophosphate accumulation in anterior pituitary gland in vitro by synthetic luteinizing hormone-releasing hormone/follicle-stimulating hormone-releasing hormone (LH-RH/FSH-RH) *Proc. Natl. Acad. Sci. U.S.A.,* 69:2677–2681.

Borgeat, P., Labrie, F., Poirier, G., Chavancy, G., and Schally, A. V. (1973): Stimulation of adenosine 3′,5′-cyclic monophosphate accumulation in anterior pituitary gland by purified growth hormone-releasing hormone. *Trans. Assoc. Am. Physicians,* 86:284–299.

Borgeat, P., Labrie, F., Côté, J., Ruel, F., Schally, A. V., Coy, D. H., Coy, E. J., and Yanaihara, N. (1974a): Parallel stimulation of cyclic AMP accumulation and LH and FSH release by analogs of LH-RH in vitro. *J. Mol. Cell. Endocrinol.,* 1:7–20.

Borgeat, P., Labrie, F., Drouin, J., Bélanger, A., Immer, I., Sestanj, K., Nelson, V., Gotz, M., Schally, A. V., Coy, D. H., and Coy, E. J. (1974b): Inhibition of adenosine 3′,5′-monophosphate accumulation in anterior pituitary gland in vitro by growth hormone-release inhibiting hormone. *Biochem. Biophys. Res. Commun.,* 56:1052–1059.

Borgeat, P., Garneau, P., and Labrie, F. (1975): Characteristics of action of prostaglandins on cyclic AMP accumulation in rat anterior pituitary gland. *Can. J. Biochem. (in press).*

Bowers, C. Y. (1971): The role of cyclic AMP in the release of anterior pituitary hormones. *Ann. N.Y. Acad. Sci.,* 185:263–290.

Brazeau, P., Vale, W., Burgus, R., Ling, V., Butcher, M., Rivier, J., and Guillemin, R. (1973): Hypothalamic polypeptide that inhibits the secretion of immunoreactive pituitary growth hormone. *Science,* 179:77–79.

Brown, M. R., and Hedge, G. A. (1974): In vivo effects of prostaglandins on TRH-induced TSH secretion. *Endocrinology,* 95:1392–1397.

Brown-Grant, K., Exley, D., and Naftolin, F. (1970): Peripheral plasma oestradiol and luteinizing hormone concentrations during the oestrous cycle of the rat. *J. Endocrinol.,* 48:295–296.

Burgus, R., Dunn, T. F., Desiderio, D., and Guillemin, R. (1969): Structure moléculaire du facteur hypothalamique TRF d'origine ovine: Mise en évidence par spectrométrie de masse de la séquence PCA-His-Pro-NH₂. *C. R. Acad. Sci. [D] (Paris),* 269:1870–1873.

Burgus, R., Butcher, M., Ling, N., Monahan, M., Rivier, J., Fellows, R., Amoss, M.,

Blackwell, R., Vale, W., and Guillemin, R. (1971): Structure moléculaire du facteur hypothalamique (LRF) d'origine ovine contrôlant la sécrétion de l'hormone de gonadotrope hypophysaire de lutéinisation. *C. R. Acad. Sci.* [D] (*Paris*), 273:1611–1613.

Burke, G., Kowalski, K., and Babiarz, D. (1971): Effects of thyrotropin, prostaglandin E_1 and a prostaglandin antagonist on iodide trapping in isolated thyroid cells. *Life Sci.*, Part II:513–521.

Carlson, J. C., Barcikowski, B., and McCracken, J. A. (1973): Prostaglandin $F_{2\alpha}$ and the release of LH in sheep. *J. Reprod. Fertil.*, 34:357–361.

Channing, C. P. (1972): Stimulatory effects of prostaglandins upon luteinization of rhesus monkey granulosa cell cultures. *Prostaglandins*, 2:331–349.

Chatterjee, A. (1972): The possible mode of action of prostaglandins II: Failure of prostaglandin $F_{2\alpha}$ in the prevention of compensatory ovulation and ovarian hypertrophy following unilateral ovariectomy in rat. *Acta Endocrinol. (Kbh.)*, 70:786–790.

Chobsieng, P., Naor, F., Koch, Y., Zor, U., and Lindner, H. R. (1975): Stimulatory effect of prostaglandin E_2 on LH release in the rat: Evidence for hypothalamic site of action. *Neuroendocrinology* (*in press*).

Cooper, R. H., McPherson, M., and Schofield, J. G. (1972): The effect of prostaglandins on ox pituitary content of adenosine 3',5'-cyclic monophosphate and the release of growth hormone. *Biochem. J.*, 127:143–154.

DeLéan, A., Beaulieu, D., and Labrie, F. (1974): Modulation of the level of the TRH receptor in rat anterior pituitary by estrogens and thyroid hormone. *Clin. Res.*, 22:730A.

DeVane, G. W., Siler, T. M., and Yen, S. S. C. (1974): Acute suppression of insulin and glucose levels by synthetic somatostatin in normal human subjects. *J. Clin. Endocrinol. Metab.*, 38:913–915.

De Wied, D., Witter, A., Versteeg, D. H. G., and Mulder, A. H. (1969): Release of ACTH by substances of central nervous system origin. *Endocrinology*, 85:561–569.

Dowd, A. J., Hoffman, D. C., and Speroff, L. (1973): Direct effects of prostaglandins and prostaglandin inhibitors on pituitary LH release demonstrated by in vitro perfusion. *Endocrinology*, 92:135A (abstract).

Drouin, J., and Labrie, F. (1975): Specificity of the stimulatory effect of prostaglandins on hormone release in rat anterior pituitary cells in culture (*in preparation*).

Drouin, J., De Léan, A., Rainville, D., Lachance, R., and Labrie, F. (1975): Characteristics of the interaction between TRH and somatostatin for thyrotropin and prolactin release (*submitted for publication*).

Dupont, A., and Redding, T. W. (1975): Purification and characterization of PIF from pig hypothalami. *Endocrinology*, 96:93A (abstract).

Everett, J. W. (1948): Progesterone and estrogen in the experimental control of ovulation time and other features of the estrous cycle in the rat. *Endocrinology*, 43:389–405.

Ferin, M., Tempone, Z., Zimmering, P. E., and Vande-Wiele, R L. (1969). Effect of antibodies to 17_β-estradiol and progesterone on the estrous cycle of the rat. *Endocrinology*, 85:1070–1078.

Ferland, L., Labrie, F., Coy, D. H., Coy, E. J., and Schally, A. V. (1975a): Inhibitory activity of four analogs of luteinizing hormone-releasing hormone in vivo. *Fertil. Steril.* (*in press*).

Ferland, L., Borgeat, P., Labrie, F., Bernard, J., De Léan, A., and Raynaud, J. P. (1975b): Changes of pituitary sensitivity to LH-RH during the rat estrous cycle. *Mol. Cell. Endocrinol.*, 2:107–115.

Flack, J. D., Jessup, R., and Ramwell, P. W. (1969): Prostaglandin stimulation of rat corticosteroidogenesis. *Science*, 163:691–692.

Gerich, J. E., Lorenzi, M., Schneider, V., Karam, J. H., Rivier, J., Guillemin, R., and Forsham, P. H. (1974): Effect of somatostatin on plasma glucose and glucagon levels in human diabetes mellitus. *N. Engl. J. Med.*, 291:544–547.

Grant, G., Vale, W., and Guillemin, R. (1973): Characteristics of the pituitary binding sites for thyrotropin-releasing factor. *Endocrinology*, 92:1629–1633.

Hall, R., Besser, G. M., Schally, A. V., Coy, D. H., Evered, D., Goldie, D. J., Kastin, A. J., McNeilly, A. S., Mortimer, C. H., Phenekos, C., Tunbridge, W., and Weightman, D. (1973): Action of growth hormone release inhibitory hormone in healthy men and in acromegalics. *Lancet*, 2:581–584.

Harms, P. G., Ojeda, S. R., and McCann, S. M. (1973): Prostaglandin involvement in hypothalamic control of gonadotropin and prolactin release. *Science*, 181:760–761.

Harms, P. G., Ojeda, S. R., and McCann, S. M. (1974): Prostaglandin-induced release of pituitary gonadotropins: Central nervous system and pituitary sites of action. *Endocrinology*, 94:1459–1464.

Hedge, G. A. (1972): The effects of prostaglandins on ACTH secretion. *Endocrinology*, 91:925–933.

Hertelendy, F. (1971): Studies on growth hormone secretion II. Stimulation by prostaglandins in vitro. *Acta Endocrinol. (Kbh.)*, 68:355–362.

Hertelendy, F., Peake, G. T., and Todd, H. (1971): Studies on growth hormone secretion: Inhibition of prostaglandin, theophylline and cyclic AMP stimulated growth hormone release by valinomycin in vitro. *Biochem. Biophys. Res. Commun.*, 44:253–260.

Hertelendy, F., Todd, H., Ehrhart, K., and Blute, R. (1972): Studies on growth hormone secretion. IV. In vivo effects of prostaglandin E_1. *Prostaglandins*, 2:79–91.

Hinkle, P. M., and Tashjian, A. H., Jr. (1973): Receptors for thyrotropin-releasing hormone in prolactin-producing rat pituitary cells in culture. *J. Biol. Chem.*, 248:6180–6186.

Hinkle, P. M., Woroch, E. L., and Tashjian, A. H., Jr. (1974): Receptor-binding affinities and biological activities of analogs of thyrotropin-releasing hormone in prolactin-producing pituitary cells in culture. *J. Biol. Chem.*, 249:3085–3090.

Holmes, S. W., and Horton, E. W. (1968): The identification of four prostaglandins in dog brain and their regional distribution in the central nervous system. *J. Physiol. (Lond.)*, 195:731–741.

Hucker, H. B., Zacchei, A. G., Cox, S. V., Brodie, D. A., and Cantwell, N. H. R. (1966): Studies on the absorption, distribution and excretion of indomethacin in various species. *J. Pharmacol. Exp. Ther.*, 153:237–249.

Ito, H., Momose, G., Katayama, T., Takagishi, H., Ito, L., Nakajima, H., and Takei, Y. (1971): Effect of prostaglandin on the secretion of human growth hormone. *J. Clin. Endocrinol. Metab.*, 32:857–859.

Jutisz, M., Kerdelhue, G., Berault, A., and Paloma de la Llosa, M. (1972): On the mechanism of action of the hypothalamic gonadotropin releasing factors. In: *Gonadotropins*, edited by B. B. Saxena, C. G. Beling, and H. M. Gandy, pp. 64–71. Wiley Interscience, New York.

Kaneko, T., Saito, S., Oka, H., Oda, T., and Yanaihara, N. (1973): Effects of synthetic LH-RH and its analogs on rat anterior pituitary cyclic AMP and LH and FSH release. *Metabolism*, 22:77–78.

Kato, Y., Dupre, J., and Beck, J. C. (1973): Plasma growth hormone in the anesthetized rat: Effects of dibutyryl cyclic AMP, prostaglandin E, adrenergic agents, vasopressin, chlorpromazine, amphetamine and L-dopa. *Endocrinology*, 93:135–146.

Kuehl, F. A., Humes, J. L., Tarnoff, J., Cirillo, V. J., and Ham, E. A. (1970): Prostaglandin receptor site: Evidence for an essential role in the action of luteinizing hormone. *Science*, 169:883–886.

Labhsetwar, A. P. (1973): Neuroendocrine basis of ovulation in hamsters treated with prostaglandin F_{2a}. *Endocrinology*, 92:606–610.

Labhsetwar, A. P., and Zolovick, A. (1973): Hypothalamic interaction between prostaglandins and catecholamines in promoting gonadotropin secretion for ovulation. *Nature [New Biol.]*, 246:55–56.

Labrie, F., Barden, N., Poirier, G., and De Léan, A. (1972): Characteristics of binding of [^{3}H] thyrotropin-releasing hormone to plasma membranes of bovine anterior pituitary gland. *Proc. Natl. Acad. Sci. U.S.A.*, 69:283–287.

Labrie, F., Pelletier, G., Lemay, A., Borgeat, P., Barden, N., Dupont, A., Savary, M., Côté, J., and Boucher, R. (1973): Control of protein synthesis in anterior pituitary gland. *Research Methods in Reproductive Endocrinology*, Geneva, pp. 301–340.

Labrie, F., Borgeat, P., Lemay, A., Lemaire, S., Barden, N., Drouin, J., and Bélanger, A. (1975a): Role of cyclic AMP in the action of hypothalamic regulatory hormones in the anterior pituitary gland. *Adv. Cyclic Nucleotide Res. (in press)*.

Labrie, F., Savary, M., Coy, D. H., Coy, E. J., and Schally, A. V. (1975b): Inhibition of LH release by analogs of LH releasing hormone (LH-RH) in vitro (submitted for publication).

Labrie, F., De Léan, A., Borgeat, P., Barden, N., Poirier, G., and Drouin, J. (1975c): Polypeptide receptor mechanisms in anterior pituitary gland. In: Anatomical Neuroendocrinology, edited by W. E. S. Stumpf and L. D. Grant. Karger, Basel (in press).

LeMaire, W. J., Yang, N. S. T., Behrman, H. H., and Marsh, J. M. (1973): Preovulatory changes in the concentration of prostaglandins in rabbit graafian follicles. Prostaglandins, 3:367–376.

MacLeod, R. M., and Lehmeyer, J. E. (1970): Release of pituitary growth hormone by prostaglandins and dibutyryl adenosine cyclic 3',5'-monophosphate in the absence of protein synthesis. Proc. Natl. Acad. Sci. U.S.A., 67:1172–1179.

MacLeod, R. M., and Lehmeyer, J. E. (1974): Studies on the mechanism of the dopamine-mediated inhibition of prolactin secretion. Endocrinology, 94:1077–1085.

Makino, T. (1973): Study of the intracellular mechanism of LH release in the anterior pituitary. Am. J. Obstet. Gynecol., 115:606–614.

Matsuo, H., Baba, Y., Nair, R. M. G., Arimura, A., and Schally, A. V. (1971): Structure of the porcine LH- and FSH-releasing hormone. I. The proposed amino acid sequence. Biochem. Biophys. Res. Commun., 43:1334–1339.

McCann, S. M., and Porter, J. C. (1969): Hypothalamic pituitary stimulating and inhibiting hormones. Physiol. Rev., 49:240–284.

McCracken, J. A., Barcikowski, B., Carlson, J. C., Green, K., and Samuelsson, B. (1973): The physiological role of prostaglandin $F_{2\alpha}$ in corpus luteum regression. Adv. Biosci., 9:599–624.

Monahan, M., Rivier, J., Vale, W., Guillemin, R., and Burgus, R. (1972): [Gly^2] LRF and des-His^2-LRF: The synthesis, purification, and characterization of two LRF analogues antagonistic to LRF. Biochem. Biophys. Res. Commun., 47:551–556.

Monahan, M. W., Amoss, M. S., Anderson, H. A., and Vale, W. (1973): Synthetic analogs of the hypothalamic luteinizing hormone releasing factor with increased agonist or antagonist properties. Biochemistry, 12:4616–4620.

Mortimer, C. H., Carr, D., Lind, T., Bloom, S. R., Mallison, C. N., Schally, A. V., Tunbridge, W. M. G., Yeomans, L., Coy, D. H., Kastin, A. J., Besser, G. M., and Hall, R. (1974): Effect of growth-hormone release-inhibiting hormone on circulating glucagon, insulin and growth hormone in normal, diabetic, acromegalic, and hypopituitary patients. Lancet, 2:697–701.

Naftolin, F., Brown-Grant, K., and Corker, S. C. (1972): Plasma and pituitary luteinizing hormone and peripheral plasma oestradiol concentrations in the normal oestrus cycle of the rat and after experimental manipulation of the cycle. J. Endocrinol., 53:17–30.

Ojeda, S. R., Harms, P. G., and McCann, S. M. (1974a): Central effect of prostaglandin E_1 (PGE$_1$) on prolactin release. Endocrinology, 95:613–618.

Ojeda, S. R., Harms, P. G., and McCann, S. M. (1974b): Possible role of cyclic AMP and prostaglandin E_1 in the dopaminergic control of prolactin release. Endocrinology, 95:1694–1703.

Ondo, J. G., Mical, R. S., and Porter, J. C. (1972): Passage of radioactive substances from CSF to hypophysial portal blood. Endocrinology, 91:1239–1246.

Orczyk, G. P., and Behrman, H. R. (1972): Ovulation blockade by aspirin or indomethacin in vivo evidence for a role of prostaglandin in gonadotropin secretion. Prostaglandins, 1:3–21.

Pelletier, G., Dupont, A., and Puviani, R. (1975): Ultrastructural study of the uptake of peroxidase by the rat median eminence. Cell Tissue Res., 156:521.

Peng, T. S., Six, K. M., and Munson, P. L. (1970): Effects of prostaglandin E_1 on the hypothalamo-hypophyseal-adrenocortical axis in rats. Endocrinology, 86:202–206.

Poirier, G., Labrie, F., Barden, N., and Lemaire, S. (1972): Thyrotropin-releasing hormone receptor: Its partial purification from bovine anterior pituitary gland and its close association with adenyl cyclase. FEBS Lett., 20:283–286.

Ratner, A., Wilson, M. C., Srivastava, L., and Peake, G. T. (1974): Stimulatory effects of prostaglandin E_1 on rat anterior pituitary cyclic AMP and luteinizing hormone release. Prostaglandins, 5:165–174.

Rees, R. W., Foell, T. J., Chai, S. Y., and Grant, N. (1974): Synthesis and biological activities of analogs of the luteinizing hormone-releasing hormone (LH-RH) modified in position 2. *J. Med. Chem.,* 17:1016–1019.

Rivier, C., and Vale, W. (1974): In vivo stimulation of prolactin secretion in the rat by thyrotropin releasing factor, related peptides and hypothalamic extracts. *Endocrinology,* 95:978–983.

Robison, G. A., Butcher, R. W., and Sutherland, E. W. (1968): Cyclic AMP. *Annu. Rev. Biochem.,* 37:149–174.

Sato, T., Taya, K., Jyujyo, T., Hirono, M., and Igarashi, M. (1974a): The stimulatory effect of prostaglandins on luteinizing hormone release. *Am. J. Obstet. Gynecol.,* 118:875–876.

Sato, T., Jyujo, T., Iesaka, T., Ishikawa, J., and Igarashi, M. (1974b): Follicle stimulating hormone and prolactin release induced by prostaglandins in rat. *Prostaglandins,* 5:483–490.

Sato, T., Hirono, M., Jyujo, T., Iesaka, T., Taya, K., and Igarashi, M. (1975): Direct action of prostaglandins on the rat pituitary. *Endocrinology,* 96:45–49.

Schally, A. V., Arimura, A., and Kastin, A. J. (1974): Hypothalamic regulatory hormones. *Science,* 179:341–350.

Schally, A. V., Dupont, A., Arimura, A., Redding, T. W., and Linthicom, G. L. (1975): Isolation of porcine GH-release inhibiting hormone (GH-RIH): The existence of 3 hours of GH-RIH. *Fed. Proc.,* 34:584.

Schofield, J. G. (1970): Prostaglandin E_1 and the release of growth hormone in vitro. *Nature (Lond.),* 228:179–180.

Siler, T. M., Yen, S. S. C., Vale, W., and Guillemin, R. (1974): Inhibition by somatostatin on the release of TSH-induced in man by thyrotropin-releasing factor. *J. Clin. Endocrinol. Metab.,* 38:742–745.

Spies, H. G., and Norman, R. L. (1973): Luteinizing hormone release and ovulation induced by the intraventricular infusion of prostaglandin E_1 into pentobarbital-blocked rats. *Prostaglandins,* 4:131–142.

Steiner, A. L., Peake, G. T., Utiger, R. D., Karl, I. E., and Kipnis, D. M. (1970): Hypothalamic stimulation of growth hormone and thyrotropin release in vitro and pituitary of 3'5'-adenosine cyclic monophosphate. *Endocrinology,* 86:1354–1360.

Tal, E., Szabo, M., and Burke, G. (1974): TRH and prostaglandin action on rat anterior pituitary: Dissociation between cyclic AMP levels and TSH release. *Prostaglandins,* 5:175–182.

Tsafiri, A., Lindner, H. R., Zor, U., and Lamprecht, S. A. (1972): Physiological role of prostaglandins in the induction of ovulation. *Prostaglandins,* 2:1–11.

Tsafiri, A., Koch, Y., and Lindner, H. R. (1973): Ovulation rate and serum LH levels in rats treated with indomethacin or prostaglandin E_2. *Prostaglandins,* 3:461–467.

Vale, W., Rivier, C., and Guillemin, R. (1971): A "prostaglandin receptor" in the mechanisms involved in the secretion of anterior pituitary hormones. *Fed. Proc.,* 30:363 (abstract).

Vale, W., Brazeau, P., Scout, S., Nussey, A., Burgus, R., Rivier, J., Ling, N., and Guillemin, R. (1972): Premières observations sur le mode d'action de la somatostatine, un facteur hypothalamique qui inhibe la sécrétion de l'hormone de croissance. *C. R. Acad. Sci. [D] (Paris),* 275:2913–2916.

Vale, W., Rivier, C., Brazeau, P., and Guillemin, R. (1974): Effects of somatostatin on the secretion of thyrotropin and prolactin. *Endocrinology,* 95:968–977.

Vane, J. R. (1971): Inhibition of prostaglandin synthesis or a mechanism of action for aspirin-like drugs. *Nature [New Biol.],* 231:232–235.

Vermouth, N. T., and Deis, R. P. (1972): Prolactin release induced by prostaglandin $F_{2\alpha}$ in pregnant rats. *Nature [New Biol.],* 238:248–250.

Vilchez-Martinez, J. A., Schally, A. V., Coy, D. H., Coy, E. J., Debeljuk, L., and Arimura, A. (1974): In vivo inhibition of LH release by a synthetic antagonist of LH-releasing hormone (LH-RH). *Endocrinology,* 95:213–218.

Vilhardt, H., and Hedquist, P. (1970): A possible role of prostaglandin E_2 in the regulation of vasopressin secretion in rats. *Life Sci.,* 9:825–830.

Wilson, D. E., Philips, C., and Levine, R. A. (1971): Inhibition of gastric secretion in man by prostaglandin A. *Gastroenterology,* 61:201–206.

Yang, N. S. T., Marsh, J. M., and LeMaire, W. J. (1973): Prostaglandin changes induced by ovulatory stimuli in rabbit graafian follicles: The effect of indomethacin. *Prostaglandins*, 4:395–404.

Yen, S. S. C., Siler, T., and De Vane, G. (1974): Effect of somatostatin in patient with acromegaly: Suppression of growth hormone, prolactin, insulin and glucose levels. *N. Engl. J. Med.*, 290:935–938.

Zor, U., Kaneko, T., Schneider, H. P. G., McCann, S. M., Lowe, I. P., Bloom, S., Borland, B., and Field, J. B. (1969): Stimulation of anterior pituitary adenyl cyclase activity and adenosine 3′,5′-cyclic phosphate by hypothalamic extract and prostaglandin E_1. *Proc. Natl. Acad. Sci. U.S.A.*, 63:918–925.

Zor, U., Kaneko, T., Schneider, H. P. G., McCann, S. M., and Field, J. B. (1970): Further studies of stimulation of anterior pituitary cyclic adenosine 3′,5′-monophosphate formation by hypothalamic extract and prostaglandins. *J. Biol. Chem.*, 245:2883–2888.

Frontiers in Neuroendocrinology, Vol. 4,
edited by L. Martini and W. F. Ganong.
Raven Press, New York © 1976.

Chapter 4

Unit Responses in Preoptic and Arcuate Neurons Related to Anterior Pituitary Function

Robert L. Moss

Department of Physiology, University of Texas Health Science Center at Dallas, Southwestern Medical School, Dallas, Texas 75235

The diencephalon has been shown to be actively involved in the regulation of pituitary function, but, the role of hypothalamic neurons in mediating the conversion of neural to hormonal signals has received relatively little attention. Neurosecretory neurons were first identified within the central nervous system (CNS) of invertebrates (Dahlgren, 1914; Kandel, 1964). These specialized nerve cells have also been observed within the CNS of many vertebrates, including the mammalian hypothalamus (Stutinsky, 1970; Pawlikowski and Karasek, 1971; Smith, 1971; Hayward, 1974). The functional significance of the neurosecretory cell as an integral unit in hormone synthesis and release is widely accepted, especially when considering the hypothalamoneurohypophyseal system.

The author's interest in the electrophysiology of neuroendocrine transducer-type nerve cells originated with studies in which electrical stimulation of specific neural sites within the CNS resulted in hormone release. For instance, electrical stimulation along the hypothalamoneurohypophyseal tract has been shown to release both vasopressin and oxytocin. These studies were based on the assumption that stimulation mimics the endogenous changes in neural activity that precede pituitary secretion. Accordingly, experiments were performed to identify and determine pharmacological sensitivity of neurons involved in the release of posterior pituitary hormones. The combined techniques of electrophysiological recording, antidromic identification, and microelectrophoresis were utilized and developed during a period of research with Professor B. A. Cross and his colleagues (Drs. Dyball, Dyer, and Lincoln) in Bristol, England.

The initial experiments demonstrated the existence of an excitatory (cholinergic) and an inhibitory (noradrenergic) input into neurosecretory paraventricular (PV) neurons responsible for neurohypophyseal hormone release (Cross et al., 1971; Moss et al., 1971, 1972a). These data are summarized in Fig. 4–1. It is clear from subsequent studies that a relationship does exist between action potentials in PV neurosecretory nerve cells and

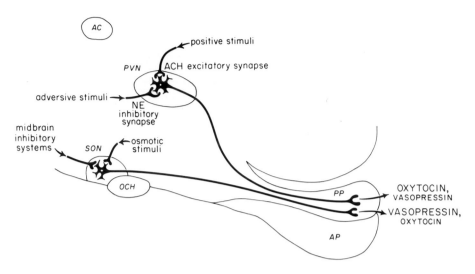

FIG. 4–1. Hypothalamoneurohypophyseal system, emphasizing the relationships between the paraventricular nucleus (PVN), supraoptic nucleus (SON), and the posterior pituitary gland (PP). OCH, optic chiasma. AP, anterior pituitary gland. AC, anterior commissure, ACH, acetylcholine. NE, norepinephrine.

release of oxytocin from the neurohypophysis (Wakerley and Lincoln, 1971a,b, 1973a,b; Lincoln and Wakerley, 1972). Oxytocin and vasopressin are produced in the PV and supraoptic nuclei (Cross and Green, 1959; Bisset et al., 1971; Dyball, 1971; Kalino and Reinne, 1972; Burford et al., 1974; Clattenburg, 1974). Several excellent reviews broader in scope than the present one present a complete survey of the literature dealing with neurophysiological correlates of neurohypophyseal hormone release (Cross, 1973a,b; Cross and Dyball, 1974): Consequently no attempt is made in the present chapter to review this field.

In contrast to the hypothalamoneurohypophyseal model, the precise localization and function of hypothalamic neurons responsible for the synthesis and release of the neurohormones that control adenohypophyseal activity remains uncertain. The present chapter summarizes recent findings from the author's laboratory on the possible relationship between neurons, their electrical and chemical activity, and adenohypophyseal function, with special consideration given to the neural mechanism(s) regulating release of luteinizing hormone-releasing hormone (LRH). An attempt is made to comment on areas of significant controversy and unsolved problems, as well as to present the limitations and future strategy for the electrophysiological approach in neuroendocrine investigation. References to much of the relevant background literature can be found in several excellent reviews (Beyer and Sawyer, 1969; Sawyer, 1970a,b; Komisaruk, 1971; Cross, 1973a,b; Cross and Dyball, 1974; Dyer, 1974a).

EVIDENCE FOR A NEURAL LINK IN THE CONTROL OF ANTERIOR PITUITARY ACTIVITY

There is little doubt that the posterior pituitary hormone secretion rate is directly related to action potentials arriving at nerve terminals in the neural lobe. A similar neurosecretory system may also exist within the hypothalamo-adenohypophyseal axis. The problem that needs to be resolved in essence is whether nerve fibers terminating in the median eminence are purely secretory in function or if they also conduct nerve impulses.

The following facts are known about the link between the hypothalamus and anterior pituitary gland (Fig. 4–2):

1. Although pituitary functions are subject to hypothalamic control, direct neural regulation is not present.

2. There is a specialized vascular connection—the hypophyseal portal system of blood vessels—between the median eminence of the hypothalamus and the anterior pituitary gland.

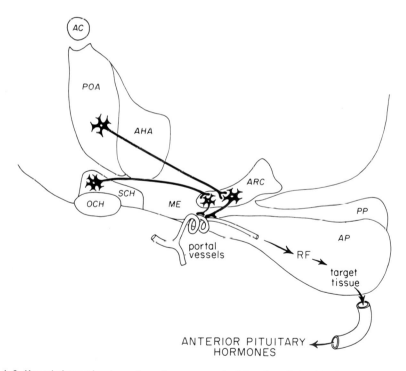

FIG. 4–2. Hypothalamoadenohypophyseal system, emphasizing the relationships between the preoptic area (POA), suprachiasmatic region (SCH), arcuate nucleus (ARC), median eminence (ME), and the anterior pituitary gland (AP). Neurons in the preoptic area and suprachiasmatic region are pictured as projecting to the arcuate nucleus while arcuate neurons are pictured as projecting to the proximal capillary plexus of the portal system. OCH, optic chiasma. PP, posterior pituitary lobe. AC, anterior commissure. AHA, anterior hypothalamic area, RF, releasing hormones.

3. Hypothalamic control over the pituitary is mediated by a variety of neurohormones, i.e., hypothalamic releasing and inhibiting hormones.

4. Release of releasing hormones into the portal circulation of the median eminence results in hormone secretion from the anterior pituitary gland (Harris, 1948, 1955; Scharrer and Scharrer, 1963; Szentagóthai et al., 1968; McCann and Porter, 1969; Greep and Porter, 1973; McCann et al., 1974).

The first notion of a humoral connection between the hypothalamus and the anterior pituitary gland emerged from the studies of Hinsey and Markee (1933), Harris (1937), and others. However, it was not until 1947 that Green and Harris fully recognized the significance of the hypophyseal portal system and promulgated the "portal vessel-chemotransmitter hypothesis" (neurohumoral hypothesis). This hypothesis proposes that neurohormones produced in the hypothalamus, which are specific for each pituitary hormone, travel via the portal vessels to stimulate specific adenohypophyseal target cells. It is thought that such a system is comprised of neurosecretory neurons in which neural events are translated into biochemical events, resulting in the production and release of specific neurohormones.

Histological examination of the hypophysiotropic area of the hypothalamus has revealed that axons from cells located in the arcuate (ARC) nucleus, ventromedial nucleus (VM), and the ventral aspect of the anterior periventricular nucleus terminate in the external layer of the median eminence (Szentagóthai et al., 1968; Rethelyi and Halász, 1970). Such neurons are distinct from the classic neurosecretory neurons of the neurohypophysis and are called tuberoinfundibular neurons (Szentagóthai et al., 1968; Rethelyi and Halász, 1970).

More recently the hypophysiotropic area (Halász et al., 1962; Halasz, 1969) has been extended to include the preoptic-suprachiasmatic (PO-SCH) region as well as the mediobasal hypothalamus (MBH), as seen in Fig. 4–2. The results of a number of experiments using a wide variety of techniques support the suggested role of PO-SCH as well as ARC-VM neurons in controlling LRH release. These two hypothalamic areas have been shown to influence the functional activity of the adenohypophysis (Critchlow, 1958; Flerkó and Bardos, 1959; Taleisnik and McCann, 1961; Everett, 1965; Butler and Donovan, 1971). They also contain LRH as measured by bioassay, radioimmunoassay, and immunohistochemistry (Schneider et al., 1969; Barry et al., 1973, 1974; Kordon et al., 1974; Palkovits et al., 1974; Zimmerman et al., 1974; McCann et al., 1975; Sétáló et al., 1975; Wheaton et al., 1975). In addition, a number of neurons located near capillaries of the PO-SCH and ARC-VM nuclei have been shown to exhibit ultrastructural changes suggestive of enhanced synthetic activity following mating, castration, and laparotomy (Clattenburg, 1974).

In addition to being localized in the PO-SCH region and the ARC-VM complex, LRH may be found in ependymal cells and in the organum vasculosum of the lamina terminalis (OVLT; Zimmerman et al., 1974). Thus it is possible that systems other than neurosecretory neurons secrete LRH into the proximal plexus of the portal system. For instance, LRH may be released by the OVLT into the ventricular cerebrospinal fluid (CSF) and be delivered to portal capillaries via the ependymal cells at the base of the third ventricle (Knowles and Anand Kumar, 1969; Anand Kumar, 1973; Knigge et al., 1973; Porter, 1973; Zimmerman et al., 1974).

It is obvious from the aforementioned that the precise mechanism regulating release of releasing hormones from the hypothalamus remains uncertain. Nonetheless, it is clear that many neurons of the ARC nucleus send their axons toward the median eminence (Spatz, 1951; Szentagóthai et al., 1962, 1968) where they contact the perivascular spaces of the hypophyseal portal capillaries (Fuxe and Hökfelt, 1967; Szentagóthai et al., 1968; Zambrano and DeRobertis, 1968). In view of the reported increase in luteinizing hormone (LH) releasing activity in portal blood following electrical stimulation of the PO area (Burger et al., 1972), the role of neurons terminating on or near the portal vessels becomes extremely important.

NEUROPHYSIOLOGICAL CORRELATES OF ADENOHYPOPHYSEAL FUNCTION

Several basic assumptions are made with respect to the nature of the "neurohumoral hypothesis." One such underlying assumption is that if the secretion of hormones from the adenohypophysis is controlled by hypothalamic neurons, changes in the electrical and neurotransmitter activity of these neurons should cause alterations in anterior pituitary secretion. Substantiating this assumption is the fact that electrical stimulation of the PO-SCH region in anesthetized rats induces an increase in LRH activity in the hypophyseal portal plasma (Harris and Ruf, 1970), an elevation of plasma LH level (Clemens et al., 1971; Keller and Lichtensteiger, 1971), and ovulation (Critchlow, 1958; Barraclough and Gorski, 1961; Everett, 1965; Barraclough, 1966; Harris and Ruf, 1970; McDonald and Gilmore, 1971). This suggests that an increase in electrical activity of the PO SCH neurons enhances gonadotropin secretion by the adenohypophysis. Accordingly, it has been proposed that an increase in hypothalamic neuronal activity might be a prerequisite for various reproductive events, such as ovulation (Terasawa and Sawyer, 1969) and/or the onset of sexual behavior (Law and Moss, 1969).

This concept prompted a number of laboratories to utilize electrophysiological recording techniques in an attempt to relate changes in the electrical activity of the hypothalamus to endocrine function. The macrorecording procedures measured electroencephalography (EEG), multicell activity, and direct-current potentials; and the microrecording methods measured single-cell activity. Some years ago in the laboratory of Dr. O. T. Law, I demonstrated a correlation between single-cell activity and the stages of the estrous cycle (Moss and Law, 1971). More specifically, 778 extracellular potentials were recorded from either the PO area, anterior hypothalamic area (AHA), cingulate cortex (CC), or the lateral septum (LS) in regular 4-day cyclic female rats anesthetized with urethane. Changes in single-cell activity in the PO area, AHA, and CC were correlated with the different stages of the estrous cycle (Fig. 4–3). No apparent change in unit activity was observed in the LS over this period. An increase was observed in CC unit activity during the afternoon of the metestrous-diestrous phase, which may reflect the importance of this structure in reproductive behavior. It was previously reported that hemidecortication of the female rat results in alterations in cyclicity and other endocrine changes (Covian et al., 1959; Rodriquez, 1959).

In contrast, an increase in unit activity in the PO area and the AHA was observed on the afternoon of proestrus (Fig. 4–3). These findings support previous observations in the intact animal using macrorecording techniques (Terasawa and Timiras, 1968, 1969) and in hypothalamic deafferentation experiments in unanesthetized animals utilizing microelectrode recording techniques (Cross and Dyer, 1970a,b). The latter experiments suggest that the hypothalamoadenohypophyseal system functions independently of extra-hypothalamic influences.

Our observations were confirmed and extended by the work of Dyer and Cross (Cross and Dyer, 1971a,b; Dyer and Cross, 1972a,b; Dyer et al., 1972). The increase in PO-AHA unit activity observed during the afternoon of proestrus was pinpointed to the ventral rather than the dorsal aspect of

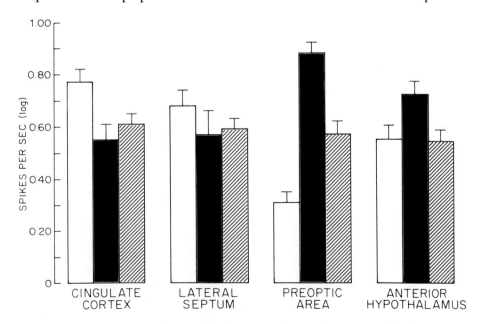

FIG. 4–3. Effect of the estrous cycle on single-cell activity in the cingulate cortex and the lateral septal, preoptic, and anterior hypothalamic areas. *Open bars, diestrus. Solid bars, proestrus. Cross-hatched bars, estrus.* (Adapted from Moss and Law. 1971.)

the PO-AHA. This finding seems to correlate with the localization of LRH in the PO-SCH region (Wheaton et al., 1975).

Recently Yagi and Sawaki (1971, 1973) reported single-cell activity in PO-SCH and ARC nuclei of cyclic and castrated female rats anesthetized with urethane. A summary of the results is shown in Fig. 4–4. Single-unit activity in the PO-SCH region was high during diestrus day 2 and proestrus (Fig. 4a), whereas ovariectomy lowered the unit activity. On the other hand, the cell activity in the ARC nucleus was high during the day of proestrus and in the castrated rat (Fig. 4b), both of which have high levels of serum LH (Ramirez and McCann, 1964).

In experiments utilizing multiunit recording techniques, Kawakami and his co-workers (Kawakami et al., 1973; Kawakami and Terasawa, 1974) demonstrated an increase in the electrical activity in the septum, PO area, and the ARC nucleus on the afternoon of proestrus. Moreover, in a recent communication Wuttke (1974) reported a rise in the level of multiunit activity during the "critical period" of the estrous cycle on the afternoon of proestrus in unanesthetized rats. Accompanying this increase in electrical activity was a rise in the plasma concentration of LH and prolactin. The hormone levels remained high after the elevated activity had subsided. A similar increase in activity and in serum LH levels was observed following vaginal stimulation on the evening of proestrus (Wuttke, 1974). Thus it appears that on the afternoon of proestrus in both the anesthetized and un-anesthetized rat there is an increase in single-cell and multiunit electrical activity of the PO area. Furthermore, the increase in PO cell activity is associated with a substantial rise in serum LH levels.

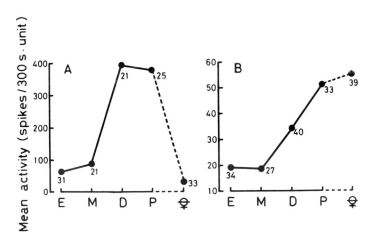

FIG. 4–4. Mean activity levels of spontaneously firing unit during the estrous cycle and after castration. A: Preoptic units. B: Arcuate units. The mean values were calculated based on the normalized data. Ovariectomy depressed the activity of the preoptic units and augmented the activity of the arcuate neurons. E, estrus. M, metestrus. D, diestrus. P, proestrus. ♀, ovariectomized. (From Yagi and Sawaki. 1973.)

In addition to the aforementioned studies, a number of investigators have used electrophysiological recording techniques to demonstrate neural correlates of endocrine function. Terasawa and Sawyer (1969) demonstrated an increase in ARC multiunit activity following ovulation-inducing electrochemical stimulation of the PO region. In subsequent studies these investigators (Terasawa et al., 1969; Terasawa and Sawyer, 1970) showed a similar increase in ARC multiunit activity following ovulation-advancing treatment with progesterone on the morning of proestrus and following treatment with exogenous LH. Moreover, Weiner et al. (1971) recorded a biphasic increase-decrease in median eminence multiunit activity following the intraventricular infusion of epinephrine or norepinephrine but not dopamine. Recently Carrer and Sawyer (1974) observed elevated multiunit activity in the PO area following ovulation-inhibiting electrochemical stimulation of the midbrain raphe nuclei. In studies by Gallo et al. (1971), electrochemical stimulation of the hippocampus decreased plasma LH levels in ovariectomized rats, blocked spontaneous ovulation in proestrous animals, and induced a rise in multiunit activity in the ventromedial hypothalamus. Thus changes in ARC, PO, and median eminence multiunit activity have been correlated with chemical or electrochemical stimulation of "ovulation-inducing" systems.

Many studies investigating the relationship between hypothalamic unit activity in the hypothalamus and reproductive functions have been correlative in nature. For example, Moss and Law (1971) demonstrated a significant increase in neuronal activity in the PO area on the day of proestrus as compared with the day of estrus and metestrus-diestrus. However, it is not known whether these neurons are involved in the release of LRH and/or the reported increase in electrical activity is related to the initiation and onset of sexual behavior.

Although application of single-unit recording techniques has enabled a closer scrutiny of neural mechanisms underlying many hypothalamic functions, there are many problems in electrophysiological research in this area. A recurrent problem is that many of the neurons in the hypothalamus are small interneurons. Single-unit recording techniques sample mostly large neurons, and so an extremely selective population is obtained. The effect of the anesthetic is a known variable which obviously modifies neural activity as well as adenohypophyseal function. Finally it is difficult to select those neurons responsible for a specific neuroendocrine function.

NEURAL CONNECTION BETWEEN HYPOTHALAMIC NUCLEI AND MEDIAN EMINENCE

The technique of antidromic identification or activation of individual nerve cells *in vivo* has recently been adapted for neuroendocrine research (Novin et al., 1970; Koizumi and Yamashita, 1972). Antidromic identification involves the electrical stimulation or activation of the terminal endings of neurons *in vivo*. The stimulation pulse initiates an antidromic action potential, which propagates up the axon toward the cell body. A recording electrode placed on or near the soma records the antidromic spike. The poststimulation latency of the spike reflects the conduction velocity (Yagi and Sawaki, 1970*a;* Makara et al., 1972; Dyer, 1974*b*). Direct antidromic activation of neurons can be distinguished from synaptic (indirect) excitation using two criteria: (1) a constant latency to the onset of the evoked spike; and (2) cancellation after collision with a "spontaneously" occurring orthodromic spike. The technique of antidromic identification showing constant latency and collision is outlined in Fig. 4–5.

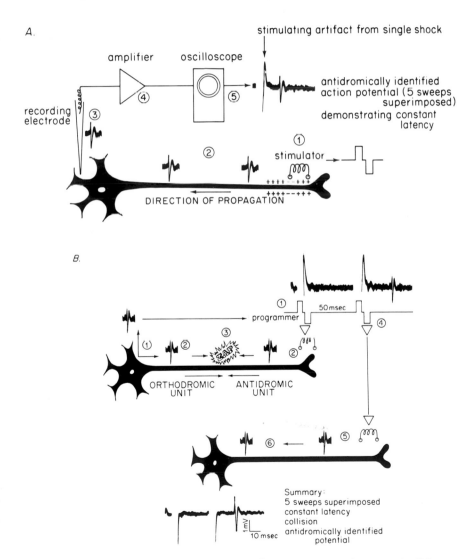

FIG. 4–5. A and B. Technique of antidromic identification with constant latency and collision.

A number of laboratories including my own have reported the electro-physiological identification of neurons with cell bodies in the ARC-VM complex and axons ending in the external layer of the median eminence (Yagi and Sawaki, 1970a; Harris et al., 1971; Makara et al., 1972; Moss and Riskind, 1973; Moss et al., 1974a, 1975a). In my experiments the parapharyngeal approach was used to expose the ventral surface of the brain and anterior pituitary gland (Fink et al., 1967; Porter and Smith, 1967). Prior to single-cell recording and antidromic identification, a bipolar stainless steel stimulating electrode was placed at the junction of the median eminence and pituitary (Fig. 4–6). Balanced biphasic pulses (0.2 msec duration) were administered to the junction at a frequency of one pulse every 5 sec and an intensity of 0.05 to 6 mA, while exploring with a record-ing microelectrode for antidromic single-cell activity in the basal hypo-thalamus.

Of the 149 single cells recorded, 79 were found to be antidromically activated in response to electrical stimulation of the median eminence. The

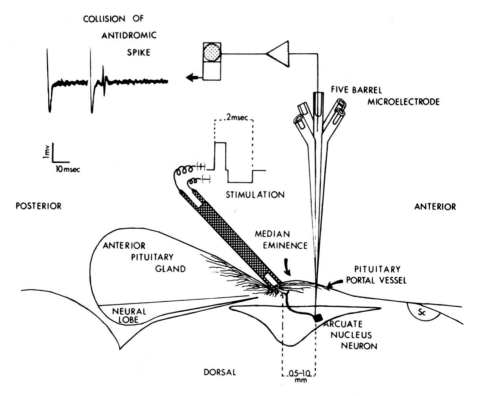

FIG. 4–6. Method for *in vivo* identification and pharmacological study of arcuate neurons using the ventral approach. Five superimposed oscilloscope traces (*top left*) show collision of orthodromic and antidromic action potentials of a recorded arcuate neuron. The positive deflection is upward. Sc, suprachiasmatic nucleus. (From Moss et al., 1975.)

cell bodies of these neurons were located in the ARC nucleus, with a few lying on the border between the ARC and VM nuclei. The mean latency of the antidromically identified potentials was 9.5 msec. The latency of the response was 8 to 14 msec with the average conduction velocity estimated to be 0.05 meters/sec. Thirty-six of the 79 units were not discharging spontaneously and would have been undetected in the absence of antidromic stimulation; these neurons were called silent cells. Forty-seven percent of the neurons recorded ($N = 70$) could not be driven antidromically but were spontaneously active. The spontaneous firing rate of antidromically identified ARC neurons ($N = 43$) varied from less than 1 to 8/sec while unidentified cells with axons that do not project to the median eminence ($N = 70$) discharged at rates that ranged from less than 3 to 10/sec. These findings are in agreement with the data of Yagi and Sawaki (1970a) and Makara et al. (1972). They provide evidence for the existence of neurons in the ARC nucleus which are capable of conducting nerve impulses and send their axons into the external layer of the median eminence (Fig. 4–7A). This suggests that ARC neurosecretory neurons are capable of conducting action potentials (Yagi et al., 1966, 1971; Novin et al., 1970; Yagi and Sawaki, 1970a,b; Yamashita et al., 1970; Sawaki and Yagi, 1973) and terminate on or near portal capillaries in the external layer of the median eminence (Kobayashi et al., 1967; Keller and Lichtensteiger, 1971; Björklund et al., 1973). In addition, their slow conduction rate suggests that their axons are small-diameter, unmyelinated C-fibers.

Yagi and Sawaki (1975a,b) presented some interesting evidence for the existence in the rat tuberoinfundibular system of inhibitory and facilitatory neural circuits activated by recurrent axon collaterals. Figure 4–7B indicates a possible recurrent neural circuit in this system. Recurrent inhibition of identified hypothalamoneurohypophyseal neuroendocrine neurons was previously found in the PO nucleus of goldfish (Kandel, 1964) and in the supraoptic (SO) and PV nuclei of rats, cats, dogs, and monkeys (Barker et al., 1971; Nicoll and Barker, 1971; Dreifuss and Kelly, 1972; Koizumi and Yamashita, 1972; Negoro and Holland, 1972; Negoro et al., 1973; Dreifuss et al., 1974; Dyball, 1974; Hayward and Jennings, 1974a,b). On the other hand, recurrent facilitation has been demonstrated in the cat (Koizumi et al., 1973). The physiological significance of recurrent neural circuits in the hypothalamoadenohypophyseal system is not currently known, but they may play a role in modulating neurosecretory activity by inhibiting or facilitating the neuronal discharge.

Recently Harris and Sanghera (1974) and Makara and Hodács (1975) demonstrated that neurons with cell bodies in the ARC, VM, and periventricular area can be antidromically activated by electrical stimulation applied to the PO and AH areas. Thus the axons of these neurons project to the PO-AH areas. The neurons are often found adjacent to other neurons, which are antidromically activated only by stimulating the junction of the pituitary stalk and the median eminence. These neural connections are represented in Fig. 4–7C. The neural connections from the ARC-VM complex to the PO-AH areas may have great physiological significance especially when considering the possible recurrent neural circuit in the tuberoinfundibular system. Certainly feedback mechanisms of all sorts can be postulated to explain a number of reproductive events. Most intriguing would be one that

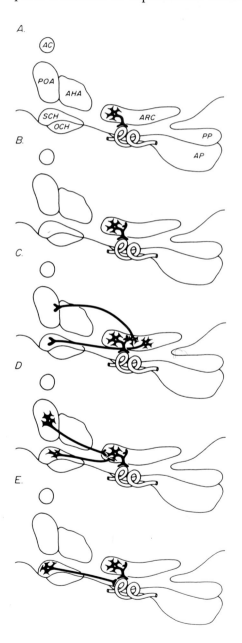

FIG. 4–7. A: Neural connection between the arcuate (ARC) nucleus and the portal vessels in the median eminence. B: Recurrent collateral in ARC-median eminence system. C: Neural connections between the ARC and preoptic area (POA) and suprachiasmatic area (SCH). D: Projections from the PO-SCH area to ARC; and E: Projections from the PO-SCH area to portal vessels. OCH, optic chiasm. PP, posterior pituitary gland. AP, anterior pituitary gland. AC, anterior commisure. AHA, anterior hypothalamic area.

offers a possible explanation for the LRH-induced facilitation of lordosis behavior in the rat (Moss and McCann, 1973, 1975). For example, if tuberoinfundibular neurons released LRH from their axonal endings, LRH would also be released from their recurrent collaterals. These collaterals could then modulate the neural activity of neurons which project from the ARC to the PO area. In turn, the PO area, which has been implicated in the neural control of sexual behavior (Powers and Valenstein, 1972; Moss et al., 1974b; Pfaff et al., 1974), could facilitate the lordotic response.

The method of identifying neurons by antidromic activation has also been utilized in my laboratory to identify PO neurons with axons that pass directly into the ARC-VM complex (Fig. 4–8). To accomplish this task, a concentric, bipolar stimulating electrode was lowered through the brain into the ARC-VM complex. The recording electrode was lowered into the PO in search of antidromically activated potentials resulting from ARC-VM stimulation; 220 units were recorded from the PO area. Antidromic action potentials with a constant latency were evoked in 34 of the cells by stimuli applied to the ARC-VM complex. In each case, when the stimulator was triggered by a spontaneous action potential the orthodromic and antidromic

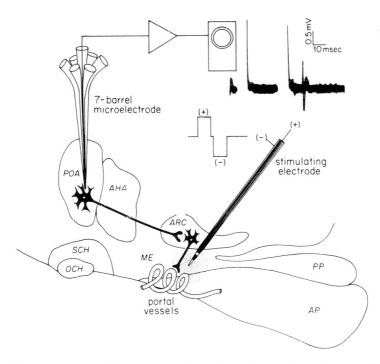

FIG. 4–8. Method for *in vivo* identification and pharmacological study of preoptic neurons. Five super-imposed oscilloscope traces (*top right*) show collision of orthodromic and antidromic action potentials of a recorded preoptic neuron. Positive deflection is upward. POA, preoptic area. AHA, anterior hypothalamic area. SCH, suprachiasmatic area. OCH, optic chiasm. ARC, arcuate nucleus. ME, median eminence. PP, posterior pituitary gland. AP, anterior pituitary gland.

spikes canceled each other (Fig. 4–8). This suggests that the neuron projects directly to the mediobasal hypothalamus without the intervention of a synapse. The average latency of the antidromic spike was 12.0 msec (range 6.0 to 28.9 msec). Assuming an average distance of 3.0 mm between recording and stimulating electrodes, the average conduction velocity was 0.25 meters/sec. This conduction velocity is similar to that obtained for the tuberoinfundibular neurons (Moss et al., 1975*b*).

These findings confirm the data of Dyer (1973). In a very detailed study Dyer showed that approximately 41% of the PO neurons (type A) projected directly to the mediobasal hypothalamus without a synapse. The remaining 59% of the PO neurons were of two types: neurons which projected through a synapse to the mediobasal hypothalamus (type B, 32%) and those that projected elsewhere (type C, 27%). The majority of PO neurons that were connected indirectly (type B) or not connected at all to the mediobasal hypothalamus (type C) showed an increase in firing rate during the proestrous phase of the estrous cycle. The activity of the fibers that connected directly to the mediobasal hypothalamus (type A) did not increase during proestrus.

Several studies suggest that neurons which appear to be involved in the secretion of LRH have cell bodies in the ventral aspect of the PO area and/or SCH region and axonal endings in the median eminence (Mess, 1969; Schneider et al., 1969; Quijada et al., 1971; Motta et al., 1973). This projection is shown in Fig. 4–7E. Electrophysiological experiments have not determined the existence of such a pathway. Antidromic potentials have been identified in SCH neurons by electrical stimulation of the median eminence. However, it cannot be proved that electrical stimulation was localized only to the median eminence; axonal endings in the ARC nucleus could also have been activated. Interestingly, experiments that have demonstrated the presence of LRH in the SCH and the median eminence have also shown a low level of LRH activity extending from the SCH region to the median eminence (Sétáló et al., 1975; Wheaton et al., 1975). This suggests the possibility of a fiber system from the SCH region to the median eminence, but more evidence is needed to confirm the existence of this pathway.

Information obtained from identified neurons is important in terms of establishing the neural connection between hypothalamic sites. However, this information does not aid in determining the function of individual neurons.

INFLUENCE OF HORMONES AND PHARMACOLOGICAL AGENTS ON NEURAL ACTIVITY RELATED TO ANTERIOR PITUITARY FUNCTION

In order to establish the functional properties of hypothalamic neurons that may be involved in neuroendocrine control of anterior pituitary activity, a number of investigators have tried to determine the sensitivity of these neurons to hormones and neurotransmitters. For instance, the possible existence of a neural circuit for estrogen feedback in the PO-SCH area, AHA, and mediobasal hypothalamus (Taleisnik and McCann, 1961; McCann and Ramirez, 1964; Halász and Gorski, 1967; Davidson, 1969; Koves and Halásez, 1969; Lisk et al., 1972; Smith and Davidson, 1974) has led to the expectation that some neurons would change their electrical activity following elevation or reduction of peripheral plasma estrogen levels (Yagi and Sawaki, 1973). Estrogen-responsive neurons have been found in these areas (Law and Sacket, 1965–1966; Lincoln, 1967; Lincoln and Cross, 1967; Law and Moss, 1969). Yagi (1970, 1973) demonstrated the existence of single neurons which significantly increased their firing rate in response to massive intravenous doses of estrogen (5 or 50 μg). Ten of 26 neurons in the PO-SCH, nine of 23 in the AHA, and four of 21 in the ARC areas responded in this fashion (Fig. 4–9A). Ten PO-SCH and nine ARC neurons decreased their firing rate after the estrogen injection (Fig. 4–9B), but the remaining neurons were unaffected. However, the large quantities of estrogen injected cast doubt on the physiological significance of the results. Injections of glucocorticoids did not modify the firing rates of the hypothalamic neurons that were excited or inhibited by estrogen.

A number of studies reported similar effects on neural activity with exogenous progesterone (Ramirez et al., 1967; Terasawa and Sawyer, 1970) and LH (Terasawa et al., 1969; Dufy et al., 1973; Faure and Vincent, 1973). In a more recent experiment, Dufy et al. (1974) correlated increased unit activity with an increase in LH levels. They reported that rabbits with premammillary neuronal activity peaking at 30 min following vaginal stimulation also showed an increase in serum LH (but not FSH), peaking at 90 min after stimulation. Thus neurons responsive to changes in plasma estrogen or progesterone do exist in the PO-SCH and ARC nuclei. It is probable that these neurons regulate hypothalamic control of the adenohypophyseal-ovarian system.

The action of hormones (Ruf and Steiner, 1967; Steiner et al., 1969) and putative neurotransmitters (Bloom et al., 1963; Oomura et al., 1969), on hypothalamic neurons has been further analyzed with the technique of microelectrophoresis. This technique offers many advantages to the neuroendocrinologist in studying brain-pituitary interrelationships, the most notable of which is elimination of the blood-brain barrier (Curtis and Crawford, 1969). Furthermore, the sites of drug action are restricted to the immediate vicinity of the neuron under observation. Recently the technique of microelectrophoresis has been combined with antidromic identification to provide a powerful tool in neuroendocrine research (Barker et al., 1971; Cross et al., 1971; Moss et al., 1971, 1972a,b). A number of studies have demonstrated the sensitivity or insensitivity of hypothalamic neurons to microelectrophoretically applied cortisol, corticosterone, dexamethasone, cyclic AMP, and prostaglandins (Feldman and Sarne, 1970; Steiner, 1972; Mandelbrod et al., 1974; Poulain and Carette, 1974).

Research in my laboratory has focused on the effect of microelectrophoresis of putative neurotransmitters and hormones on tuberoinfundibular neurons as well as on PO neurons that project their axons to the ARC-VM complex. In a recent series of experiments (Moss et al., 1975a), my associates and I studied the effects of microelectrophoretically applied norepinephrine (NE), dopamine (DA), and glutamate on antidromically identified

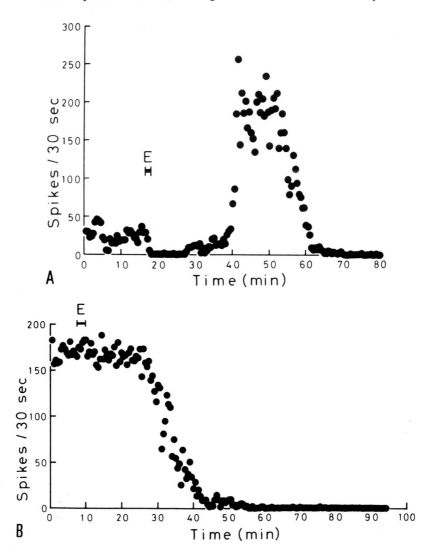

FIG. 4–9. A: Increase in firing rate following intravenous injection of 50 μg 17β-estradiol in a unit recorded from the arcuate nucleus of the hypothalamus in a female rat 2 weeks after ovariectomy. E, time of injection. Total volume of the injected solution was 0.2 ml. (From Yagi, 1973.) B: Decrease in firing rate following intravenous injection of 50 μg 17β-estradiol. The unit was recorded from the medial preoptic nucleus of the ovariectomized rat. The inhibition continued throughout the observation period of up to 150 min. (From Yagi, 1973.)

tuberoinfundibular neurons, i.e., neurons with cell bodies in the ARC nucleus and axons terminating in the external layer of the median eminence. We also studied neurons that could not be antidromically identified by stimulating the median eminence (referred to as "other ARC neurons"). The stimulation and recording procedures are outlined in Fig. 4–6. The spontaneously active, antidromically identified ARC neurons were divided into two populations based on their responsiveness to electrophoretically applied NE and DA (Fig. 4–10). Tuberoinfundibular neurons excited by NE $(N = 23)$ were either reproducibly inhibited $(N = 10)$ or nonresponsive $(N = 13)$ to DA; no NE-sensitive ARC neurons were excited by DA. The second population

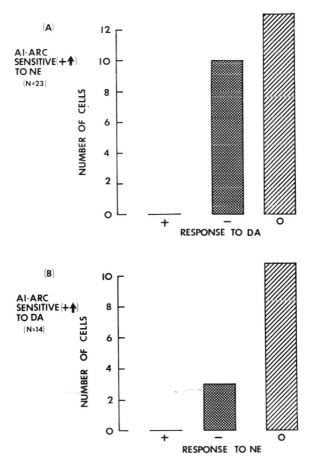

FIG. 4–10. A: Histographic analysis showing responsiveness of antidromically identified (AI) norepinephrine (NE)-sensitive arcuate (ARC) neurons to iontophoretic application of dopamine (DA). B, Histographic analysis showing responsiveness of antidromically identified dopamine sensitive arcuate neurons to iontophoretic application of norepinephrine. (From Moss et al., 1975c.)

of ARC neurons were excited by DA ($N = 14$). These neurons when tested with NE were either reproducibly inhibited ($N = 3$) or nonresponsive ($N = 11$); no DA-sensitive neurons were excited by NE. The unidentified or other ARC neurons did not show this interrelationship between NE and DA; just as many ARC neurons were reproducibly excited, inhibited, or nonresponsive to either NE or DA.

Figures 4–11 through 4–13 illustrate the pharmacological responsiveness of three antidromically identified ARC neurons selected from a population of either NE- or DA-sensitive neurons. In preliminary experiments DA excitation but not NE excitation was blocked by electrophoretic administration of the DA receptor blocker pimozide. Electrophoretic application of phentolamine, an α-adrenergic receptor blocker, blocked both DA and NE excitation.

In a similar study by Kawakami and Sakuma, reported in the first Geoffrey Harris Memorial Lecture by Sawyer (1975) a slight overlap was demonstrated in the excitatory effects of NE and DA on antidromically identified neurons. Of the 40 units excited by NE and the 27 units by DA, only 12 were excited by both amines. The difference between these findings and our results may be found in the criteria used to establish whether an effect is excitatory, inhibitory, or nonresponsive. In my laboratory a change of 30% from the baseline firing rate is considered meaningful.

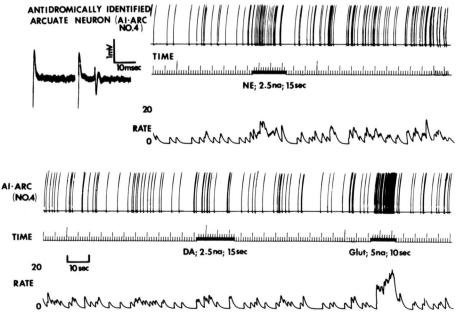

FIG. 4–11. Responses of a single antidromically identified (AI) arcuate (ARC) neuron to iontophoretically applied norepinephrine (NE), dopamine (DA), and glutamate (Glut). (From Moss et al., 1975c.)

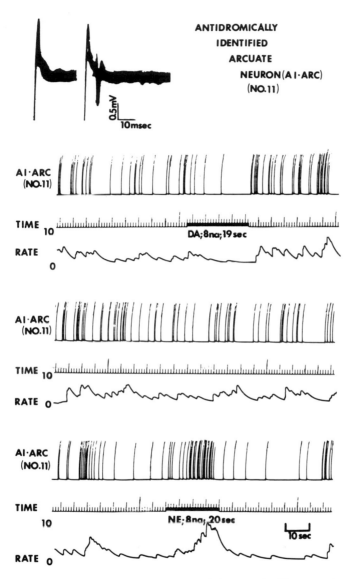

FIG. 4–12. Responses of a single antidromically identified (AI) arcuate (ARC) neuron to iontophoretic application of dopamine (DA) and norepinephrine (NE). (From Moss et al., 1975c.)

In any case, the findings indicate that the NE and DA present in the medio-basal hypothalamus (Björklund et al., 1968; Keller and Lichtensteiger, 1971) may modulate the activity of ARC neurons with axons that project to the median eminence. These results appear compatible with the postulated functional roles for both NE and DA in modulating activity of hypophysio-tropic neurons (Everett, 1964; Kordon and Glowinski, 1969; Lichtensteiger, 1969; Kalra and McCann, 1973).

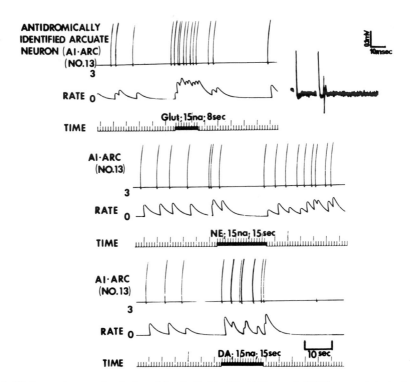

FIG. 4–13. Responsiveness of a single antidromically identified (AI) arcuate (ARC) neuron to iontophoretic application of glutamate (Glut), norepinephrine (NE), and dopamine (DA). (From Moss et al., 1975c.)

Research on the pharmacological sensitivity of PO neurons that project to the ARC-VM complex was begun in our laboratory some time ago. Unfortunately the results are anything but clear. The procedures for stimulation and recording are shown in Fig. 4–8. In our initial experiments 202 PO neurons were tested with microelectrophoretically applied NE, DA, LRH, and glutamate. Thirty-four neurons were identified by antidromic stimulation of the ARC-VM complex. A summary of the results is presented in Table 4–1 (Kelly et al., 1975; Moss et al., 1975b). The results show that the catecholamines (NE and DA), as well as LRH, reproducibly inhibit just as many antidromically identified PO neurons as they reproducibly excite. However, most of the neurons were unresponsive to the chemicals tested. Glutamate generally had an excitatory action on both identified and unidentified PO neurons, i.e., PO neurons that do not project to the ARC-VM complex. The neural activity in the unidentified PO neurons was predominantly unaffected by the electrophoretic application of NE, DA, and LRH.

In subsequent studies antidromically identified PO neurons were tested with microelectrophoretically applied NE, DA, glutamate, and LRH, as well as with thyrotropin-releasing hormone (TRH), estrogen (E_2), corticosterone (CS), serotonin (5-HT), and acetylcholine (ACh). The results from 65

TABLE 4–1. *Percentage of antidromically identified and unidentified preoptic neurons responding to iontophoretically applied substances*

Iontophorically applied substance	Antidromically identified preoptic neurons			Unidentified preoptic neurons		
	+	0	—	+	0	—
Norepinephrine	14	69	17	33	40	27
Dopamine	21	50	29	31	47	22
Luteinizing hormone-releasing hormone	19	69	12	33	50	17
Glutamate	50	45	5	59	24	17

+, excitation. 0, no effect. —, inhibition.

antidromically identified neurons are summarized in Table 4–2 (Moss et al., 1975*b*). The monoamines (NE, DA, 5–HT), glutamate, ovarian hormones (E$_2$), and neurohormones (LRH, TRH) reproducibly inhibited just as many antidromically identified PO neurons as they reproducibly excited, but most of these neurons were unresponsive to the chemicals tested. Most of the PO neurons tested were unresponsive to ACh; of the remaining neurons, more were excited than inhibited by ACh. Interpretation of these results is extremely difficult, but the findings are similar to the studies of Whitehead and Ruf (1974) and Dyball et al. (1974). The former study concludes that PO neurons which project to the mediobasal hypothalamus are inhibited by DA and NE but not by ACh. In addition, estrogen injections did not modify the responsiveness of the antidromically identified PO neurons to iontophoretically applied DA, NE, and ACh. The latter study (Dyball et al., 1974) suggests that NE and DA have little or no excitatory action on the neurons which project from the PO and AH areas to the mediobasal hypothalamus.

The aforementioned findings on the action of electrophoretically applied LRH substantiate the findings of Dyer and Dyball (1974) and Dyer (1974*a,b*). They found that the majority of antidromically identified PO-SCH neurons were unresponsive to LRH. Oxytocin was also without effect on

TABLE 4–2. *Percentage of antidromically identified preoptic-suprachiasmatic neurons responding to the iontophoretic application of releasing hormones, steroids, and neurohumoral agents*

Response	NE	DA	5-HT	ACh	Glut	LRH	TRH	E$_2$	CS
+	14	12	9	31	35	11	12	20	0
0	60	68	82	63	55	52	63	60	100
—	25	20	9	6	10	37	25	20	0

NE, norepinephrine. DA, dopamine. 5-HT, serotonin. ACh, acetylcholine. Glut, glutamate. LRH, luteinizing hormone-releasing hormone. TRH, thyrotropin-releasing hormone. E$_2$, estrogen. CS, cortisol.

+, excitation. 0, no effect. —, inhibition.

the neurons tested. On the other hand, TRH excited one neuron, inhibited seven, and had no effect on nine (Fig. 4–14). Steiner (1972) also found that hypothalamic neurons were relatively insensitive to microelectrophoretically applied TRH. These findings have been confirmed and extended by Kawakami and Sakuma (1974). They demonstrated that only two of 45 antidromically identified PO neurons responded to the electrophoretic administration of LRH, whereas 12 neurons responded with excitation to LH. None of these neurons showed inhibition to either LRH or LH. Fourteen neurons were tested with FSH; five were excited, and one was inhibited. Forty-four of 74 antidromically identified ARC-VM neurons altered their electrical activity to LRH (Fig. 4–15). Excitation and inhibition were seen in 33 neurons and 11 neurons, respectively. Responses to LH were seen in 33 of 48 units—28 neurons showing excitation and five inhibition. Sixteen of 41 neurons tested responded to FSH. Of these 16, excitation and inhibition were seen in 12 and four, respectively. These authors concluded that microelectrophoresis of LH and FSH caused no significant changes in unit activity in the ARC and PO neurons. In addition, they suggested that LRH itself may play a feedback role in the neural control of LRH secretion.

The effectiveness of LRH in inducing changes in the unit activity of PO and ARC neurons fits well with previous observations on LRH-induced

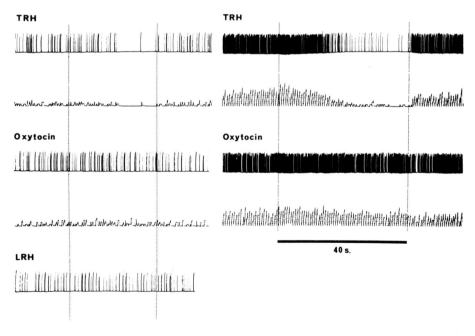

FIG. 4–14. *Left:* Polygraph record and integrated firing rate of a preoptic neuron that was inhibited by TRH (5 nA) but not LRH or oxytocin (8 nA). *Right:* Record of another unit inhibited by TRH and unaffected by oxytocin (both 7 nA). This second cell was not adequately tested with LRH. (From Dyer and Dyball, 1974.)

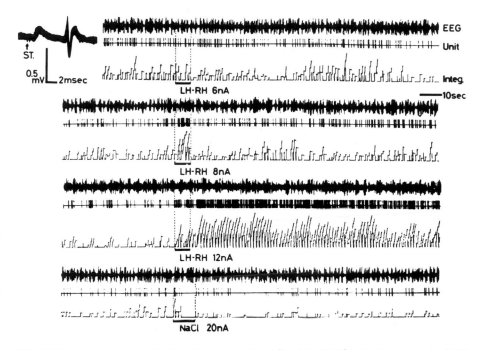

FIG. 4–15. Responses of a medial basal hypothalamic unit (*top left;* ✕ 20) to the iontophoresis of LRH (LH-RH). 100 μg/ml solution, at different intensities of anodal current. Note the dose-response relationship between the rate of the unit and the intensity of current flow. The stronger current delivered by the 0.15 M NaCl barrel was without effect. (From Kawakami and Sakuma, 1974.)

lordosis behavior in female rats (Moss and McCann, 1973, 1975; Pfaff, 1973; Moss et al., 1975c,d; Moss and Dudley, *unpublished observations*). In these experiments 500 ng LRH administered systemically facilitated lordosis behavior. In subsequent experiments Moss and Foreman (1975) infused 50 ng LRH, a dose found to be ineffective when given systemically, directly into the PO or ARC nucleus. LRH infused into either of these sites potentiated lordosis behavior in the estrogen-primed ovariectomized female rat, whereas LRH infused into the cortex did not initiate similar behavioral patterns. Thus it is suggested that the PO and ARC nuclei may serve as sites at which LRH activates neurons involved in the induction of sexual behavior.

CONCLUDING REMARKS

The use of microelectrophoresis in the field of neuroendocrinology provides a means of testing the sensitivity of hypothalamic neurons to hormones and neurotransmitters. Minute quantities of these substances can be applied directly to the surface of single hypothalamic neurons to circumvent the blood-brain barrier. However, this technique is not without problems. These include the possible complicating effects of anesthetics on the activity of neurons and/or pituitary function, as well as the inability to determine drug concentration at the nerve cell receptor. The effects of anesthetics on pituitary function have been clearly demonstrated (Blake and Sawyer, 1972; Lincoln and Kelly, 1972; Whitehead and Ruf, 1974) and at the present time cannot be avoided. Thus in the interpretation of electrophysiological data, the experimenter must take into account the possible effects of the anesthetic used and ensure that the neuroendocrine mechanism under study is still operational. On the other hand, one can theoretically determine the concentration of putative neurotransmitters microelectrophoresed from glass micropipettes (Bradley and Candy, 1970; Hoffer et al., 1971; Candy et al., 1974; Zieglgansberger et al., 1974). LRH can in fact be iontophoretically released from a glass micropipette (Fig. 4–16). In addition, the released material is biologically active when injected into estrone-primed ovariectomized female

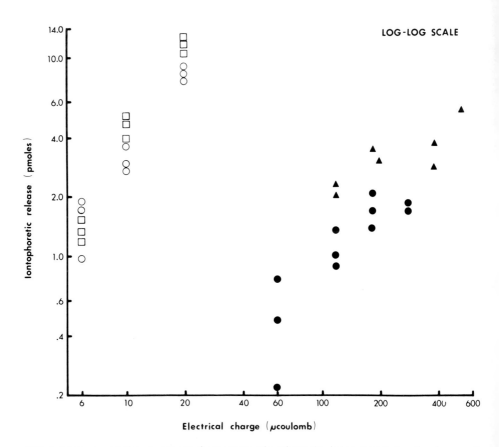

FIG. 4–16. Representative experiments demonstrating the relationship between iontophoretic release and electrical charge for norepinephrine. (○, experiment 25: 3 μm diameter, 120 MΩ chemical barrel impedance, and experiment 24: 5 μm, 60 M; norepinephrine values have been divided by a factor of 10 in order to graph them on the same scale) and for luteinizing hormone-releasing hormone (●, experiment 38: 2 μ, 600 M and △, experiment 32: 3 μ, 425 M; experiment 38 luteinizing hormone-releasing hormone values have been multiplied by a factor of 10).

rats (Kelly and Moss, 1975). Two important findings should be noted: (1) A higher charge was needed in order to obtain a detectable quantity of LRH as compared to the charge required to release NE; and (2) a relationship between the charge and the quantity of LRH released was established.

Even though PO-SCH and ARC neurons have been localized by antidromic identification and tested chemically by microelectrophoresis, the question still remains: Are these identified neurons involved in releasing LRH? To answer this question, we are performing two types of experiments. In the first we attempt to demonstrate an increase in unit activity in the identified tuberoinfundibular neuron and at the same time to measure LRH activity in portal blood. One neuron cannot be expected to release an easily measurable quantity of LRH, but the possibility does exist that neurons which have been found via histochemical techniques to contain LRH can be recruited by electrical stimulation from the surrounding area to produce hormone release. The second experiment is to establish, by use of a fluorescent dye and antibodies to LRH, where the identified neuron actually terminates in the median eminence and whether the neuron contains neurosecretory granules and/or the catecholamines. It is already known that tuberoinfundibular neurons can be injected with Procion yellow (Dyer, 1974*b*). A multidisciplinary approach utilizing such techniques as microelectrophoresis, antidromic identification, fluorescence microscopy, and radioimmunoassay, will allow proper investigation of monoaminergic systems of the PO-SCH region and of the ARC nucleus, which are thought to be involved in the synthesis and release of LRH.

The question posed at the beginning of this chapter concerning the precise physiological role of hypothalamic neurons in the control of gonadotropin secretion has not been answered. However, some important generalizations emerge from the studies discussed in the preceding pages: (1) Variations in hypothalamic unit activity can be correlated with altered gonadotropin release. (2) The existence of neural connections between the PO-SCH area and the ARC-VM complex, and the ARC nucleus and the external layer of the median eminence has been demonstrated. (3) Some of the tuberoinfundibular neurons are NE-sensitive, and some are DA-sensitive. (4) PO neurons for the most part are unresponsive to microelectrophoretically applied NE, DA, ACh, 5-HT, LRH, TRH, CS, and E_2 (5) LRH administered microelectrophoretically appears to modify substantially the electrical activity of tuberoinfundibular neurons but not that of PO neurons. These observations lay the foundation for further investigations of the role of hypothalamic neurons in the control of anterior pituitary function.

ACKNOWLEDGMENTS

The author is greatly indebted to his colleagues S. M. McCann, J. E. Wheaton, M. J. Kelly, M. M. Foreman, and C. A Dudley for helpful criticism and comments during the preparation of the manuscript. The author also wishes to acknowledge with special thanks the editorial assistance and typing of Miss D. S. Zavislan, the technical assistance of Miss P. R. Chapus, the photography of Mr. R. A. Cooper, and the artistry of Mrs. M. L. Nelson. Synthetic LRH was obtained through the courtesy of Drs. Gotz and Rochefort of Ayerst Research Laboratories, Quebec, Canada; and the synthetic TRH was obtained through the generosity of Drs. Dorn and Weinstein and Mr. Flanagan of Abbott Laboratories, North Chicago, Illinois.

For permission to copy figures of their published work, the author wishes to thank Drs. Dyer, Dyball, Kawakami, Sakuma, Sawaki, and Yagi.

This review and the author's research discussed in it were supported by Research Grant NIH-USPHS-NS 10434-END.

REFERENCES

Anand Kumar, T. C. (1973): Cellular and humoral pathways in the neuroendocrine regulation of reproductive function. *J. Reprod. Fertil. [Suppl.]*, 20:11–25.

Barker, J. L., Crayton, J. W., and Nicoll, R. A. (1971): Supraoptic neurosecretory cells: Adrenergic and cholinergic sensitivity. *Science*, 171:208–210.

Barraclough, C. A. (1966): Modification in the CNS regulation of reproduction after exposure of prepubertal rats to steroid hormones. *Recent Prog. Horm. Res.*, 22:503–539.

Barraclough, C. A., and Gorski, R. A. (1961): Evidence that the hypothalamus is responsible for androgen-induced sterility in the female rat. *Endocrinology*, 68:68–79.

Barry, J., Dubois, M. P., and Carette, B. (1974): Immunofluorescence study of the preoptico-infundibular LRF neurosecretory pathway in the normal, castrated or testosterone-treated male guinea pig. *Endocrinology*, 95:1416–1423.

Barry, J., Dubois, M. P., and Poulain, P. (1973): LRF producing cells of the mammalian hypothalamus. *Z. Zellforsch. Mikrosk. Anat.*, 146:351–366.

Beyer, C., and Sawyer, C. H. (1969): Hypothalamic unit activity related to control of the pituitary gland. In: *Frontiers in Neuroendocrinology 1969*, edited by W. F. Ganong and L. Martini, pp. 255–287. Oxford University Press, New York.

Bissett, G. W., Clark, B. J., and Errington, M. L. (1971): The hypothalamic neurosecretory pathways for the release of oxytocin and vasopressin in the cat. *J. Physiol. (Lond.)*, 217:111–131.

Björklund, A., Falck, B., Homek, F., Owen, C., and West, K. A. (1968): Identification and terminal distribution of the tubero-hypophyseal monoamine fiber system in the rat by means of stereotaxic and microspectrofluorimetric techniques. *Brain Res.*, 17:1–3.

Björklund, A., Moore, R. L., Nobin, A., and Stenevi, U. (1973): The organization of tubero-hypophyseal and reticulo-infundibular catecholamine neuron systems in the rat brain. *Brain Res.*, 51:171–191.

Blake, C. A., and Sawyer, C. H. (1972): Ovulation blocking actions of urethane in the rat. *Endocrinology*, 91:87–94.

Bloom, F. E., Oliver, A. P., and Salmoiraghi, G. C. (1963): The responsiveness of individual hypothalamic neurons to microelectrophoretically administered endogenous amines. *Int. J. Neuropharmacol.*, 2:181–193.

Bradley, P. B., and Candy, J. M. (1970): Iontophoretic release of ACh, NE, 5-HT, and LSD from micropipettes. *Br. J. Pharmacol.*, 40:194–201.

Burford, G. D., Dyball, R. E. J., Moss, R. L., and Pickering, B. T. (1974): Synthesis of both neurohypophysial hormones in both the paraventricular and supraoptic nuclei of the art. *J. Anat.*, 117:261–269.

Burger, H. G., Fink, G., and Lee, V. W. K. (1972): Luteinizing hormone releasing factor in ultrafiltrates of blood collected from the pituitary stalk of ovariectomized rats and rats subjected to electrical stimulation of the preoptic area. *J. Endocrinol.,* 54:227–234.

Butler, J. E. M., and Donovan, B. T. (1971): The effect of surgical isolation of the hypothalamus on reproductive function in the female rat. *J. Endocrinol.,* 49:293–304.

Candy, J. M., Boakes, R. J., Key, B. J., and Worton, E. (1974): Correlation of the release of amines and antagonists with their effects. *Neuropharmacology,* 13:423–439.

Carrer, H. F., and Sawyer, C. H. (1974): Changes in multiunit spike activity in the preoptic area induced by midbrain stimulation. *Program and Abstracts of the Fourth Annual Meeting of the Society for Neuroscience,* St. Louis, p. 162.

Clattenburg, R. E. (1974): Ultrastructure of hypothalamic neurons and of the median eminence. *Can. J. Neurol. Sci.,* 1:40–58.

Clemens, J. A., Shaar, C. J., Kleber, J. W., and Tandy, W. A. (1971): Areas of the brain stimulatory to LH and FSH secretion. *Endocrinology,* 88:180–184.

Covian, M. R., Migliorini, R. H., and Tramezzani, J. H. (1959): Endocrine changes in hemidecorticate rats. *Acta Physiol. Lat. Am.,* 9:24–34.

Critchlow, V. (1958): Ovulation induced by hypothalamic stimulation in the anesthetized rat. *Am. J. Physiol.,* 195:171–174.

Cross, B. A. (1973a): Unit responses in the hypothalamus. In: *Frontiers in Neuroendocrinology 1973,* edited by W. F. Ganong and L. Martini, pp. 133–171. Oxford University Press, New York.

Cross, B. A. (1973b): Towards a neurophysiological basis for ovulation. *J. Reprod. Fertil.* [*Suppl.*], 20:97–117.

Cross, B. A., and Dyball, R. E. J. (1974): Central pathways for neurohypophysial hormone release. In: *Handbook of Physiology, Section 7: Endocrinology,* Vol. 4, Part 1, edited by R. O. Greep and E. B. Astwood, pp. 269–285. American Physiology Society, New York.

Cross, B. A., and Dyer, R. G. (1970a): Characterization of unit activity in hypothalamic islands with special reference to hormone effects. In: *The Hypothalamus,* edited by L. Martini, M. Motta, and F. Fraschini, pp. 115–122. Academic Press, New York.

Cross, B. A., and Dyer, R. G. (1970b): Effect of hypophysectomy on firing rates of hypothalamic neurones in diencephalic islands. *J. Endocrinol.,* 48:475–476.

Cross, B. A., and Dyer, R. G. (1971a): Unit activity in diencephalic islands: The effect of anaesthetics. *J. Physiol. (Lond.),* 212:467–481.

Cross, B. A., and Dyer, R. G. (1971b): Cyclic changes in neurones of the anterior hypothalamus during the oestrous cycle, and the effects of anesthesia. In: *Steroid Hormones and Brain Function,* edited by R. Gorski and C. H. Sawyer, pp. 95–102. University of California Press, Los Angeles.

Cross, B. A., and Green, J. D. (1959): Activity of single neurones in the hypothalamus: Effect of osmotic and other stimuli. *J. Physiol. (Lond.),* 148:554–569.

Cross, B. A., Moss, R. L., and Urban, I (1971): Effects of iontophoretic application of acetylcholine and noradrenaline to antidromically identified paraventricular neurones. *J. Physiol. (Lond.),* 214:28P–30P.

Curtis, D. R., and Crawford, J. M. (1969): Central synaptic transmission microelectrophoretic studies. *Ann. Rev. Pharmacol.,* 9:209–240.

Dahlgren, U. (1914): The electric motor nerve centers in the skates (Rajidae). *Science,* 40:862–863.

Davidson, J. M. (1969): Feedback control of gonadotropin secretion. In: *Frontiers in Neuroendocrinology 1969,* edited by W. F. Ganong and L. Martini, pp. 343–388. Oxford University Press, New York.

Dreifuss, J. J., and Kelly, J. S. (1972): Recurrent inhibition of antidromically identified rat supraoptic neurones. *J. Physiol. (Lond.),* 220:87–103.

Dreifuss, J. J., Nordmann, J. J., and Vincent, J. D. (1974): Recurrent inhibition of supraoptic neurosecretory cells in homozygous Brattleboro rats. *J. Physiol. (Lond.),* 237:25P–27P (abstract).

Dufy, B., Vincent, J. D., Bensch, C., and Faure, J. M. A. (1973): Effects of vaginal stimulation and luteinizing hormone on hypothalamic single units in the freely moving rabbit. *Neuroendocrinology,* 11:119–129.

Dufy, B., Dufy-Barbe, L., and Poulain, D. (1974): Gonadotropin release in relation to electrical activity in hypothalamic neurons. *J. Neurol. Trans.*, 35:47–52.

Dyball, R. E. J. (1971): Oxytocin and ADH secretion in relation to electrical activity in antidromically identified supraoptic and paraventricular units. *J. Physiol. (Lond.)*, 214:245–256.

Dyball, R. E. J. (1974): Single unit activity in the hypothalamo-neurohypophysial system of Brattleboro rats. *J. Endocrinol.*, 60:135–143.

Dyball, R. E. J., Dyer, R. G., and Drewett, R. F. (1974): Chemical sensitivity of preoptic neurons which project to the medial basal hypothalamus. *Brain Res.*, 71:140–143.

Dyer, R. G. (1973): An electrophysiological dissection of the hypothalamic regions which regulate the pre-ovulatory secretion of luteinizing hormone in the rat. *J. Physiol. (Lond.)*, 234:421–442.

Dyer, R. G. (1974a): The electrophysiology of the hypothalamus and its endocrinological implications. In: *Progress in Brain Research, Vol. 41: Integrative Hypothalamic Activity*, edited by D. F. Swaab and J. P. Schadé, pp. 133–147. Elsevier, Oxford.

Dyer, R. G. (1974b): Characteristics of neurons projecting directly to the region of the median eminence. *Proceedings of the International Symposium on Hypothalamic Hormones*, Milan, Italy. Academic Press, New York (*in press*).

Dyer, R. G., and Cross, B. A. (1972a): Antidromic identification of units in the preoptic and anterior hypothalamic areas projecting directly to the ventromedial and arcuate nuclei. *Brain Res.*, 43:254–258.

Dyer, R. G., and Cross, B. A. (1972b): Location of preoptic neurons projecting to the medial basal hypothalamus. *J. Anat.*, 114:307–308.

Dyer, R. G., and Dyball, R. E. J. (1974): Evidence for a direct effect of LRF and TRF on single unit activity in the rostral hypothalamus. *Nature (Lond.)*, 252:486–488.

Dyer, R. G., Pritchett, C. J., and Cross, B. A. (1972): Unit activity in the diencephalon of female rats during the oestrous cycle. *J. Endocrinol.*, 53:151–160.

Everett, J. W. (1964): Central neural control of reproductive functions of the adenohypophysis. *Physiol. Rev.*, 44:373–431.

Everett, J. W. (1965): Ovulation in rats from preoptic stimulation through platinum electrodes: Importance of duration and spread of stimulus. *Endocrinology*, 76:1195–1201.

Faure, J. M. A., and Vincent, J. D. (1973): Approche electrophysiologique de la function gonadotrope de l'hypothalamus. *Arch. Ital. Biol.*, 111:686–697.

Feldman, S., and Sarne, Y. (1970): Effect of cortisol on single cell activity in hypothalamic islands. *Brain Res.*, 23:67–75.

Fink, G., Nallar, R., and Worthington, W. C., Jr. (1967): The demonstration of luteinizing hormone releasing factor in hypophysial portal blood of pro-oestrous and hypophysectomized rats. *J. Physiol. (Lond.)*, 191:407–415.

Flerkó, B., and Bardos, V. (1959): Zwei verschiedene effekte experimenteller lasion dis hypothalamus auf die gonaden. *Acta Neuroveg. (Wien)*, 20:248–262.

Fuxe, K., and Hökfelt, T. (1967): The influence of central catecholamine neurons on the hormone secretion from the anterior and posterior pituitary. In: *Neurosecretion*, edited by F. Stutinsky, pp. 165–177. Springer, Berlin.

Gallo, R. V., Johnson, J. H., Goldman, B. D., Whitmoyer, D. I., and Sawyer, C. H. (1971): Effects of electrochemical stimulation of the ventral hippocampus on hypothalamic electrical activity and pituitary gonadotropin secretion in female rats. *Endocrinology*, 89:704–713.

Green, J. D., and Harris, G. W. (1947): The neurovascular link between the neurohypophysis and adenohypophysis. *J. Endocrinol.*, 5:136–145.

Greep, R. O., and Porter, J. F., editors (1973): Hypothalamic control of fertility. *J. Reprod. Fertil.* [*Suppl.*], 20.

Halász, B. (1969): The endocrine effects of isolation of the hypothalamus from the rest of the brain. In: *Frontiers in Neuroendocrinology 1969*, edited by F. Ganong and L. Martini, pp. 307–342. Oxford University Press, New York.

Halász, B., and Gorski, R. A. (1967): Gonadotrophin hormone secretion in female rats after partial or total interruption of neural afferents to the medial basal hypothalamus. *Endocrinology,* 80:608–622.

Halász, B., Pupp, L., and Uhlarik, S. (1962): Hypophysiotropic area in the hypothalamus. *J. Endocrinol.,* 25:147–154.

Harris, G. W. (1937): The induction of ovulation in the rabbit by electrical stimulation of the hypothalamo-hypophyseal mechanism. *Proc. R. Soc. Lond. [Biol.],* 122:374–394.

Harris, G. W. (1948): Neural control of the pituitary gland. *Physiol. Rev.,* 28:139–179.

Harris, G. W. (1955): *Neural Control of the Pituitary Gland.* Arnold, London.

Harris, G. W., and Ruf, K. B. (1970): Luteinizing hormone releasing factor in the rat hypophysial portal blood collected during electrical stimulation of the hypothalamus. *J. Physiol. (Lond.),* 208:243–250.

Harris, M. C., and Sanghera, M. (1974): Projection of medial basal hypothalamic neurons to the preoptic anterior hypothalamic areas and the paraventricular nucleus in the rat. *Brain Res.,* 81:401–411.

Harris, M. C., Makara, G. B., and Spyer, K. M. (1971): Electrophysiological identification of neurones of the tuberoinfundibular system. *J. Physiol. (Lond.),* 218:86–87.

Hayward, J. N. (1974): Physiological and morphological identification of hypothalamic magnocellular neuroendocrine cells in goldfish preoptic nucleus. *J. Physiol. (Lond.),* 239:103–124.

Hayward, J. N., and Jennings, D. P. (1974a): Activity of magnocellular neuroendocrine cells in the hypothalamus of unanaesthetized monkeys. I. Functional cell types and their anatomical distribution in the supraoptic nucleus and the internuclear zone. *J. Physiol. (Lond.),* 232:515–543.

Hayward, J. N., and Jennings, D. P. (1974b): Activity of magnocellular neuroendocrine cells in the hypothalamus of unanaesthetized monkeys. II. Osmo-sensitivity of functional cell types in the supraoptic nucleus and the internuclear zone. *J. Physiol. (Lond.),* 232:545–572.

Hinsey, J. C., and Markee, J. E. (1933): Pregnancy following bilateral section of the cervical sympathetic trunks in the rabbit. *Proc. Soc. Exp. Biol. Med.,* 31:270–271.

Hoffer, B. J., Niff, N. H., and Siggins, G. R. (1971): Microiontophoretic release of norepinephrine from micropipettes. *Neuropharmacology,* 10:175–180.

Kalino, H., and Reinne, U. K. (1972): Ultrastructural studies on the hypothalamic neurosecretory neurons of the rat. II. The hypothalamo-neurohypophysial system in rats with hereditary hypothalamic diabetes insipidus. *Z. Zellforsch. Mikrosk. Anat.,* 134:205–225.

Kalra, S. P., and McCann, S. M. (1973): Effect of drugs modifying catecholamine synthesis on LH release induced by preoptic stimulation in the rat. *Endocrinology,* 93:356–362.

Kandel, E. R. (1964): Electrical properties of hypothalamic neuroendocrine cells. *J. Gen. Physiol.,* 47:691–717.

Kawakami, M., and Sakuma, Y. (1974): Responses of hypothalamic neurons to the microiontophoresis of LH-RH, LH and FSH under various levels of circulating ovarian hormones. *Neuroendocrinology,* 15:290–307.

Kawakami, M., and Terasawa, E. (1974): Role of limbic structure on reproductive cycles. In: *Biological Rhythms in Neuroendocrine Activity,* edited by M. Kawakami, pp. 197–219. Igaku Shoin, Tokyo.

Kawakami, M., Terasawa, E., Kimura, F., and Kubo, K. (1973): Correlated changes in gonadotropin release and electrical activity of the hypothalamus induced by electrical stimulation of the hippocampus in immature and mature rats. In: *Hormones and Brain Function,* edited by K. Lissák, pp. 347–374. Plenum Press, New York.

Keller, P. J., and Lichtensteiger, W. (1971): Stimulation of tubero-infundibular neurones and gonadotrophin secretion. *J. Physiol. (Lond.),* 219:385–401.

Kelly, M. J., and Moss, R. L. (1975): Quantitative evaluation and determination of the biologic potency of iontophoretically applied luteinizing hormone-releasing hormone (LRH).

Kelly, M. J., Dudley, C., and Moss, R. L. (1975): Responsiveness of hypothalamic neurons to iontophoretically applied releasing factors and monoamines. Presented at the Eighth Annual Winter Conference on Brain Research, January 1975, Steamboat Springs, Colorado.

Knigge, K. M., Joseph, S. A., Silverman, A. J., and Vaala, S. (1973): Further observations on the structure and function of the median eminence, with reference to the organization of RF-producing elements in the endocrine hypothalamus: *Prog. Brain Res.,* 39:7–20.

Knowles, F., and Anand Kumar, T. C. (1969): Structural changes related to reproduction in the hypothalamus and in the pars tuberalis of the rhesus monkey. *Philos. Trans. R. Soc. Lond. [Biol. Sci.]*, 256:357–375.

Kobayashi, T., Kobayashi, T., Yammamoto, K., and Kaibara, M. (1967): Electron microscopic observation on the hypothalamo-hypophysial system in the rat. II. Ultrafine structure of the median eminence and of the nerve cells of the arcuate nucleus. *Endocrinol. Jap.,* 14:158–177.

Koizumi, K., and Yamashita, H. (1972): Studies of antidromically identified neurosecretory cells of the hypothalamus by intracellular and extracellular recordings. *J. Physiol. (Lond.)*, 221:683–705.

Koizumi, K., Ishikawa, T., and Brooks, C. McC. (1973): The existence of facilitatory axon collaterals in neurosecretory cells of the hypothalamus. *Brain Res.,* 63:408–413.

Komisaruk, B. R. (1971): Strategies in neuroendocrine neurophysiology. *Am. Zool.,* 11:741–754.

Kordon, C., and Glowinski, J. (1969): Selective inhibition of superovulation by blockade of dopamine synthesis during the "critical period" in the immature rat. *Endocrinology,* 85:924–931.

Kordon, C., Kerdelhué, B., Pattou, E., and Jutisz, M. (1974): Immunocytochemical localization of LH-RH in axons and nerve terminals of the rat median eminence. *Proc. Soc. Exp. Biol. Med.,* 147:122–127.

Köves, K., and Halász, B. (1969): Data on the location of the neural structures indispensable for the occurrence of ovarian compensatory hypertrophy. *Neuroendocrinology,* 4:1–11.

Law, O. T., and Moss, R. L. (1969): Sex and the single neuron. Presented at the Annual Meeting of the Western Psychological Association, Vancouver, B. C.

Law, O. T., and Sacket, G. P. (1965–1966): Hypothalamic potentials in female rats evoked by hormones and vaginal stimulation. *Neuroendocrinology,* 1:31–34.

Lichtensteiger, W. (1969): Cyclic variations of catecholamine content in hypothalamic nerve cells during the estrous cycle of the rat, with a concomitant study of the substantia nigra. *J. Pharmacol. Exp. Ther.,* 165:204–215.

Lincoln, D. W. (1967): Unit activity in the hypothalamus, septum and preoptic area of the rat: Characteristics of spontaneous activity and the effect of oestrogen. *J. Endocrinol.,* 37:177–189.

Lincoln, D. W., and Cross, B. A. (1967): Effect of oestrogen on the responsiveness of neurones in the hypothalamus, septum and preoptic area of rats with light-induced persistent oestrus. *J. Endocrinol.,* 37:191–203.

Lincoln, D. W., and Kelly, W. A. (1972): The influence of urethane on ovulation in the rat. *Endocrinology,* 90:1594–1599.

Lincoln, D. W., and Wakerley, J. B. (1972): Accelerated discharge of paraventricular neurosecretory cells correlated with reflex release of oxytocin during suckling. *J. Physiol. (Lond.)*, 222:23–24.

Lisk, R. D., Ciaccio, L. A., and Reuter, L. A. (1972): Neural centers of estrogen and progesterone action in the regulation of reproduction. In: *III Panamerican Congress of Anatomy,* edited by J. T. Velardo, and B. A. Kasprow, pp. 71–87.

Makara, G. B., and Hodács, L. (1975): Rostral projections from the hypothalamic arcuate nucleus. *Brain Res.,* 84:23–29.

Makara, G. B., Harris, M. C., and Spyer, K. M. (1972): Identification and distribution of tuberoinfundibular neurones. *Brain Res.,* 40:283–290.

Mandelbrod, I., Feldman, S., and Werman, R. (1974): Inhibition of firing is the primary effect of microelectrophoresis of cortisol of units in the rat tuberal hypothalamus. *Brain Res.,* 80:303–315.

McCann, S. M., and Porter, J. C. (1969): Hypothalamic pituitary stimulating and inhibiting hormones. *Physiol. Rev.,* 49:240–284.

McCann, S. M., and Ramirez, V. D. (1964): The neuroendocrine regulation of hypophyseal luteinizing hormone secretion. *Recent Prog. Horm. Res.,* 20:131–170.

McCann, S. M., Fawcett, C. P., and Krulich, L. (1974): Hypothalamic hypophysial releasing and inhibiting hormones. In: *MTP International Review of Science, Endocrine Physiology, Vol. 5: Physiology Series One,* edited by S. M. McCann, pp. 31–65. University Park Press, Baltimore.

McCann, S. M., Krulich, L., Quijada, M., Wheaton, J. E., and Moss, R. L. (1975): *Anatomical Neuroendocrinology,* edited by W. E. Stumpf and L. D. Grant. Karger, Basel (*in press*).

McDonald, P. G., and Gilmore, D. P. (1971): The effect of ovarian steroids on hypothalamic thresholds for ovulation in the female rat. *J. Endocrinol.,* 49:421–429.

Mess, B. (1969): Site and onset of production of releasing factors. In: *Progress in Endocrinology,* edited by C. Gual and F. J. G. Ebling, pp. 564–570. Excerpta Medica, Amsterdam.

Moss, R. L., and Foreman, M. M. (1975): Facilitation of lordosis behavior by intrahypothalamic infusion of LRH. *Endocrinology,* 96:A45.

Moss, R. L., and Law, O. T. (1971): The estrous cycle: Its influence on single unit activity in the forebrain. *Brain Res.,* 30:435 438.

Moss, R. L., and McCann, S. M. (1973): Induction of mating behavior in rats by luteinizing hormone-releasing factor. *Science,* 181:177–179.

Moss, R. L., and McCann, S. M. (1975): Action of luteinizing hormone-releasing factor (LRF) in the initiation of lordosis behavior in the estrone-primed ovariectomized female rat. *Neuroendocrinology,* 17(4):309–318.

Moss, R. L., and Riskind, P. (1973): Some electrical and chemical properties of arcuate neurons antidromically identified by stimulation of the median eminence. *Proceedings of the 3rd Annual Neuroscience Meeting,* Vol. 3, p. 31 (abstract).

Moss, R. L., Dyball, R. E. J., and Cross, B. A. (1971): Response of antidromically identified supraoptic and paraventricular units to acetylcholine, noradrenaline and glutamate applied iontophoretically. *Brain Res.,* 35:573 575.

Moss, R. L., Dyball, R. E. J., and Cross, B. A. (1972a): Excitation of antidromically identified neurosecretory cells of the paraventricular nucleus by oxytocin applied iontophoretically. *Exp. Neurol.,* 34:95–102.

Moss, R. L., Urban, I., and Cross, B. A. (1972b): Microelectrophoresis of cholinergic and aminergic drugs on paraventricular neurons. *Am. J. Physiol.,* 223:310–318.

Moss, R. L., Kelly, M. J., and Danhof, I. E. (1974a): Neuropharmacology of antidromically identified neurons of the arcuate nucleus. *Fed. Proc.,* 33:288 (abstract).

Moss, R. L., Paloutzian, R. F., and Law, O. T. (1974b): Electrical stimulation of forebrain structures and its effect on copulatory as well as stimulus-bound behavior in ovariectomized hormone-primed rats. *Physiol. Behav.,* 12:997–1004.

Moss, R. L., Kelly, M. J., and Riskind, P. (1975a): Tuberoinfundibular neurons: Dopaminergic and norepinephrinergic sensitivity. *Brain Res.,* 89(2):265–277.

Moss, R. L., Kelly, M. J., and Dudley, C. A. (1975b): Responsiveness of medialpreoptic neurons to releasing hormones and neurohumoral agents. *Proc. Soc. Exp. Biol. Med.,* 5:9.

Moss, R. L., Dudley, C. A., Foreman, M. M., and McCann, S. M. (1975c): Synthetic LRF: a potentiator of sexual behavior in the rat. In: *Proceedings of the International Society of Neuroendocrinology.* Academic Press, New York.

Moss, R. L., McCann, S. M., and Dudley, C. A. (1975d): Releasing hormones and sexual behavior. *Prog. Brain Res.,* 42:37–46.

Motta, M., Piva, F., and Martini, L. (1973): New findings on the central control of gonadotrophin secretion. *J. Reprod. Fertil. [Suppl.],* 20:27–42.

Negoro, H., and Holland, R. C. (1972): Inhibition of unit activity in the hypothalamic paraventricular nucleus following antidromic activation. *Brain Res.,* 42:385–402.

Negoro, H., Visessuwan, S., and Holland, R. C. (1973): Inhibition and excitation in paraventricular nucleus after stimulation of the septum, amygdala and neurohypophysis. *Brain Res.,* 57:479–483.

Nicoll, R. A., and Barker, J. L. (1971): Excitation of supraoptic neurosecretory cells by angiotensin II. *Nature [New Biol.],* 233:172–174.

Novin, D., Sundsten, J. W., and Cross, B. A. (1970): Some properties of antidromically activated units in the paraventricular nucleus of the hypothalamus. *Exp. Neurol.*, 26:330–341.

Oomura, Y., Ooyama, H., Yamamoto, T., Ono, T., and Kobayashi, N. (1969): Behavior of hypothalamic unit activity during electrophoretic application of drug. *Ann. N.Y. Acad. Sci.*, 157:642–665.

Palkovits, M., Arimura, A., Brownstein, M., Schally, A. V., and Saavedra, J. M. (1974): Luteinizing hormone-releasing hormone (LH-RH) content of hypothalamic nuclei in rat. *Endocrinology*, 95:554–558.

Pawlikowski, M., and Karasek, M. (1971): Ultrastructural basis of neurosecretion. *Acta. Physiol. Pol. [Suppl. 3]*, 22:755–766.

Pfaff, D. W. (1973): Luteinizing hormone-releasing factor potentiates lordosis behavior in hypophysectomized ovariectomized female rats. *Science*, 182:1148–1149.

Pfaff, D. W., Diakow, C., Zigmond, R. E., and Kow, L. M. (1974): Neural and hormonal determinants of female mating behavior in rats. In: *The Neurosciences, III Study Program*, edited by F. O. Schmitt and F. G. Worden, pp. 621–646. MIT Press, Cambridge, Mass.

Porter, J. C. (1973): Neuroendocrine systems: The need for precise identification and rigorous description of their operations. *Prog. Brain Res.*, 39:1–6.

Porter, J. C., and Smith, K. R. (1967): Collection of hypophysial stalk blood in rats. *Endocrinology*, 81:1182–1185.

Poulain, P., and Carette, B. (1974): Iontophoresis of prostaglandins on hypothalamic neurons. *Brain Res.*, 79:311–314.

Powers, B., and Valenstein, E. S. (1972): Sexual receptivity: Facilitation by medial preoptic lesions in female rats. *Science*, 175:1003–1005.

Quijada, M., Krulich, L., Fawcett, C. P., Sundberg, D., and McCann, S. M. (1971): Localization of TSH-releasing factor (TRF), LH-RF and FSH-RF in rat hypothalamus. *Fed. Proc.*, 30:197 (abstract).

Ramirez, V. D., and McCann, S. M. (1964): Comparison of the regulation of luteinizing hormone (LH) secretion in immature and adult rats. *Endocrinology*, 72:452–464.

Ramirez, V. D., Komisaruk, B. R., Whitmoyer, D. I., and Sawyer, C. H. (1967): Effects of hormones and vaginal stimulation on the EEG and hypothalamic units in rats. *Am. J. Physiol.*, 212:1376–1384.

Rethelyi, M., and Halász, B. (1970): Origin of the nerve endings in the surface zone of the median eminence of the rat hypothalamus. *Exp. Brain Res.*, 11:145–158.

Rodriquez, E. M. (1959): Influencia de la corteza cerbral sobre el ciclo sexuel de la rats blance. *Rev. Soc. Argent. Biol.*, 35:5–15.

Ruf, K., and Steiner, F. A. (1967): Steroid-sensitive single neurons in rat hypothalamus and midbrain: Identification by microelectrophoresis. *Science*, 156:667–669.

Sawaki, Y., and Yagi, K. (1973): Electrophysiological identification of cell bodies of tubero-infundibular neurones in the rat. *J. Physiol. (Lond.)*, 230:75–85.

Sawyer, C. H. (1970a): Some endocrine applications of electrophysiology. In: *The Hypothalamus*, edited by L. Martini, M. Motta, and F. Fraschini, pp. 83–101. Academic Press, New York.

Sawyer, C. H. (1970b): Electrophysiological correlates of release of pituitary ovulating hormones. *Fed. Proc.*, 29:1895–1899.

Sawyer, C. H. (1975): Some recent developments in brain-pituitary-ovarian physiology: First Geoffrey Harris Memorial Lecture. *Neuroendocrinology*, 17:97–124.

Scharrer, E., and Scharrer, B., editors (1963): *Neuroendocrinology*. Columbia University Press, New York.

Schneider, H. P. G., Crighton, D. B., and McCann, S. M. (1969): Suprachiasmatic LH-releasing factor. *Neuroendocrinology*, 5:271–280.

Sétáló, G., Vigh, S., Schally, A. V., Arimura, A., and Flerko, B. (1975): LH-RH-containing neural elements in the rat hypothalamus. *Endocrinology*, 96:135–142.

Smith, A. D. (1971): Summing up: Some implications of the neuron as a secreting cell. *Philos. Trans. R. Soc. Lond. [Biol. Sci.]*, 261:423–437.

Smith, E. R., and Davidson, J. M. (1974): Feedback suppression of LH with maintained pituitary sensitivity: Evidence for a cerebral action of estrogen. *Neuroendocrinology*, 14:369–373.

Spatz, H. (1951): Neues uber die verknupfung von hypophyse und hypothalamus. *Acta Neuroveg. (Wein)*, 3:5–49.

Steiner, F. A. (1972): Effects of locally applied hormones and neurotransmitters on hypothalamic neurons. In: *Proceedings of the IV International Congress of Endocrinology*, pp. 202–204. Excerpta Medica, Amsterdam.

Steiner, F. A., Ruf, K., and Akert, K. (1969): Steroid-sensitive neurones in rat brain: Anatomical localization and responses to neurohumors and ACTH. *Brain Res.*, 12:74–85.

Stutinsky, F. S. (1970): Hypothalamic neurosecretion. In: *The Hypothalamus*, edited by L. Martini, M. Motta, and F. Fraschini, pp. 1–23. Academic Press, New York.

Szentagóthai, J., Flerkó, B., Mess, B., and Halász, B., editors (1962): Hypothalamic control of hypophyseal gonadotrophic function. In: *Hypothalamic Control of the Anterior Pituitary*, pp. 192–264. Akademiai Kiado, Budapest.

Szentagóthai, J., Flerkó, B., Mess, B., and Halász, B. (1968): *Hypothalamic Control of the Anterior Pituitary*, Ed. 3. Akademiai Kiado, Budapest.

Taleisnik, S., and McCann, S. M. (1961): Effects of hypothalamic lesions on the secretion and storage of hypophyseal luteinizing hormone. *Endocrinology*, 68:263–272.

Terasawa, E., and Sawyer, C. H. (1969): Changes in electrical activity in the rat hypothalamus related to electrochemical stimulation of adenohypophyseal function. *Endocrinology*, 85:143–149.

Terasawa, E., and Sawyer, C. H. (1970): Diurnal variation in the effects of progesterone on multiple unit activity in the rat hypothalamus. *Exp. Neurol.*, 27:359–374.

Terasawa, E., and Timiras, P. S. (1968): Electrical activity during the estrous cycle of the rat; cyclic changes in limbic structures. *Endocrinology*, 83:207–216.

Terasawa, E., and Timiras, P. S. (1969): Cyclic changes in electrical activity of the rat midbrain reticular formation during the estrous cycle. *Brain Res.*, 14:189–198.

Terasawa, E., Whitmoyer, D. I., and Sawyer, C. H. (1969): Effects of luteinizing hormone (LH) on multiple-unit activity in the rat hypothalamus. *Am. J. Physiol.*, 217:1119–1126.

Wakerley, J. B., and Lincoln, D. W. (1971a): Phasic discharge of antidromically identified units in the paraventricular nucleus of the hypothalamus. *Brain Res.*, 25:192–194.

Wakerley, J. B., and Lincoln, D. W. (1971b): Intermittent release of oxytocin during suckling in the rat. *Nature [New Biol.]*, 233:180–181.

Wakerley, J. B., and Lincoln, D. W. (1973a): Unit activity in the supraoptic nucleus during reflex milk ejection. *J. Endocrinol.*, 59:xlvi–xlvii.

Wakerley, J. B., and Lincoln, D. W. (1973b): The milk-ejection reflex of the rat: A 20- to 40-fold acceleration in the firing of paraventricular neurones during oxytocin release. *J. Endocrinol.*, 57:477–493.

Weiner, R. I., Blake, C. A., Rubinstein, L., and Sawyer, C. H. (1971): Electrical activity of the hypothalamus: Effects of intraventricular catecholamines. *Science*, 171:411–412.

Wheaton, J. E., Krulich, L., and McCann, S. M. (1975): Localization of luteinizing hormone-releasing hormone in the preoptic area and hypothalamus of the rat using radioimmunoassay. *Endocrinology*, 97:30–38.

Whitehead, S. A., and Ruf, K. B. (1974): Responses of antidromically identified preoptic neurons in the rat to neurotransmitters and to estrogen. *Brain Res.*, 79:185–198.

Wuttke, W. (1974): Preoptic unit activity and gonadotropin release. *Exp. Brain Res.*, 19:205–216.

Yagi, K. (1970): Effects of estrogen on the unit activity of the rat hypothalamus. *J. Physiol. Soc. Jap.*, 32:692–693.

Yagi, K. (1973): Changes in firing rates of single preoptic and hypothalamic units following an intravenous administration of estrogen in the castrated female rat. *Brain Res.*, 53:343–352.

Yagi, K., and Sawaki, Y. (1970a): On the localization of neurosecretory cells controlling adenohypophysial function. *J. Physiol. Soc. Jap.*, 32:621–622.

Yagi, K., and Sawaki, Y. (1970b): Neural mechanism in the rat hypothalamus. *J. Physiol. Soc. Jap.*, 32:496.

Yagi, K., and Sawaki, Y. (1971): Changes in the electrical activity of the hypothalamus during sexual cycle and the effect of castration on it in the female rat. *J. Physiol. Soc. Jap.,* 33:546–547.

Yagi, K., and Sawaki, Y. (1973): Feedback of estrogen in the hypothalamic control of gonadotrophin secretion. In: *Neuroendocrine Control,* edited by K. Yagi and Y. Sawaki, pp. 297–325. University of Tokyo Press, Japan.

Yagi, K., and Sawaki, Y. (1975a): Recurrent inhibition and facilitation: Demonstration in the tubero-infundibular system and effects of strychnine and picrotoxin. *Brain Res.,* 84:155–159.

Yagi, K., and Sawaki, Y. (1975b): Recurrent neural control in the tubero-infundibular system. *Brain Res.,* 84:155–159.

Yagi, K., Azuma, T., and Matsuda, K. (1966): Neurosecretory cell: Capable of conducting impulse in rats. *Science,* 142:778–779.

Yagi, K., Iwasaki, S., Sawaki, Y., and Satow, Y. (1971): Electrophysiological studies on the neurosecretory neuron. *Med. J. Osaka Univ.,* 21:75–90.

Yamashita, H., Koizumi, K., and Brooks, C. McC. (1970): Electrophysiological studies of neurosecretory cells in the cat hypothalamus. *Brain Res.,* 20:462–466.

Zambrano, D., and DeRobertis, E. (1968): The effect of castration upon the ultrastructure of the rat hypothalamus. II. Arcuate nucleus and outer zone of the median eminence. *Z. Zellforsch. Mikrosk. Anat.,* 73:405–413.

Zieglgansberger, W., Sothman, G., and Herz, A. (1974): Iontophoretic release of substances from micropipettes in vitro. *Neuropharmacology,* 13:417–422.

Zimmerman, E. A., Hsu, K. C., Ferin, M., and Kozlowski, G. P. (1974): Localization of gonadotropin-releasing hormone (Gn-RH) in the hypothalamus of the mouse by immunoperoxidase technique. *Endocrinology,* 95:1–6.

Frontiers in Neuroendocrinology, Vol. 4,
edited by L. Martini and W. F. Ganong.
Raven Press, New York © 1976.

Chapter 5

Brain Regulation of Growth Hormone Secretion

Joseph B. Martin

*Departments of Neurology and Experimental Medicine, Montreal General Hospital and McGill
University, Montreal, Quebec, Canada*

> The causes are not fully understood, but it is conceivable, such is the complex
> interconnection of mind and body, that some people may be able to choose
> not to grow up, like Peter Pan, though perhaps not so consciously.

Alison Lurie: *New York Review of Books,* Feb. 6, 1975

The secretion of growth hormone (GH), like prolactin, is precisely regulated by a complex interaction of neural influences, both stimulatory and
inhibitory. There is convincing evidence that this control is achieved by at
least two hypothalamic hormones: GH-releasing hormone (GRH), the structure of which is still unknown, and GH-release-inhibiting hormone (GIH, or
somatostatin[1]), which has now been isolated and structurally identified.
These hormones are believed to be synthesized in and released from neurons
of the mediobasal hypothalamus (peptidergic neurons). In addition to these
neurohormones, there is evidence that monoamines, notably dopamine (DA),
norepinephrine (NE), and serotonin, act at a neural level to modulate the
release of the hypothalamic hormones, perhaps acting as neurotransmitters in
monoaminergic neuron systems. Such a remarkably complex neural regulatory system appears to have developed for the control of those pituitary hormones which lack specific peripheral target organs and whose regulation may
not crucially depend on a feedback system comparable to that of thyrotropin
(TSH), adrenocorticotropin (ACTH), and the gonadotropins.

The objective of this chapter is to provide a critical review of recent developments in the area of neural control of GH secretion. Particular attention is given to the function of hypothalamic and higher centers, the effects
of stress and sleep, the role of monoamines, and evidence supporting short-
loop feedback control of GH secretion. Several other reviews on various
aspects of GH control have been published during the last few years (Brown
and Reichlin, 1972; Martin, 1973; Müller, 1973; Reichlin, 1974).

---

[1] The terms GIH and somatostatin are used interchangeably in this chapter.

PATTERNS OF GROWTH HORMONE SECRETION

Plasma levels of radioimmunoassayable GH measured at frequent intervals throughout the day and night show striking variations in both man and experimental animals. In the case of man, plasma GH levels may surge as high as 40 to 60 ng/ml, the largest bursts occurring during the first part of night sleep (Quabbe et al., 1966; Takahashi et al., 1968; Finkelstein et al., 1972).

The number and the magnitude of the spontaneous bursts of GH secretion in man are partly age-dependent. Finkelstein et al. (1972) showed that the transition from early puberty to adolescence is associated with an increased number of GH surges, occurring as frequently as eight times during each 24-hr period; similar observations were made by Parker and Rossman (1974). The surges in GH during the first few hours of the night were the largest, reaching levels of over 60 ng/ml plasma in some subjects (Fig. 5–1). This study indicated a close correlation between age and total 24-hr secretory rates of GH. Adolescents had a mean GH secretory rate of 690 μg/24 hr compared to 385 μg/24 hr in young adults. Daytime pulses also occurred more frequently during adolescence. Such bursts of secretion occur with sufficient frequency at all ages to cause some difficulty in assessing effects of stimulatory agents on GH release (Quabbe et al., 1966; Best et al., 1968; Glick and Goldsmith, 1968; Merimee et al., 1969; Spitz et al., 1972; Parker and Rossman, 1973).

A host of investigations have been undertaken to determine the basis of these physiological variations in GH secretion. Factors such as sleep (Taka-

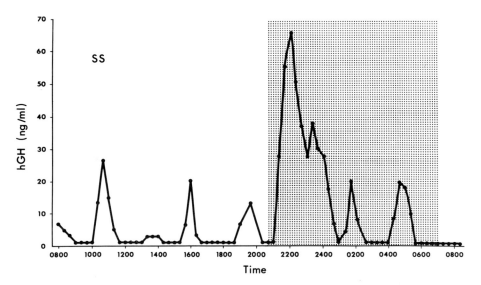

FIG. 5–1. Twenty-four-hour profile of GH secretory bursts in an adolescent male. (After Finkelstein et al., 1972, with permission).

hashi et al., 1968; Parker and Rossman, 1973), exercise, (Hunter et al., 1965; Schalch and Reichlin, 1968), stress (Schalch and Reichlin, 1968; Reichlin, 1974), and postprandial glucose decline (Parker and Rossman, 1973) account for some of these fluctuations, but a careful review of the available data indicates that many of the surges are spontaneous (Spitz et al., 1972).

Despite a considerable body of data relating plasma GH levels to changes in glucose, amino acids, or free fatty acids (FFA), it is evident that gross pharmacological and not physiological changes in these metabolites are required before GH levels are appreciably affected (Reichlin, 1974). Glick and Goldsmith (1968) showed that hyperglycemia only temporarily suppresses the daytime surges of GH secretion, and nocturnal GH rises are not affected by fasting or hyperglycemia (Parker and Rossman, 1971). Parker and Rossman (1973, 1974) described alteration in the timing and amplitude of the daytime pulses with shifts of mealtimes and daytime naps. They argued that glucose caused suppression of GH during the early postprandial period but could not account for all late postprandial GH surges on this basis. More frequent pulses did occur during fasting, as was previously observed (Glick and Goldsmith, 1968; Goldsmith and Glick, 1970). Daytime surges were enhanced by concurrent sleep.

The evidence for a role of glucose, amino acids, and lipids in the metabolic control of GH secretion was extensively reviewed by Reichlin (1974). With respect to glucose homeostasis he concludes: "These observations provide relatively weak evidence to support the thesis that reflex alterations in GH secretion are important in glucose homeostasis except possibly as an emergency mechanism, as in immature organisms. Even if it could be shown that minor degrees of hypoglycemia induced greater GH responses the effects of exercise, sleep, psychological stress, random GH bursts, and postprandial glucose decline, are so much more important in determining the secretion rate of GH that these factors, and not the demands of glucose homeostasis, dominate the controlling mechanisms of GH secretion." Similar conclusions were made after a detailed consideration of the role of amino acids and lipids in GH control in man.

A certain degree of species variability may occur, however, particularly with respect to the role of FFA in GH regulation. Ruminants such as the sheep and cow, which depend primarily on FFA for energy requirements, show prominent physiological GH fluctuations in relation to changes in these plasma metabolites (Hertelendy and Kipnis, 1973). On the other hand, the available evidence does not indicate any major role of glucose, proteins, or lipids in GH regulation in the pig (Machlin et al., 1968), cat (Kokka et al., 1971), or rat (Müller et al., 1972).

The profile of the secretory bursts of GH in man and their nonsuppressibility by potential metabolic regulators of GH secretion suggest that the surges are the result of primary activation of GH release induced by neural mechanisms. The pulses often show a striking, acute profile (Fig. 5–1) with rapid rises in plasma GH followed by a decline consistent with the known half-life of the hormone. The duration of active secretion may therefore be quite brief. In this respect the GH secretory pattern resembles the episodic secretion of ACTH (Weitzman et al., 1971), prolactin (Sassin et al., 1972;

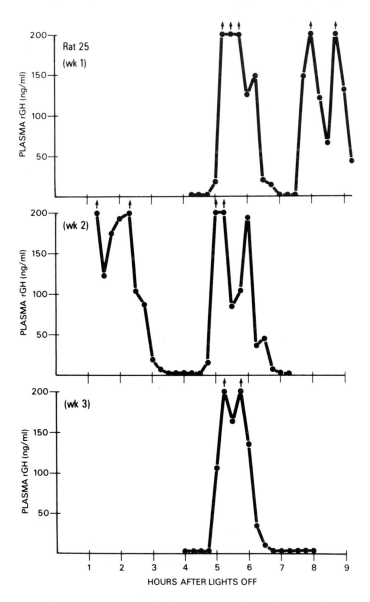

FIG. 5–2. Pulsatile GH secretion in a normal male rat sampled during dark cycle. The pulses occur at a similar time on three separate occasions, 1 week apart. Arrows indicate GH values greater than 200 ng/ml. (From Tannenbaum and Martin, 1975b.)

Parker et al., 1973), TSH (van Haelst et al., 1972), and the gonadotropins (Boyar et al., 1972). The surges of GH secretion in humans continue during long-term anesthesia (Werder et al., 1970).

Similar profiles of GH secretion have been documented in experimental animals. Chair-adapted rhesus monkeys (Sassin et al., 1971; G. Brown, *personal communication*) show episodic secretion of GH unrelated to feeding, stress, or blood glucose levels. The baboon, like man, shows a prominent rise during sleep (Parker et al., 1972). Unanesthetized rabbits also show surges of GH secretion (McIntyre and Odell, 1974).

We recently showed that previously observed marked variations in plasma GH obtained with random sampling in the rat (Garcia and Geschwind, 1968; Schalch and Reichlin, 1968; Dunn et al., 1973/1974; Brown and Martin, 1974) are due to prominent, high-amplitude secretory bursts of GH (Fig. 5–2) that may reach levels of 300 to 400 ng/ml (Martin et al., 1974a, 1975a). The pulses of GH secretion in this species show a regular 3 to 4-hr

TABLE 5–1. *Factors that stimulate GH secretion in primates*

Physiological	Pharmacological	Pathological
1. Episodic, spontaneous	1. Hypoglycemia	1. Acromegaly
2. Exercise	a. 2-Deoxyglucose	a. TRH
3. Stress	b. Insulin	b. LRH
a. Physical	2. Amino acid infusions	c. Glucose
b. Psychological	a. Arginine	d. Arginine
4. Sleep	b. Leucine	2. Pyrogens
5. Postprandial glucose	c. Lysine, etc.	3. Protein depletion
decline	3. Small peptides	4. Fasting and starvation
	a. Vasopressin	5. Anorexia nervosa
	b. α-MSH	
	c. ACTH (1–24)	
	d. Glucagon	
	4. Monoaminergic stimuli	
	a. Epinephrine, α-receptor	
	stimulation	
	b. L-DOPA	
	c. Apomorphine	
	d. 2-Bromo-α-ergocryptine	
	e. Clonidine	
	f. 5-Hydroxytryptophan	
	g. Fusaric acid (DOPA-β-	
	hydroxylase inhibitor)	
	(Hidaka et al. 1973)	
	h. Propranolol	
	i. Melatonin	
	5. Nonpeptide hormones	
	a. Estrogens	
	b. Diethylstilbestrol	
	6. Potassium infusion,	
	(Dluhy et al. 1972)	
	7. Dibutyryl cyclic AMP	

pattern, often with complex double or triple secretory peaks that are entrained to the light-dark cycle (Tannenbaum and Martin, 1975). The bursts of GH release occur independently of fluctuations in corticosterone (Martin et al., 1974a), prolactin (Willoughby et al., 1975), or TSH (Martin and Willoughby, *unpublished observations*) and are not related to stress.

Pulsatile GH secretion in the rat is significantly reduced by bilateral lesions of the hypothalamic ventromedial nuclei (VMN; Martin et al., 1974a), indicating a probable hypothalamic regulatory mechanism. As in man, episodic secretion of GH in the rat is not primarily regulated by glucose requirements since it is not affected by fasting, feeding, or glucose infusions (Tannenbaum and Martin, 1975a). The timing of the bursts show no correlation with either slow-wave or rapid eye movement (REM) sleep (Martin et al., 1975a;

TABLE 5–2. *Factors that inhibit GH secretion in primates*[a]

Physiological	Pharmacological	Pathological
1. Postprandial hyperglycemia	1. Melatonin	1. Acromegaly
2. Elevated free fatty acids	2. Serotonin antagonists	a. L-DOPA
(? pharmacological)	a. Methysergide	b. Apomorphine
3. Elevated GH levels	b. Cyproheptadine	c. Phentolamine
	3. Phentolamine	d. 2-Bromo-α-
	4. Chlorpromazine	ergocryptine
	5. Morphine	2. Hyperthyroidism
	6. Zinc tetracosactin	3. Hypothyroidism
	7. Progesterone	
	8. Theophylline	

[a] In many instances the inhibition can be demonstrated only as a suppression of GH release induced by a pharmacological stimulus.

Willoughby et al., 1975); we concluded that this secretory GH pattern is regulated by an intrinsic central nervous system (CNS) rhythm cued by the light-dark cycle but unaffected by sleep-wake rhythms.

Although spontaneous GH bursts may be the predominant form of GH secretion, particularly during growth, a number of other stimuli have been shown to affect GH release in primates. Certain of these physiological, pharmacological, and pathological factors are summarized in Table 5–1. Factors that inhibit GH secretion appear in Table 5–2.

Sleep-Associated GH Release

After the early descriptions of nighttime serum GH rises by Quabbe et al. (1966) and the suggestion by Takahashi et al. (1968) that they coincide with slow-wave sleep (SWS), there have been a number of studies undertaken to determine the mechanism and significance of this GH surge. There is considerable evidence that the nocturnal rise is a true nyctohemeral secretory response, related to sleep and not simply a diurnal variation. Evidence for this includes the following: (1) The most prominent phase of nocturnal GH secretion usually occurs during the first 2 hr of night sleep, coincident with a predominant electroencephalographic (EEG) pattern of stage 3 and 4 sleep (SWS). (2) Bursts of GH may occur later in the night but are less prominent. (3) Delay of sleep onset is associated with a delay in GH secretion. (4) Arousal during the night followed by return to deep sleep may be accompanied by a further burst of GH secretion. (5) Daytime naps with stage 3 and 4 sleep are associated with GH release. (6) Blind persons who show less sleep-associated GH release also have less SWS. (7) There is a coincident ontogenetic development of the nocturnal GH secretory pattern which correlates to some degree with the appearance of stage 3 and 4 sleep. (8) Narcoleptics who frequently enter directly into REM sleep may fail to secrete GH early in sleep (Martin, 1973; Reichlin, 1974). Given this evidence, most investigators have concluded that GH release and SWS are strongly associated, although a critical review of the relationship of SWS and nocturnal GH release has led to the conclusion that this association has been overemphasized (Willoughby et al., 1975).

The salient question here is whether the two events—nocturnal GH release and SWS—are interdependent or only temporally associated. A review of the available data shows that conclusions are based on evidence drawn from a very select population, usually males 20 to 30 yr of age, although some data are available on young, aged, and female subjects. Most series contain normal subjects who occasionally or regularly fail to secrete GH during sleep. This was also observed in the baboon (Parker et al., 1973).

If there is a common neural mechanism that simultaneously triggers SWS and release of GRH (or inhibits release of GIH) with resulting GH secretion, then GH should appear consistently with each SWS episode and in some constant temporal relation to it. Some correlation between SWS duration and GH levels might be expected also. There are no reports that specifically examine GH profiles with respect to all episodes of SWS (as distinct from all sleep cycles containing SWS). Only one specifically examined the temporal relation of GH to SWS (Pawel et al., 1972): Seven subjects were observed for two nights; on two occasions there was no sleep-associated GH secretion (one subject), whereas in two others (one occasion each) GH was released *before* sleep onset. Of the remaining 10 occasions, the first epoch of SWS preceded GH secretion by 0 to 60 min. A review of these data shows that SWS can be calculated to have commenced *after* GH release on four occasions. These findings do not support the authors' conclusion that there is a *consistent* temporal relation between SWS and GH release.

Furthermore, although plasma GH-sleep stage profiles in most studies show examples of concurrent GH secretion and SWS, there are many occasions when SWS episodes and GH secretory episodes occur independently.

In one study of SWS deprivation (Karacan et al., 1971), the authors concluded that "the amount of SWS does not determine the concentration of GH released during sleep." In another study with 3-hr sleep-wake cycles "no . . . relationship could be demonstrated between the initiation of GH release and the duration of stage 3–4 sleep" (Weitzman et al., 1974). These studies indicate *no* direct correlation between GH release and SWS. This is supported by the usual lack of correlation between GH release and second or third SWS cycles during a normal night's sleep. Finkelstein et al. (1972) found only five of 23 secondary secretory GH episodes to be associated with SWS-containing cycles.

Corresponding changes in GH and SWS in blind (Krieger and Glick, 1971) and SWS-deprived subjects (Sassin et al., 1969) are used as evidence for a relationship between the two. In the study of blind subjects (Krieger and Glick, 1971), SWS and GH levels were correspondingly reduced. However, two of the five subjects were aged (*vide infra*) and still produced feeble GH elevations despite absence of SWS, and another young subject produced an equal GH elevation despite significant amounts of SWS. The basal GH levels in some of these subjects appear to be higher than usual. It is thus possible that 24-hr GH secretion is actually normal in blind subjects, and that loss of a 24-hr light-dark cycle has disturbed both GH secretion and sleep patterns. The reduction in GH release in SWS-deprived subjects was not great (Sassin et al., 1969) and was shown not to be statistically significant.

Besides the absence of conclusive positive data for an association between GH and SWS, there is considerable evidence that there is no association. As noted above, individual normal controls occasionally or regularly fail to secrete GH during normal sleep despite normal SWS. A dissociation has also been described in a number of disease states in which abnormal SWS and abnormal GH secretion occur independently: Cushing's syndrome in remission (Krieger and Gewitz, 1974), Nelson's syndrome, some cases of Cushing's disease in remission, hypothalamic tumors (with or without Cushing's syndrome), systemic lupus erythematosus where the patient is taking steroids, Addison's disease (Krieger and Glick, 1974), and the maternal deprivation syndrome (Powell et al., 1973). In addition, several pharmacological agents can result in dissociation of SWS and GH secretion: imipramine, chlorpromazine and phenobarbital (Takahashi et al., 1968), flurazepam (Rubin et al., 1973a), medroxyprogesterone (Lucke and Glick, 1971a), acute high-dose glucose infusion (Lucke and Glick, 1971a,b), zinc-tetracosactrin (Evans et al., 1973), and free fatty acids (Lucke et al., 1972). The clinical dogma that GH secretory episodes and SWS are related by a common neural process does not seem to be proved and has already been criticized by Krieger and Glick (1974). Although nocturnal secretory episodes are usually strongly entrained to sleep, even this association is not obligatory.

Observations in the rhesus monkey also fail to show a relationship between SWS and episodic GH release (Sassin et al., 1971); the explanation offered was that the chair-adapted monkey shows short sleep cycles as compared to man. GH release coincident with SWS was identified in one of two baboons, but the absence of close correlation between GH secretion and SWS was attributed to the personalities of the baboons rather than to any great differences in the amount of SWS recorded (Parker et al., 1972). The prominent secretory bursts of GH observed in the rat clearly show *no* relationship to sleep cycles (Willoughby et al., 1975).

A conservative viewpoint at present is that nocturnal GH release is a sleep-related event which probably should not be considered as closely linked to or caused by the neural processes that subserve SWS. As has been noted by others (Parker and Rossman, 1974), the EEG characteristics of SWS relate to cortical electrical activity, which does not necessarily accurately reflect the changes in subcortical mechanisms involved in neuroendocrine control. A dissociation of the two phenomena (SWS and GH release) might therefore be expected to occur.

Stress-Associated GH Secretion

Several reviews discussed the mechanisms and teleology of stress-associated GH release (Brown and Reichlin, 1972; Reichlin, 1974). Species differences in the effects of stress on GH are evident: GH release secondary to stress occurs in primates, to a lesser degree in the sheep (Machlin et al., 1968) and cow (Mitra and Johnson, 1972), but not in the dog (Lovinger et al., 1974a), pig (Machlin et al., 1968), rat (Schalch and Reichlin, 1968; Brown and Martin, 1974), or mouse (Schindler et al., 1972). The GH response to major stress such as anesthesia and surgery in man is considerable but may not be as great as that of prolactin (Noel et al., 1972). Stress causes a decline in plasma GH levels in the rodent (Schalch and Reichlin, 1968; Schindler et al., 1972; Brown and Martin, 1974). Disorders such as the childhood maternal deprivation syndrome may result in chronic suppression of GH release during both sleep (without affecting SWS) and hypoglycemia or arginine infusion (Gardner and Amacher, 1973; Powell et al., 1973). This condition is reversible by placing the child in an emotionally secure environment. James Barrie, the English novelist and playwright who wrote Peter Pan, is a case in point. The seventh of eight children, he was subjected to severe maternal deprivation when his mother, after the accidental death of James' elder brother, "got into bed and stayed there for over a year." The emotionally deprived James never grew up, remaining less than 5 feet tall and sexually underdeveloped. Like Peter Pan, he may have chosen not to grow up.

Pharmacological Stimuli for GH Release

In considering the mechanisms that control GH secretion, it is important to distinguish physiological changes in GH levels from those that are pharmacologically induced. During the course of a normal day's activity, it appears that sleep, stress, exercise, and spontaneous surges in GH account for most if not all of the fluctuations in GH secretion in most species. In many studies directed toward elucidation of neural regulatory mechanisms, pharmacological stimuli such as insulin-induced hypoglycemia, amino acid infusions, or administration of L-DOPA, apomorphine, vasopressin, isoproterenol, glucagon, and the α- and β-adrenergic receptor blockers phentolamine and propranolol have been used (*vide infra*) (see Table 5–1).

This point is emphasized not to detract from the valuable information derived from such experiments but rather to suggest that physiological secretion may be controlled by different mechanisms. For example, sleep-associated GH release is not affected by prior treatment with phentolamine, an α-receptor blocker (Lucke and Glick, 1971*a*), or by chlorpromazine (Takahashi et al., 1968), although these agents do block GH secretion produced by insulin-induced hypoglycemia, vasopressin, or L-DOPA (Martin, 1973). Studies have not been reported concerning the effectiveness of such agents in blocking spontaneous daytime surges of GH release in humans. Exercise-induced GH secretion is prevented by phentolamine (Hansen, 1971). Morphine is reported to attenuate or prevent the GH release associated with major surgery (George et al., 1974). Chlorpromazine is effective in blocking pyrogen-induced GH secretion in the monkey (Rayfield et al., 1974).

Several pharmacological stimuli are also effective in eliciting GH release in the rat. Both pentobarbital (Howard and Martin, 1972; Martin, 1973/1974) and morphine (Kokka et al., 1972*a;* Martin et al., 1975*b*) are potent in this regard and seem to act at neural sites (Martin, 1973/1974; Martin et al., 1975*b*). These agents have proved useful for testing long-acting analogues of GIH.

NEURAL REGULATION OF GH SECRETION

Hypothalamic Regulation of GH Secretion

Several lines of evidence reviewed in detail elsewhere (Reichlin, 1966, 1974; Brown and Reichlin, 1972; Martin, 1973; Müller, 1973) support the importance of particular hypothalamic areas in GH regulation. Hypothalamic destruction and pituitary stalk section result in reduced plasma levels in man and in partial or complete loss of responses to hypoglycemia. Hypothalamic lesions also partially or completely block sleep-associated GH release (Krieger and Glick, 1974). Direct experimental evidence for the role of the hypothalamus has been obtained in several species. In the squirrel monkey small lesions of the median eminence and midline basal hypothalamus block insulin-induced (Abrams et al., 1966) and stress-mediated (Brown et al., 1971) GH release. Lesions of the VMN in young female rats result in growth retardation and a fall in plasma and pituitary GH levels (Frohman and Bernardis, 1968; Frohman et al., 1972). The lesions in young female rats were shown to be quantitative, larger lesions producing a greater fall in GH levels and greater growth failure. Lesions outside the VMH and arcuate nucleus are not associated with GH deficiency (Martin and Jackson, 1975). Lesions in the VMN area in adult male rats block pulsatile GH secretion but do not always affect pituitary GH levels (Martin et al., 1974a, 1975b). A form of growth retardation without altered plasma GH levels is also reported to occur with lesions of the dorsomedial hypothalamic nuclei (Bernardis and Goldman, 1972). The defect in these animals appears to be a caloric deficiency secondary to hypophagia. Taken in totality, the results with hypothalamic lesions suggest that the VMN-arcuate region contains a rather specific neural stimulatory area for GH control.

This hypothesis is strengthened further by consideration of the effects obtained with electrical stimulation. Both unilateral (Frohman et al., 1968) and bilateral (Martin, 1972) stimulation of the mediobasal hypothalamus in pentobarbital-anesthetized rats elicits GH secretion within 5 to 15 min after the onset of pulsed square waves. The effective stimulation sites are strictly confined to the VMN-arcuate complex. Stimulation of the lateral or anterior hypothalamus (Frohman et al., 1972; Martin, 1972) and of the supraoptic or paraventricular nuclei have no effect on plasma GH (Martin, 1972; Cheng et al., 1972). In fact, stimulation of the preoptic area causes significant inhibition of GH (Martin et al., 1975c), an observation that is of interest in view of prior speculation that an anterior hypothalamic or parachiasmatic inhibitory area inhibits GH secretion (Brown and Reichlin, 1972; Martin, 1973). Recent studies show that there is GIH in this region of brain (vide infra).

Observations concerning the time course of GH release after VMN stimulation are of considerable interest. In our studies the rise in plasma GH levels induced by hypothalamic stimulation invariably occurred after termination of the stimulus, as a postinhibitory rebound surge of secretion (Fig. 5–3). A similar delay was noted by Frohman et al. (1968). The peak of the response usually occurs 10 to 15 min after cessation of stimulation; longer periods of stimulation cause an appropriate further delay in the GH rise until termination of the stimulus. Before the discovery of GIH, it was difficult to interpret these findings. It now seems reasonable to speculate that hypothalamic stimulation elicits GIH release, with temporary cessation of GH secretion, and a postinhibitory rebound in secretion. The rise may be due to release of GRH, which was initially prevented from exerting its stimulatory effect by the inhibitory action of GIH. A similar postinhibitory GH surge has been described after hypothalamic stimulation in the sheep (Malven, 1974). Hypothalamic stimulation has also been reported to increase GH secretion in the monkey (Smith and Root, 1971), but it is difficult to exclude a nonspecific stress effect in these experiments since the animals were visibly distressed by the procedure. Electrical stimulation of the anterior or posterior

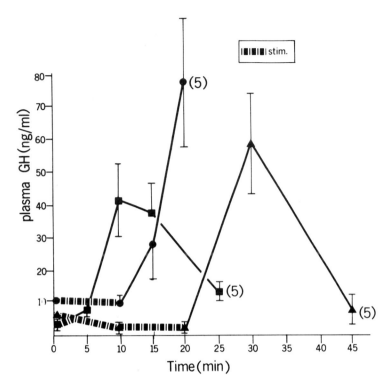

FIG. 5–3. Time course of GH release to hypothalamic VMN stimulation. GH release always occurs *after* end of stimulation. (From Martin, 1974b, with permission.)

hypothalamus in the cat (Kokka et al., 1972b) had no effect on plasma GH levels; however, the VMN and arcuate nucleus were not stimulated. Growth hormone release can also be induced by stimulation of the VMN in unanesthetized rabbits (McIntyre and Odell, 1974.)

Stimulation of these hypothalamic sites may be effective in causing GH release by direct excitation of tuberoinfundibular (TI) peptidergic neurons. Several investigators have successfully identified such cells by antidromic activation of axon terminals in the median eminence (Chapter 4). TI neurons are not restricted to the arcuate region but are considerably more widespread within the mediobasal hypothalamus. They extend as a rim of cells along the entire wall of the third ventricle, including the periventricular nucleus and the medial portion of the VMN (Martin and Renaud, 1974), as seen in Fig. 5–4. It can be argued from hypothalamic electrical stimulation experiments that a certain degree of anatomical specificity exists for regulation of individual anterior pituitary hormones. Effective sites for TSH release (Martin and Reichlin, 1972) and LH release (McCann, 1974) are much more widespread in the hypothalamus than those for GH release, presumably

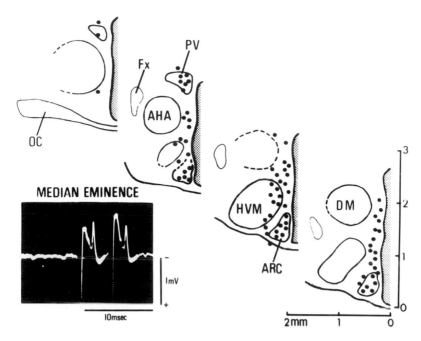

FIG. 5–4. Distribution of antidromically identified tuberoinfundibular (TI) neurons, throughout the arcuate nucleus (ARC), periventricular region, and part of the ventromedial nucleus (HVM). Dots in the paraventricular nucleus (PV) refer to magnocellular neurosecretory neurons. *Inset (lower left)*: Antidromic spikes from one TI cell in response to two median eminence shocks at 220 Hz. AHA, anterior hypothalamic area. Fx, fornix. DM, dorsomedial hypothalamic nucleus. OC, optic chiasm. (From Renaud and Martin, 1975.)

because selective populations of peptidergic neurons are excited by these stimuli.

That the hypothalamic regulatory hormones for GH are in fact localized to this region of the hypothalamus is now supported by both bioassay and radioimmunoassay data. Krulich et al. (1972) reported several years ago that the median eminence region of the hypothalamus contained GIH activity as measured by bioassay. GRH activity was localized primarily to the lateral zone of the VMN. Recent bioassay and radioimmunoassay studies confirmed that the arcuate nucleus and median eminence contain large amounts of GIH (Vale et al., 1974a; Arimura and Schally, 1975; Patel et al., 1975). Within the median eminence, GIH has been localized to axon terminals using immunohistochemical methods (Pelletier et al., 1974). It was estimated in these studies that 30% of nerve terminals on the portal capillaries contain GIH, an observation supported by the high concentrations of the peptide found in this region of hypothalamus by radioimmunoassay (Arimura et al., 1975; Patel et al., 1975). A high concentration of GIH is also found in the VMN, and significant amounts are present in the preoptic area and the amygdala. These observations are of interest because it has been shown that electrical stimulation of both the preoptic area (Martin et al., 1975c) and the corticomedial portion of the amygdala (CMA) (Martin et al., 1973; Martin, 1974a) cause significant GH inhibition in pentobarbital-anesthetized rats. Stimulation of these areas causes a fall in plasma GH without a postinhibitory rebound surge, in contrast to effects of VMN stimulation. We recently found that the corticomedial amygdala contains approximately 10-fold greater concentrations of GIH as determined by bioassay in monolayer pituitary cultures than does the basolateral amygdala complex (Brazeau and Martin, *unpublished observations*).

These data indicate a selective neural regulatory system for GH involving a specific group of hypothalamic neurons. The VMN has probably been adapted for this function by virtue of its role in homeostasis, serving as an integrative center for control of food intake, emotionality, and aggressivity. Glucoreceptors are postulated to be localized in or near the VMN. Himsworth et al. (1972) found a zone immediately lateral to the VMN in the rhesus monkey in which local applications of 2-deoxyglucose were effective in causing GH release, presumably by their effects on glucoreceptors.

Hypothalamic Regulatory Factors for GH Secretion

GRH

Evidence derived from the effects of stalk section and hypothalamic lesions indicates a predominant stimulatory influence of the brain in GH control in various species. Hypothalamic lesions in rats (Frohman and Bernardis, 1968), cats (O'Brien and Bach, 1970), monkeys (Abrams et al., 1966; Brown and Reichlin, 1972), and humans (Krieger and Glick, 1974) cause GH deficiency and/or block reflex GH secretion to various stimuli. Despite such compelling evidence for a GRH, attempts to identify this substance have thus far been unsuccessful. GRH activity has been identified by bioassay in pituitary portal blood (Wilber and Porter, 1970). In retrospect it is apparent that in some studies hypothalamic extracts were rendered biologically inactive so far as GH-releasing activity was concerned by the large concentrations of GIH now known to be present in the hypothalamus.

A major problem prior to the development of radioimmunoassays was interpreting the pituitary depletion bioassay which made use of the tibial epiphyseal assay of Greenspan et al. (1949) as a measure of GH activity. Using this assay system, Schally and collaborators (1968, 1971) isolated a decapeptide with pituitary GH-depleting activity from porcine hypothalamic fragments. This peptide, now known to be identical to a portion of the β-chain of porcine hemoglobin, has been shown to have no stimulatory effect on radioimmunoassayable levels of GH in rats (Schally et al., 1973a), monkeys (Knobil et al., 1968), or humans (Kastin et al., 1972). The current controversy surrounding the discrepancies between the bioassay and radioimmunoassay data was admirably reviewed by Reichlin (1974). It seems unlikely that the decapeptide reported by Schally and co-workers (1971) has any important physiological role in GH control. Similarly, the tripeptide described by Youdaev and Outacheva (1973) was not found to be active when tested in other laboratories (Schally et al., 1973b; Reichlin, 1974).

Despite these discouraging results, subsequent studies have confirmed that crude and semipurified extracts of hypothalamus can stimulate release of radioimmunoassayable GH in the rat and monkey. In some cases the GH-releasing activity in hypothalamic extracts may be due to vasopressin (Reichlin, 1974), although GRH activity has been demonstrated in several experimental systems where vasopressin cannot be implicated. Malacara et al. (1972) showed that methanol extracts of rat hypothalamus contain GRH activity when assayed in rats treated with estrogen and progesterone. Direct intrapituitary injection (Frohman et al., 1971) or infusion into the pituitary portal vessels (Sandow et al., 1972) of hypothalamic extracts was also effective in releasing GH in rats. Wilber and co-workers (1971) partially purified a GRH activity and found it to be effective in vitro in causing GH release from incubated rat pituitaries. However, the possibility that the GH-releasing activity may have been due at least in part to contamination with TRH was not excluded in these studies. TRH is effective in causing GH release from incubated pituitaries (Carlson et al., 1974). To exclude this possibility, Machlin et al. (1974) further characterized the GH-releasing activity of fragments of porcine hypothalamus. They found that the activity was not abolished by incubation with plasma, which should destroy TRH activity. Peake et al. (1973) also reported GRH activity in ovine hypothalamic extracts that did not release TSH and which stimulated cyclic GMP but not cyclic AMP. It should be noted that partially purified GRH material from porcine hypothalamic fragments that is active in radioimmunoassay systems has been studied in vitro in pituitary cultures (Chapter 3), although its nature has not been reported. In summary, there is a considerable body of data to support the existence of a hypothalamic GRH, but its structure remains to be defined.

Other Peptides That Stimulate GH Release

It is interesting that a number of unrelated peptides have now been shown to release GH in various species, including man. It is well known that several individual amino acids including arginine, leucine, phenylalanine, and lysine (Reichlin, 1974) can cause GH release, although the site and mechanism of action are unknown. Several small polypeptide hormones are also effective in this regard.

TRH, although ineffective in inducing GH release in normal human subjects, is a remarkably potent stimulant for GH release in patients with acromegaly (Irie and Tsushima, 1972; Faglia et al., 1973a; Tolis et al., 1975) and those with renal failure (Gonzalez-Barcena et al., 1973). TRH is a potent stimulator of GH release in the cow (Convey et al., 1972) and in incubated bovine (Machlin et al., 1974), sheep (Takahara et al., 1974), and rat (Carlson et al., 1974) pituitaries. Interestingly, TRH-induced GH release in acromegaly is not inhibited by somatostatin (Giustina et al., 1974). LRH is also reported to cause GH release in some but not all acromegalic subjects (Faglia et al., 1973*b*; Rubin et al., 1973*b*), and this effect is also not prevented by somatostatin (Giustina et al., 1974).

Vasopressin in pharmacological doses releases GH in humans (Heidingsfelder and Blackard, 1968), monkeys (Meyer and Knobil, 1966), and rats (Malacara et al., 1972). This effect was considered to be of little or no physiological significance until Zimmerman et al. (1973) observed that vasopressin (and neurophysin) are present in extremely high concentrations in the pituitary portal blood of surgically stressed rhesus monkeys. This resurrected the possibility that vasopressin might act as a "GRH" in stimulating GH release during stress.

Reichlin (1974) argues convincingly that vasopressin cannot be the only GRH since rats with hereditary vasopressin deficiency have normal plasma GH levels. We recently investigated this problem further, and our results indicate that such rats show normal GH release after electrical stimulation of the VMN (J. Martin, *unpublished observations*). Further evidence against a role of vasopressin as a GRH in the rat is the finding that stimulation of the supraoptic nuclei (Cheng et al., 1972), which is effective in releasing neurophysin (and presumably vasopressin), has no effect on GH release. The possibility remains, however, that vasopressin may have a physiological function as a GH releaser during stress in the primate.

Several papers have appeared which suggest that the active peptide sequence of ACTH may be effective in releasing GH in man (Zahnd et al., 1969; Pandos et al., 1970). Recently Girault et al. (1973) reported that *α-MSH,* which contains an amino acid sequence identical to the first 13 residues of ACTH, causes a marked rise in GH 30 to 45 min after intravenous administration. The question of the specificity of this response requires further study.

Glucagon, which contains 29 amino acids, is well known for its capacity to release GH in man (Wieland et al., 1973; Eddy et al., 1974). The site of action of glucagon is unknown, but it is not likely to be secondary to changes in plasma glucose, although this is still debated by some investigators (Parks et al., 1973). The effect of glucagon is potentiated by β-receptor blockade, suggesting that it may act on neural monoaminergic systems (Martin, 1973).

Rappaport and Grant (1973) reported a potent GRH substance of microbial origin: *cholera enterotoxin GRH*. This material, a protein of molecular weight 84,000, was isolated from cholera enterotoxin and is active *in vitro* in eliciting GH release by stimulating cyclic AMP. Its effects are blocked by somatostatin. These observations are of great interest and may result in identification of structure-activity relationships which will assist in the elucidation of native hypothalamic GRH.

GRH activity has also been reported in human lung tumor tissue (Beck et al., 1973) indicating the possibility that the peptide may be synthesized in neoplastic tissue as has been documented for other peptide hormones. It remains to be demonstrated whether the effects of these polypeptide substances act via specific receptors or are due to individual amino acids which form after breakdown of the parent molecule.

GIH

In studies aimed at characterizing GRH, Brazeau et al. (1973) were impressed by the repeated demonstration of inhibitory activity in purified fractions of sheep hypothalamic extracts. This potent inhibition of GH release was demonstrated both *in vivo* and *in vitro*. The effect was sufficiently consistent to permit purification and identification of a tetradecapeptide—subsequently named somatostatin (Fig. 5–5) for somatotropin-release-inhibiting

H-Ala-Gly-Cys-Lys-Asn-Phe-Phe-Trp-Lys-Thr-Phe-Thr-Ser-Cys-OH

FIG. 5–5. Structure of cyclic somatostatin.

factor (SRIF) or GH-release-inhibiting factor (GRIF or GIH). Earlier studies by Krulich and co-workers (1972) indicated that GIH activity was present in Sephadex fractions of hypothalamus and in frozen sections of hypothalamic tissue. These workers emphasized that the GIH activity was localized primarily to the median eminence. Stachura et al. (1972) had also reported the presence of GIH activity in bovine hypothalamic fragments. This material was shown to inhibit both the synthesis and release of GH *in vitro*.

During purification of somatostatin, Brazeau et al. (1974*a*) chose only one of several areas of GIH activity obtained from Sephadex fractions for subsequent chemical identification. It is thus possible that other hypothalamic substances with GIH activity will eventually be isolated. This possibility has also been suggested by work from Schally's laboratory (Dupont et al., 1974).

Somatostatin has widespread inhibitory effects on hormone secretion, both across species and on different hormones. Somatostatin inhibits GH secretion in rats induced pharmacologically by pentobarbital (Brazeau et al., 1973, 1974*b*), morphine (Martin et al., 1975*b*), and chlorpromazine (Kato et al., 1974), as well as by electrical stimulation of the hypothalamus and amygdala (Martin, 1974*b*). It is effective in preventing the increase in GH secretion produced by L-DOPA in humans (Siler et al., 1975), baboons (Ruch et al.,

1974), and dogs (Lovinger et al., 1974*b*), as well as that produced by insulin-induced hypoglycemia in humans (Hall et al., 1973; Yen et al., 1974) and baboons (Ruch et al., 1974), and by arginine in humans (Siler et al., 1973). The sleep-associated GH rise is prevented by somatostatin (Parker et al., 1974), which also blocks TRH-induced TSH release (Siler et al., 1974; Vale et al., 1974*b*), without affecting TRH-mediated prolactin release. It has no effect on basal secretion of prolactin, FSH, LH, TSH, or ACTH (Hall et al., 1973) and does not block LRH-induced LH or FSH release. It has been shown to be effective in suppressing elevated plasma GH levels in acromegaly (Hall et al., 1973; Yen et al., 1974) and to decrease ACTH levels in Nelson's syndrome (Tyrrell et al., 1975).

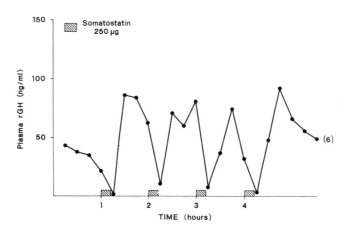

FIG. 5–6. Postinhibitory rebound secretion of GH after repeated infusions of somatostatin in the rat.

The onset of effect of GIH is rapid and may be mediated by decreased cyclic AMP generation in the pituitary somatotrops (Chapter 3). The duration of action of somatostatin is brief owing primarily to its short biological half-life, which is less than 5 min in plasma (Brazeau et al., 1974*b;* Martin, 1974*b*). Following cessation of infusion, GH levels tend to rebound and may reach levels exceeding those prior to inhibition. This has been demonstrated *in vivo* in humans (Hall et al., 1973), monkeys (Ruch et al, 1974), dogs (Lovinger et al., 1974*b*), and rats (Martin, 1974*a;* Martin et al., 1975*a*).

The mechanism of this postinhibitory rebound effect has been investigated in the rat. Infusions of large doses of somatostatin (250 μg) to rats results in GH inhibition followed within 15 min by a pronounced rebound secretion of GH (Fig. 5–6), which may reach levels as high as 200 ng/ml (Martin et al., 1975*a*). Hypothalamic VMN lesions in the rat (which do not cause a significant decrease in pituitary GH content) prevent postinhibitory rebound, suggesting that a short-loop feedback mechanism may contribute to the response (Martin et al., 1975a). On the other hand, superfused isolated rat pituitaries also show a postinhibitory rise in GH secretion, indicating that temporary cessation of GH secretion by GIH may be followed by enhanced pituitary GH release (Carlson et al., 1974).

The observation of a short inhibitory action of GIH associated with post-inhibitory rebound GH secretion has raised the question whether physiological control of GH secretion requires a GRH. In considering the total available physiological evidence, aside from the rather meager biochemical evidence described above, I conclude that compelling arguments remain for the existence of GRH:

1. The predominant hypothalamic control of GH secretion is stimulatory. The effect of interrupting the hypothalamic-pituitary continuity is decreased GH secretion. If hypothalamic control of GH secretion were due solely to tonic GIH secretion, with intermittent inhibition of GIH release to account for rises in plasma GH, then hypothalamic lesions that affect GIH neurons should result in a rise in GH. This occurs with prolactin but not with GH (Martin et al., 1974a,b).

2. Stimulation of certain extrahypothalamic regions elicits rapid GH secretion that cannot be accounted for by rebound after inhibition. Electrical stimulation of the basolateral amygdala (*vide infra*) results in a three- to fivefold rise in plasma GH within 5 min of the onset of stimulation, a response that strongly suggests a GRH releasing mechanism (Martin, 1974a). In contrast, stimulation of other regions such as the preoptic area and corticomedial amygdala causes GH inhibition without rebound, implying a specific GIH control system (Martin et al., 1975c).

3. Evidence of the mechanism of pulsatile GH secretion in the rat also seems to require a GRH drive. Hypothalamic VMN lesions obliterate pulsatile secretion and result in low baseline GH levels. Although GIH infusions in normal rats cause GH inhibition with prompt rebound, GIH infusions to VMN-lesioned rats fail to cause rebound secretion despite normal pituitary GH content (Martin et al., 1975a). These findings also indicate that GRH secretion may be regulated by a short-loop feedback system.

Other effects of somatostatin

In addition to the lack of specificity of somatostatin on GH secretion at the pituitary level, it is now documented that somatostatin inhibits insulin and glucagon secretion by direct effects on pancreatic islets (Devane et al., 1973; Koerker et al., 1974; Dobbs et al., 1975). This effect is observed following intravenous administration of pharmacological doses of somatostatin and has given rise to the possibility that somatostatin may be a widespread and nonspecific inhibitor of many endocrine glands. Further evidence for this is suggested by the recent observation that somatostatin inhibits gastrin secretion in normal human subjects and in patients with excessive gastrin secretion secondary to pancreatic delta cell adenomas: Zollinger-Ellison syndrome (Blood et al., 1974). In patients with ACTH-secreting pituitary adenomas, ACTH secretion is also inhibited after infusions of somatostatin (Tyrell et al., 1975). In recent studies of cultured pancreatic islets in the rat (P. Brazeau, *unpublished observations*), GIH activity has been demonstrated in the media. Patel et al. (1975) and Arimura et al. (1975) detected radioimmunoassayable somatostatin in normal pancreatic islets, indicating the possibility that this peptide may function physiologically as a regulator of pancreatic hormone secretion.

The implications of somatostatin in the treatment of diabetics with hyperglucagonemia have been discussed and may be of considerable importance (Gerich et al., 1974; Dobbs et al., 1975; Ungar and Orci, 1975). Many diabetics, particularly those with onset during childhood have abnormally high plasma glucagon levels or show exaggerated glucagon responses to such stimuli as hypoglycemia and arginine. Administering a combination of GIH and insulin causes glucagon suppression and results in a significant reduction in plasma glucose levels after meals with a resulting enhancement in the efficacy of insulin in such subjects (Gerich et al., 1974; Ungar and Orci, 1975).

The short duration of action of GIH and its rebound effect substantially reduce the potential effectiveness of the agent in the treatment of clinical disorders such as acromegaly and diabetes, and emphasize the necessity of obtaining a long-acting preparation. Brazeau and co-workers (1974b) reported that a suspension of somatostatin in protamine zinc (PZ) is effective in inhibiting pentobarbital-induced GH release for up to 16 hr in the rat; more recently Martin et al. (1974a) showed that PZ-somatostatin blocks pulsatile GH secretion in the rat for as long as 8 hr. In both of these studies, PZ was combined with linear somatostatin. Besser et al. (1974) reported that cyclized somatostatin combined with PZ is effective in prolonging the action of GIH for up to 4 hr in humans. Acylation of the cystine-3 position of somatostatin with acetyl, benzoyl, or other derivatives was shown by Brazeau et al. (1974c) to prolong the duration of action of somatostatin in inhibiting pentobarbital-stimulated release in the rat, but this prolonged inhibitory effect is inconstant (Brown et al., 1975; Brazeau and Martin, *unpublished data*). These various observations point to the importance and feasibility of eventually obtaining a satisfactory long-acting preparation of this important peptide.

Distribution of somatostatin in the brain

The results of both bioassay and radioimmunoassay confirm the presence of somatostatin in a number of neural regions outside the hypothalamus. Highest concentrations have been reported in the preoptic area and the amygdala, but significant amounts are also found in the cerebral cortex, thalamus, cerebellum, brainstem, spinal cord, and pineal gland (Vale et al., 1974a; Brownstein et al., 1975; Patel et al., 1975).

It is possible, given the information currently available, that the regions of the hypothalamus containing GIH are confluent with those known to contain TI peptidergic neurons. Recent electrophysiological studies provided evidence that certain of these cells have branching axon collaterals, one of which terminates on the portal vessels and the other ends in various other regions of the hypothalamus, the preoptic area, or the limbic system (Renaud and Martin, 1975a). By use of antidromic activation from the median eminence in addition to similar, concurrent activation from other brain sites, we defined a population of such cells in the VMN. These observations permit speculation that TI peptidergic neurons, like dopaminergic, noradrenergic, and serotoninergic neurons, may give rise to complex neural pathways which terminate in widespread areas of the neural axis.

Do such collaterals represent recurrent feedback loops that might function, for example, in the mediation of pulsatile secretion? Do collateral terminals which end in regions such as the preoptic area, brainstem, and amygdala—all regions that contain somatostatin—account for the widespread distribution of this peptide in extrahypothalamic tissues? Is somatostatin released from such terminals to have important biological effects on other neurons by influencing both electrophysiological and behavioral aspects of brain function? The answers to these and other intriguing questions must await further experimental evidence.

In support of a possible role of hypothalamic peptides in neuronal function is the observation that direct application of these peptides by iontophoresis onto single neurons (Dyer and Dyball, 1974; Renaud and Martin, 1975b) results in significant depression of neuronal firing rates. Somatostatin, as well as TRH and LRH, has a depressant effect on a certain population of central neurons both in the hypothalamus and in other areas such as the cerebral and cerebellar cortex and the spinal cord (Renaud et al., 1975). There is preliminary evidence that somatostatin, like TRH and LRH, may have behavioral effects (Plotnikoff et al., 1974; Segal and Mandell, 1974). The significance of these early reports of behavioral effects of GIH are difficult to assess at this time. It is apparent that further investigation of the neural effects of somatostatin will have profound significance not only in terms of our understanding the role of hypothalamic peptides in anterior pituitary regulation but also in the function of such peptides in regulating other brain mechanisms (Martin et al., 1975d).

Extrahypothalamic Regulation of GH Secretion

Physiological studies demonstrating the effects of stress and sleep on GH secretion point to a probable role of extrahypothalamic structures in GH control. The isolated hypothalamus appears capable of maintaining near-normal basal secretion of GH (Halász et al., 1971), including pulsatile release (J. Martin, *unpublished observations*); but at least in the rat the effects of selective hypothalamic cuts indicate that disconnection of specific inputs to the mediobasal hypothalamus can have differential excitatory or inhibitory effects on GH secretion.

The anatomical pathways connecting the limbic system to the mediobasal hypothalamus in general, and the VMN-arcuate complex in particular, have been most clearly defined in the rat (Fig. 5–7). Direct monosynaptic inputs

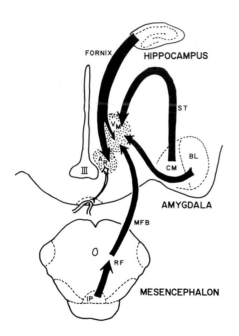

FIG. 5–7. Major afferent pathways to the VMN-arcuate complex in the rat. ST, stria terminalis. VM, ventromedial hypothalamic nucleus. AR, arcuate nucleus. CM, corticomedial amygdala. BL, basolateral amygdala. MFB, medial forebrain bundle. RF, reticular formation. IP, interpeduncular nucleus. See text for explanation. (From Martin, 1972, with permission.)

from a portion of the hippocampus reach the arcuate nucleus via the medial corticohypothalamic tract (Raisman and Field, 1971). The amygdala has a large monosynaptic connection from its corticomedial subdivision which reaches the VMN via the stria terminalis (des Olmos and Ingram, 1972). The connection(s) of the basolateral amygdala to the mediobasal hypothalamus has not been clearly defined in the rat. Electrophysiological studies in the cat (Murphy and Renaud, 1969) indicated an inhibitory pathway from the corticomedial amygdala via the stria terminalis to the VMN and a complementary excitatory pathway from the basolateral amygdaloid complex to the hypothalamic VMN. This latter pathway is postulated to be carried in the ventral amygdalohypothalamic tract.

A possible role of extrahypothalamic structures in GH control was first suggested by the studies of Eleftheriou et al. (1969) who reported that amygdaloid lesions in the deermouse increase the pituitary GH and hypo-

thalamic GRH as determined by bioassay. Lesions of the amygdala and pyriform cortex have also been reported to reduce plasma GH levels in the rat
as determined by radioimmunoassay (Newman et al., 1967).

In a series of experiments detailed elsewhere, we showed that electrical
stimulation of the hippocampal formation causes GH release (Martin, 1972,
1974; Martin et al., 1973). Stimulation of the amygdala can elicit either a
rise or a fall in plasma GH, depending on the precise site stimulated. Thus
stimulation of the basolateral amygdala causes prompt GH release. This release appears to be entrained to the stimulus, plasma levels increasing within
5 min of the onset of stimulation and declining immediately after its termination (Fig. 5–8). This response is blocked by placement of bilateral hypo-

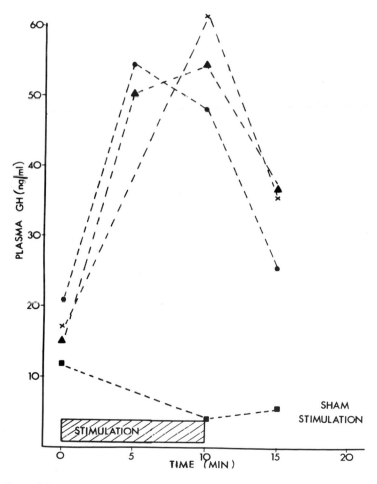

FIG. 5–8. Plasma GH response to stimulation of the basolateral amygdaloid complex in the rat. There was
a significant rise in GH *during* stimulation in three separate experiments. (From Martin, 1974b, with permission.)

thalamic VMN lesions, indicating that the effects on GH release are mediated through the mediobasal hypothalamus (Martin, 1974a). Stimulation of the corticomedial amygdala, on the other hand, causes a fall in plasma GH levels comparable to that observed with preoptic stimulation. Since an important component of the efferent system of the corticomedial amygdala travels in the stria terminalis to terminate in the septum and preoptic area (des Olmos and Ingram, 1972), it remains to be shown whether the corticomedial inhibitory response is mediated via connections in these areas. It is significant, perhaps, that coronal cuts through the anterior hypothalamus cause an increase in the rat's growth (Mitchell et al., 1972) and an elevation in plasma GH levels in some (Collu et al., 1973; Kato et al., 1974) but not all (Mitchell et al., 1972) studies. Such cuts would result in interruption of the stria terminalis but might also disconnect inhibitory effects of the preoptic area. Complete mediobasal hypothalamic deafferentation in which the VMN and arcuate nucleus are isolated from the overlying brain is reported to result in an increased growth rate and elevated plasma GH levels (Mitchell et al., 1973). Rice and Critchlow (1975) reported that preoptic lesions block stress-induced inhibition of GH secretion in the rat, permitting the emergence of a stress-induced GH release mechanism in this species. These observations suggest that extrahypothalamic inhibitory inputs to the mediobasal hypothalamus are important in maintaining a degree of tonic inhibition of GH in the rat and in the mediation of stress-induced GH suppression.

Stimulation of other brain regions can also cause a rise in plasma GH. One effective site is the ventral tegmental area of Tsai surrounding the interpeduncular nucleus (Martin, 1972). This region gives rise to dopaminergic inputs to higher brain regions. Electrical stimulation of the locus ceruleus also resulted in GH release in some but not all animals (Martin, 1974a). Stimulation of the raphe nucleus, the site of serotoninergic neurons in the brainstem, inhibits GH release during stimulation followed by a postinhibitory rebound (Fig. 5–9), a response similar to that which occurs after VMN stimulation (Martin, *unpublished observations*). Further investigation of these brain areas is required to elucidate their potential role in GH regulation. The results of locus ceruleus and raphe nucleus stimulation are of interest because both NE and serotonin have been implicated in the regulation of GH secretion (*vide infra*).

The functions of the limbic regions that affect GH secretion are complex. Experimental evidence indicates that the hippocampus is involved in several aspects of behavior such as the alerting response and in the recording of new information, as in learning or memory storage (Adey, 1967). The amygdala, on the other hand, is important in establishing emotionality and in the mediation of aggressive behavior (Mogenson and Huang, 1973). It is also important in regulation of feeding and drinking. The locus ceruleus is the origin of the ascending noradrenergic fiber system, lesions of which have been implicated in the "sham rage" associated with the "VMH syn-

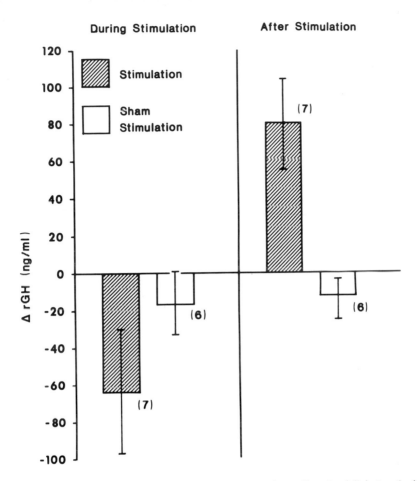

FIG. 5–9. Plasma GH response to stimulation of the raphe nuclei in the rat. There is a fall during stimulation followed by a significant rebound in plasma GH after stimulation.

drome" (Gold, 1973). The raphe nuclei have been shown to have a role in induction of SWS. Lesions of the raphe nuclei lead to insomnia as does inhibition of serotonin synthesis by p-chlorophenylalanine (Martin, 1973).

It is too simplistic to envision that complex neural structures such as the hippocampus or amygdala may mediate specific differential responses with respect to anterior pituitary hormone secretion; it is interesting to note, however, that studies from other laboratories support the role of these structures in the regulation of ACTH, TSH, and LH secretion, and that these effects are often opposite to those observed for GH. Evidence from electrical stimulation experiments indicate that the extrahypothalamic structures involved in GH control are similar to those implicated in LH regulation but with a reversal of influence. Electrochemical stimulation of the hippocampus is inhibitory (Velasco and Taleisnik, 1969a) and corticomedial amygdaloid stimulation excitatory for LH release (Velasco and Taleisnik, 1969b), effects opposite to those for GH. That this difference may have functional significance is suggested by the observation that GH is inhibited (Brown and Martin, 1974), whereas LH is released, by stress in this species (Ajika et al., 1972). The secretion of TSH, ACTH, and prolactin are reported to be inhibited by administration of pentobarbital, whereas GH is released by this agent in the rat. Studies from our laboratory (Martin, 1973/1974) indicate that pentobarbital causes activation of the hippocampus and of the basolateral amygdala, which may be one mechanism by which this agent exerts its neuroendocrine effects. Pentobarbital is also known to play a role in blocking ovulation in the female rat by causing inhibition of LH (McCann, 1974).

Short-Loop Feedback Control

Is the secretion of GH determined entirely by neural events, or is there evidence for feedback effects mediated by either GH or somatomedin? Evidence reviewed elsewhere (Motta et al., 1969; Martin, 1973; Müller, 1973; Reichlin, 1974) indicates that under certain prescribed conditions GH is capable of inhibiting its own secretion. Administration of GH, implantation of GH-secreting tumors, or direct hypothalamic placement of GH pellets reduce pituitary GH levels. These effects occur over a rather prolonged time course and may indicate only that the setpoint of the GH regulatory system is sensitive to circulating levels of GH.

Acute experiments have also shown that pharmacologically stimulated GH secretion can partially block a subsequent GH response to a second stimulus. Elevation of serum GH levels by exercise in humans prevented a further rise in response to arginine (Hagen et al., 1972). Prior GH administration to humans (Abrams et al., 1971; Hagen et al., 1972) and rhesus monkeys (Sakuma and Knobil, 1970) partially blocks GH release induced by arginine and/or insulin hypoglycemia. Although these results support a role for GH in regulating its own secretion, they do not provide an explanation of the mechanism. Since GH induces formation of somatomedin in peripheral tissue, it is relevant to ask if the feedback might be mediated via this second "hormone," although there is no direct evidence to support this mechanism. The Laron dwarf, who seems to lack normal peripheral tissue production of somatomedin, has strikingly elevated levels of GH, consistent with a failure in normal feedback regulation (Laron et al., 1966). It seems likely that the effects of somatomedin might be comparable to those of thyroid hormones in TSH regulation, acting to establish at the pituitary level the sensitivity of the pituitary somatotrop to hypothalamic regulatory factors.

Experiments in rats infested with the tapeworm *Spirometra mansonoides* have provided further evidence for a short-loop feedback control of GH (Garland and Daughaday, 1972). The tapeworm produces a substance(s) that is not immunoreactive in GH assays but which competes with GH in radioreceptor assays (Tsushima et al., 1974) and is capable of stimulating somatomedin production. Infestation with the worm leads to depletion of radioimmunoassayable GH in the pituitary, indicating a feedback effect either via the tapeworm substance or somatomedin.

In summary, it is probable that acute fluctuations in GH secretion are the result of acute neural effects; the degree of GH secretory response to neural stimuli may be determined by the previous circulating levels of GH and/or somatomedin. With further purification of somatomedin, it should be possible to test this hypothesis directly.

Monoaminergic Control

There is evidence to indicate that monoamines (DA, NE, and serotonin) are of considerable importance in the neural regulation of GH secretion. The high concentration of these monoamines in the hypothalamus, particularly in the median eminence (Chapter 1), has emphasized the possibility that they serve important regulatory functions for release of the hypothalamic hypophysiotropic hormones.

There is considerable evidence to suggest that NE, DA, and serotonin may each have a stimulatory role in GH regulation in primates. Oral administration of L-DOPA, the precursor of both NE and DA, which readily crosses the blood-brain barrier, causes release of GH in humans (Boyd et al., 1970), a response opposite to its effects on prolactin (Martin et al., 1974b). This effect could be mediated by effects on either noradrenergic or dopaminergic mechanisms. Evidence for noradrenergic control is derived from experiments which show that L-DOPA-induced GH release is blocked by phentolamine, an α-adrenergic blocking agent (Kansal et al., 1972), as GH release is induced by insulin hypoglycemia, vasopressin, and exercise (Martin, 1973).

A potential role of α-adrenergic receptors in GH control is supported further by the recent report that clonidine (Lal et al., 1974, 1975a), a central α-agonist, is effective in causing GH release in man. The GH response to clonidine was less marked than that to apomorphine. However, clonidine (presumably by its α-adrenergic effects on the liver, or on glucagon release) caused a modest rise in plasma glucose levels which preceded the GH rise and may have partly inhibited the response. The rise in glucose may have been sufficient to block partially the full central effects of clonidine on GH release.

GH is also released in man by subemetic doses of apomorphine, a centrally active dopaminergic stimulating agent, indicating that stimulation of dopaminergic receptors is also effective in GH release (Lal et al., 1973;

Brown et al., 1974). This response is not accompanied by a rise in plasma cortisol, suggesting that the effect is probably not by a nonspecific stress response (Brown et al., 1974; Lal et al., 1975b). Both L-DOPA-induced (Mims et al., 1973) and apomorphine-induced (Ettigi et al., 1975) GH release are attenuated by prior glucose administration, which indicates that glucoreceptor stimulation can partially override catecholaminergic stimuli for GH release.

Serotonin may also be involved in GH release in primates. Oral administration of L-tryptophan or 5-hydroxytryptophan (5-HTP) in man causes GH release although the response is not great (Imura et al., 1973; Müller et al., 1974). The GH response to hypoglycemia is blocked by the serotonin antagonists methysergide and cyproheptadine (Bivens et al., 1973; Smythe and Lazarus, 1974a). Administration of melatonin to man is reported both to stimulate GH release, presumably by activating serotonin receptors (Smythe and Lazarus, 1974b), and to block insulin- and exercise-induced GH release (Smythe and Lazarus, 1974b), a dual effect which may depend on the time course of melatonin effects.

Studies reported in other species point to a considerable degree of variability between species with respect to the effects of these pharmacological agents in GH regulation. In the baboon, intrahypothalamic injection of NE but not DA causes GH release, an effect blocked by phentolamine (Toivola and Gale, 1972; Toivola et al., 1972). The effects of serotonin were not reported in these studies. In the rhesus monkey intravenous administration of L-DOPA and clonidine are effective in causing GH release, whereas apomorphine was effective only when administered in a dose sufficient to cause vomiting (Brown et al., 1973). This apomorphine effect was accompanied by a rise in serum cortisol and therefore could be attributed to stress. Administration of 5-HTP was also effective in causing GH release in this species. The response was considerably more dramatic than that observed in man, but in the latter the route was oral. It is of interest that serotonin appears to be capable of eliciting GH release in all species in which it has been tested, similar to the remarkably consistent interspecies inhibitory effects of dopamine on prolactin secretion.

L-DOPA also causes GH release in dogs (Lovinger et al., 1974a), as does clonidine (Lovinger et al., 1975) but not apomorphine. L-DOPA is reported to inhibit GH secretion in response to arginine in the unanesthetized sheep (Davis and Berger, 1973). Other species differences also become apparent with respect to L-DOPA and apomorphine. L-DOPA and apomorphine both cause GH inhibition (Kato et al., 1973; Kokka and George, 1974) in the urethane-anesthetized rat. Intraventricular administration of dopamine also causes GH inhibition in this species, whereas serotonin causes GH release, an effect blocked by phenoxybenzamine, an α-receptor blocker (Collu et al., 1972). The use of urethane as an anesthetic agent is open to some question. This agent is remarkably nonphysiological, resulting in extremely elevated corticosterone levels (Ondo and Kitay, 1973) and causing alteration in blood gases and hematocrit (Blake and Sawyer, 1972). Moreover, urethane is a lethal agent, animals rarely recovering from its anesthetic effects. As GH levels are very low and show minimal fluctuations, it is likely that somatostatin release is high. Therefore, the evidence for a dopaminergic inhibitory system in such animals may only indicate a somatostatin-release system under stimulatory DA control. Further evidence for profound GH inhibition by urethane is the failure to demonstrate any GH release after VMN or amygdaloid stimulation in urethane-anesthetized rats (Martin et al., 1975c).

It should be emphasized that systemic or intraventricular administration of these pharmacologic agents provides little direct evidence of their physiologic role or site of action in GH control. With respect to prolactin, evidence has been published recently to suggest that DA may have direct effects on the pituitary to inhibit prolactin sceretion (see Chapter 5). Although there is little support for this site of action of monoamines in GH secretion, this possibility has not been entirely excluded. In electrical stimulation experiments in the rat, it has been shown that GH release after VMN stimulation is not blocked by agents which alter DA, NE, and serotonin content in rat brain (Martin, 1974b). On the other hand, GH release induced by amygdaloid and hippocampal stimulation are prevented by α-methyl-p-tyrosine, and by p-chlorophenylalanine, results consistent with the interpretation that monoamines may function as neurotransmitters in the relay of these responses from higher neural centers to hypothalamic GRH or GIH neurons. Amygdaloid-induced release of GH was prevented by α- but not β-adrenergic blockade.

In contrast to these results, evidence from intravenous administration of pharmacological agents to the urethane-anesthetized rat suggested that β-receptors are important in regulation of GH release (Kato et al., 1973). Intravenous chlorpromazine elicits GH release, an effect that is blocked by propranolol. The chlorpromazine response was attenuated by hypothalamic lesions and by posterior hypothalamic cuts, giving rise to the suggestion that neural inputs to hypothalamus are important for mediation of monoaminergic GH responses in this species (Kato et al., 1974). These observations, however, may be valid only under the effects of urethane.

Alterations in monoaminergic control may play a role in certain disease states. In acromegaly there is usually a "paradoxical" suppression of elevated GH levels by L-DOPA, apomorphine (Liuzzi et al., 1972; Chiodini et al., 1974), and by 2 bromo-α-ergocryptine, a dopaminergic-receptor stimulating agent (Liuzzi et al., 1974) that is currently used widely for its inhibitory effects on prolactin secretion. At least in some cases, this abnormality in GH regulation seems to be a secondary and not a primary disorder. In one case, successful total removal of a GH-secreting adenoma resulted in a return to normal of L-DOPA-, apomorphine-, and TRH-stimulated GH release (Hoyte and Martin, 1975). In a single case of the maternal deprivation syndrome, β-blockade with propranolol resulted in a restoration of the plasma GH responses to hypoglycemia (Imura et al., 1971). Excessive β-receptor stimulation might have induced chronic suppression of GH in this subject.

CONCLUSIONS

The secretion of GH is intermittent rather than continuous, and minute-to-minute regulation depends on neural influences that are largely independent of metabolic events. Over longer periods of time, metabolic and homeostatic perturbations such as periods of rapid growth, glucose intolerance (diabetes mellitus), protein depletion, and psychogenic disorders may affect both basal and episodic GH secretion. The mechanisms whereby these effects alter neural control and/or feedback regulation are unknown.

The neural control of GH secretion includes regulation by hypothalamic peptide hormones, monoamines, and extrahypothalamic influences, each component of which can enhance or reduce GH secretion. It is evident that full elucidation of this complex control system will not come easily.

ACKNOWLEDGMENTS

The author thanks the hormone distribution officer, National Institute of Arthritis and Metabolic Diseases, for generous supplies of radioimmunoassay materials. The assistance of Dr. John O. Willoughby in the review of sleep-associated GH release is gratefully acknowledged. The collaboration of Leo Renaud, Paul Brazeau and Gloria Shaffer Tannenbaum was of major importance in the authors' studies. Skillful typing assistance was given by Gail Hannaford and Sandra Harrington. The work reported herein was supported by the Medical Research Council of Canada.

REFERENCES

Abrams, R. L., Parker, M. L., Blanco, S., Reichlin, S., and Daughaday, W. H. (1966): Hypothalamic regulation of growth hormone secretion. *Endocrinology,* 78:605–613.
Abrams, R. L., Kaplan, S., and Grumbach, M. (1971): The effect of administration of human growth hormone on the plasma GH, cortisol, glucose, and free fatty acid response to insulin: Evidence for growth hormone autoregulation in man. *J. Clin. Invest.,* 50:940–950.
Adey, W. R. (1967): Intensive organization of cerebral tissue in alert, orienting and discriminative response. In: *The Neurosciences—A Study Program,* edited by G. C. Quarton, T. Melnechuk, and F. O. Schmitt, pp. 615–633. Rockefeller University Press, New York.
Ajika, K., Kalra, S. P., Fawcett, C. P., Krulich, L., and McCann, S. M. (1972): The effect of stress and Nembutal on plasma levels of gonadotropins and prolactin in ovariectomized rats. *Endocrinology,* 90:707–715.
Arimura, A., Sato, H., DuPont, A., Nishi, A., and Schally, A. V. (1975): Abundance of

immunoreactive GH-release inhibiting hormone in the stomach and pancreas of rat. *Fed. Proc.,* 34:273.

Beck, C., Larkins, R. G., Martin, T. J., and Burger, H. G. (1973): Stimulation of growth hormone release from superfused rat pituitary by extracts of hypothalamus and of human lung tumors. *J. Endocrinol.,* 59:325–333.

Bernardis, L. L., and Goldman, J. K. (1972): Growth and metabolic changes in weanling rats with lesions in the dorsomedial hypothalamic nuclei. *Exp. Brain Res.,* 15:424–429.

Besser, G. M., Mortimer, C. H., McNeilly, A. A., Thorner, M. D., Batistoni, G. A., Bloom, S. R., Kastrup, K. W., Hansen, R. F., Hall, R., Coy, D. H., Kastin, A. J., and Schally, A. V. (1974): Long term infusion of growth hormone release inhibiting hormone in acromegaly: Effects on pituitary and pancreatic hormones. *Br. Med. J.,* 4:622–627.

Best, J., Catt, K. J., and Burger, H. G. (1968): Non-specificity of arginine infusion as a test for growth hormone secretion. *Lancet,* 2:124–126.

Bivens, C. H., Lebovitz, H. E., and Feldman, J. M. (1973): Inhibition of hypoglycemia-induced growth hormone secretion by the serotonin antagonists cyproheptadine and methysergide. *N. Engl. J. Med.,* 289:236–239.

Blake, C. A., and Sawyer, C. H. (1972): Ovulation blocking actions of urethane in the rat. *Endocrinology,* 91:87–94.

Blood, S. R., Mortimer, C. H., Thorner, M. O., Besser, G. M., Hall, R., Gomez-Pan, A., Roy, V. M., Russell, R. C. G., Coy, D. H., Kastin, A. J., and Schally, A. V. (1974): Inhibition of gastrin and gastric-acid secretion by growth-hormone release-inhibiting hormone. *Lancet,* 2:1106–1109.

Boyar, R., Perlow, M., Hellman, L., Kapen, S., and Weitzman, E. (1972): Twenty-four hour pattern of luteinizing hormone secretion in normal men with sleep stage recording. *J. Clin. Endocrinol. Metab.,* 35:73–81.

Boyd, A. E., Lebovitz, H. E., and Pfeiffer, J. B. (1970): Stimulation of growth hormone secretion by L-DOPA. *N. Engl. J. Med.,* 283:1425–1429.

Brazeau, P., Vale, W., Burgus, R., Ling, N., Butcher, M., Rivier, J., and Guillemin, R. (1973): Hypothalamic polypeptide that inhibits the secretion of immunoreactive pituitary growth hormone. *Science,* 179:77–79.

Brazeau, P., Vale, W., Burgus, R., and Guillemin, R. (1974a): Isolation of somatostatin (a somatotropin release inhibiting factor) of ovine hypothalamic origin. *Can. J. Biochem.,* 52:1067–1072.

Brazeau, P., Rivier, J., Vale, W., and Guillemin, R. (1974b): Inhibition of growth hormone secretion in the rat by synthetic somatostatin. *Endocrinology,* 94:184–187.

Brazeau, P., Vale, W., Rivier, J., and Guillemin, R. (1974c): Acylated des [ALA^1-GLY^2]-somatostatin analogs: Prolonged inhibition of growth hormone secretion. *Biochem. Biophys. Res. Commun.,* 60:1202–1207.

Brown, G. M., and Martin, J. B. (1974): Corticosterone, prolactin and growth hormone responses to handling and new environment in the rat. *Psychosom. Med.,* 36:241–247.

Brown, G. M., and Reichlin, S. (1972): Psychological and neural regulation of growth hormone secretion. *Psychosom. Med.,* 34:45–61.

Brown, G. M., Schlach, D. S., and Reichlin, S. (1971): Hypothalamic mediation of growth hormone and adrenal stress response in the squirrel monkey. *Endocrinology,* 89:694–703.

Brown, G. M., Chambers, J. W., and Feldman, J. (1973): Neurotransmitter regulation of growth hormone release. In: *3rd Annual Meeting Society for Neuroscience,* p. 404.

Brown, W. A., Krieger, D. T., van Woert, M. H., and Ambani, L. M. (1974): Dissociation of growth hormone and cortisol release following apomorphine. *J. Clin. Endocrinol. Metab.,* 38:1127–1130.

Brown, M., Vale, W., Rivier, J., and Guillemin, R. (1975); Effects of TRF, somatostatin and H$_2$ somatostatin analogs on the secretion of growth hormone (GH), insulin and glucagon in the rat. *Endocrinology,* 96:A202.

Brownstein, M., Arimura, A., Sato, H., Schally, A. V., and Kizer, J. S. (1975): The regional distribution of somatostatin in the rat brain. *Endocrinology,* 96:1456–1461.

Carlson, H. E., Mariz, I. K., and Daughaday, W. H. (1974): Thyrotropin-releasing hormone stimulation and somatostatin inhibition of growth hormone secretion. *Endocrinology,* 94:1709–1913.

Cheng, K. W., Martin, J. B., and Friesen, H. G. (1972): Studies of neurophysin release. *Endocrinology,* 91:177–184.

Chiodini, P. G., Liuzzi, A., Botalla, L., Cremascoli, G., and Silverstrini, F. (1974): Inhibitory effect of dopaminergic stimulation on GH release in acromegaly. *J. Clin. Endocrinol. Metab.,* 38:200–206.

Collu, R., Fraschini, F., Visconti, P., and Martini, L. (1972): Adrenergic and serotoninergic control of growth hormone secretion in adult male rats. *Endocrinology,* 90:1231–1237.

Collu, R., Jéquier, J-C., Letarte, J., Leboeuf, G., and Ducharme, J. R. (1973): Effect of stress and hypothalamic deafferentation on the secretion of growth hormone in the rat. *Neuroendocrinology,* 11:183–190.

Convey, E. M., Tucker, H. A., Smith, V. G., and Zolman, J. (1972): Bovine prolactin, growth hormone, thyroxine and corticoid responses to thyrotropin-releasing hormone. *Endocrinology,* 92:471–476.

Davis, S. L., and Berger, M. L. (1973): Hypothalamic catecholamine effects on plasma levels of prolactin and growth hormone in sheep. *Endocrinology,* 92:303–309.

des Olmos, J. S., and Ingram, S. R. (1972): The projection field of the stria terminalis in the rat brain: An experimental study. *J. Comp. Neurol.,* 146:303–334.

DeVane, G. W., Siler, T. M., and Yen, S. S. C. (1973): Acute suppression of insulin and glucose levels by synthetic somatostatin in normal human subjects. *J. Clin. Endocrinol. Metab.,* 38:913–915.

Dluhy, R. G., Axelrod, L., and Williams, G. H. (1972): Serum immunoreactive insulin and growth hormone response to potassium infusion in normal man. *J. Appl. Physiol.,* 33:22–26.

Dobbs, R., Sakurai, H., Sasaki, H., Valverde, I., Baetens, D., Orci, L., and Unger, R. (1975): Glucagon: Role in the hyperglycemia of diabetes mellitus. *Science,* 187:544–547.

Dunn, J. D., Schindler, W. J., Hutchins, M. D., Scheving, L. E., and Turpen, C. (1973/1974): Daily variation in rat growth hormone concentration and the effect of stress on periodicity. *Neuroendocrinology,* 13:69–78.

Dupont, A., Schally, A. V., Takahara, J., Redding, T. W., and Locke, W. (1974): The presence of several peptides with GIF activity in pig hypothalamus. *Endocrinology,* 94:A156.

Dyer, R. G., and Dyball, R. E. J. (1974): Evidence for a direct effect of LRF and TRF on single unit activity in the rostral hypothalamus. *Nature (Lond.),* 252:486–488.

Eddy, R. L., Gilliland, P. F., Ibarra, J. D., McMurray, J. F., Jr., and Thompson, J. Q. (1974): Human growth hormone release—comparison of provocative test procedures. *Am. J. Med.,* 56:179–185.

Eleftheriou, B. E., Desjardins, C., Pattison, M. L., Norman, R. L., and Zolovick, A. J. (1969): Effects of amygdaloid lesions on hypothalamic-hypophyseal growth-hormone activity. *Neuroendocrinology,* 5:132–139.

Ettigi, P., Lal, S., Martin, J. B., and Friesen, H. G. (1975): Effects of sex, oral contraceptives and glucose loading on apomorphine-induced growth hormone secretion. *J. Clin. Endocrinol. Metab.,* 40:1094–1098.

Evans, J. I., Glass, D., Daly, J. R., and McLean, A. W. (1973): The effect of Zn-tetracosactrin on growth hormone release during sleep. *J. Clin. Endocrinol. Metab.,* 36:36–41.

Faglia, G., Beck-Peccoz, P., Ferrari, C., Travaglini, P., Ambrossi, B., and Spada, A. (1973a): Plasma growth hormone response to thyrotropin-releasing hormone in patients with active acromegaly. *J. Clin. Endocrinol. Metab.,* 36:1259–1262.

Faglia, G., Beck-Peccoz, P., Travaglini, P., Paracchi, A., Spada, A., and Lewin, A. (1973b): Elevations in plasma growth hormone concentration after luteinizing hormone-releasing hormone (LRH) in patients with active acromegaly. *J. Clin. Endocrinol. Metab.,* 37:336–340.

Finklestein, J. W., Anders, T. F., Sachar, E. J., Roffwarg, H. P., and Hellman, L. D. (1971): Behavioural state, sleep stage and growth hormone levels in human infants. *J. Clin. Endocrinol. Metab.,* 32:368–371.

Finklestein, J. W., Roffwarg, H. P., Boyar, R. M., Kream, J., and Hellman, L. (1972): Aged-related changes in the twenty-four-hour spontaneous secretion of growth hormone. *J. Clin. Endocrinol. Metab.*, 35:665–670.

Frohman, L. A., and Bernardis, L. L. (1968): Growth hormone and insulin levels in weanling rats with ventromedial hypothalamic lesions. *Endocrinology*, 82:1125–1132.

Frohman, L. A., Bernardis, L. L., and Kant, K. (1968): Hypothalamic stimulation of growth hormone secretion. *Science*, 162:580–582.

Frohman, L. A., Maran, J. W., and Dhariwal, A. P. S. (1971): Plasma growth hormone responses to intrapituitary injections of GH-RF in the rat. *Endocrinology*, 88:1483–1488.

Frohman, L. A., Bernardis, L. D., Burck, L., Maran, J. W., and Dhariwal, A. P. S., (1972): Hypothalamic control of growth hormone secretion in the rat. In: *Growth and Growth Hormone,* edited by A. Pecile and E. E. Müller, pp. 271–282. Excerpta Medica, Amsterdam.

Garcia, J. F., and Geschwind, I. I. (1968): Investigation of growth hormone secretion in selected mammalian species. In: *Growth Hormone,* edited by A. Pecile and E. F. Müller, pp. 267–291. Excerpta Medica, Amsterdam.

Gardner, L. I., and Amacher, P. (1973): *Endocrine Aspects of Malnutrition.* Kroc Foundation, Santa Ynez, California.

Garland, J. T., and Daughaday, W. H. (1972): Feedback inhibition of pituitary growth hormone in rats infected with Spirometra mansenoides. *Proc. Soc. Exp. Biol. Med.,* 139:497–499.

George, J. M., Reier, C. E., Lanese, R. R., and Rower, J. M. (1974): Morphine anesthesia blocks cortisol and growth hormone response to surgical stress in humans. *J. Clin. Endocrinol. Metab.,* 38:736–741.

Gerich, J. E., Lorenzi, M., Schneider, W., Karam, J. H., Rivier, J., Guillemin, R., and Forsham, P. H., (1974): Effects of somatostatin on plasma glucose and glucagon levels in human diabetes mellitus. *N. Engl. J. Med.,* 291:544–547.

Girault, D., Strauch, G., Rifai, M., and Bricaire, H. (1973): Alpha-MSH stimulation of growth hormone release. *J. Clin. Endocrinol. Metab.,* 37:990–993.

Giustina, G., Reschini, E., Peracchi, M., Cantalamessa, L., Cavagnin, F., Pinto, M., and Bulgheroni, P. (1974): Failure of somatostatin to suppress thyrotropin releasing factor and luteinizing hormone releasing factor-induced growth hormone release in acromegaly. *J. Clin. Endocrinol. Metab.,* 38:906–909.

Glick, S. M., and Goldsmith, S. (1968): The physiology of growth hormone secretion. In: *Growth Hormone,* edited by A. Pecile and E. E. Müller, pp. 84–88. Excerpta Medica, Amsterdam.

Gold, R. M. (1973): Hypothalamic obesity: The myth of the ventromedial nucleus. *Science,* 182:488–490.

Goldsmith, S. J., and Glick, S. M. (1970): Rhythmicity of human growth hormone secretion. *J. Mt. Sinai Hosp.,* 37:501–509.

Gonzalez-Barcena, D., Kastin, A. J., Schalch, D. S., Torres-Zamora, M., Perez-Pasten, E., Kato, A., and Schally, A. V. (1973): Responses to thyrotropin-releasing hormone in patients with renal failure and after infusion in normal men. *J. Clin. Endocrinol. Metab.,* 36:117–120.

Greenspan, F. S., Li, C. H., Simpson, M. E., and Evans, H. M. (1949): Bioassay of hypophyseal growth hormone; tibia test. *Endocrinology,* 45:455–463.

Hagen, T. C., Lawrence, A. M., and Kirsteins, L. (1972): Autoregulation of growth hormone secretion in normal subjects. *Metabolism,* 21:603–610.

Halasz, B., Schalch, D. S., and Gorski, R. A. (1971): GH secretion in young rats after partial or total interruption of neural afferents to the medial basal hypothalamus. *Endocrinology,* 89:198–203.

Hall, R., Besser, G. M., Schally, A. V., Coy, D. H., Evered, D., Goldie, D. J., Kastin, A. J., McNeilly, A. S., Mortimer, C. H., Phenekos, C., Tunbridge, W. M. G., and Weightman, D. (1973): Action of growth-hormone-release inhibitory hormone in healthy men and in acromegaly. *Lancet,* 2:581–586.

Hansen, A. P. (1971): The effect of adrenergic receptor blockade on the exercise-induced serum growth hormone rise in normals and juvenile diabetics. *J. Clin. Endocrinol. Metab.,* 33:807–812.

Heidingsfelder, S., and Blackard, W. H. (1968): Adrenergic control mechanism for vasopressin induced plasma growth hormone response. *Metabolism*, 17:1019–1024.

Hertelendy, F., and Kipnis, D. M. (1973): Studies on growth hormone secretion. V. Influence of plasma free fatty acid levels. *Endocrinology*, 92:402–410.

Hidaka, H., Nagasaka, A., and Takeda, A. (1973): Fusaric (5-butylpicolinic) acid: Its effect on plasma growth hormone. *J. Clin. Endocrinol. Metab.*, 37:145–147.

Himsworth, R. L., Carmel, P. W., and Frantz, A. G. (1972): The location of the chemoreceptor controlling growth hormone secretion during hypoglycemia in primates. *Endocrinology*, 91:217–226.

Howard, N. J., and Martin, J. M. (1972): Sodium pentobarbital and rat growth hormone secretion in vitro. *Endocrinology*, 91: 1513–1515.

Hoyte, K., and Martin, J. B. (1975): Recovery from paradoxical GH responses in acromegaly after transphenoidal selective adenonectomy. *J. Clin. Endocrinol. Metab. (in press).*

Hunter, W. M., Fonseka, C. C., and Passmore, R. (1965): The role of growth hormone in mobilization of fuel for muscular exercise. *Q. J. Exp. Physiol.* 50:406–416.

Imura, H., Yoshimi, T., and Ikekubo, K. (1971): Growth hormone secretion in a patient with deprivation dwarfism. *Endocrinol. Jap.*, 18:301–304.

Imura, H., Nakai, Y., and Hoshimi, T. (1973): Effect of 5-hydroxytryptophan (5-HTP) on growth hormone and ACTH release in man. *J. Clin. Endocrinol. Metab.*, 36:204–206.

Irie, M., and Tsushima, T. (1972): Increase of serum growth hormone concentration following thyrotropin-releasing hormone injection in patients with acromegaly or gigantism. *J. Clin. Endocrinol. Metab.*, 35:97–100.

Kansal, P. C., Buse, J., Talbert, O. R., and Base, M. G. (1972): The effect of L-dopa on plasma growth hormone, insulin, and thyroxine. *J. Clin. Endocrinol. Metab.*, 34:99–105.

Karacan, I., Rosenbloom, A. L., Williams, R. L., Finley, W. W., and Hursch, C. J. (1971): Slow wave sleep deprivation in relation to plasma growth hormone concentration. *Behav. Neuropsychiatry*, 2:11–14.

Kastin, A. J., Schally, A. V., Gual, C., Glick, S., and Arimura, A. (1972): Clinical evaluation in men of a substance with growth hormone-releasing activity in rats. *J. Clin. Endocrinol. Metab.*, 35:326–529.

Kato, Y., Dupre, J., and Beck, J. C. (1973): Plasma growth hormone in the anesthetized rat: Effects of dibutyryl cyclic AMP, prostaglandin E, adrenergic agents, vasopressin, chlorpromazine, amphetamine and L-dopa. *Endocrinology*, 93:135–145.

Kato, Y., Chihara, K., Ohgo, S., and Imura, H. (1974): Effects of hypothalamic surgery and somatostatin on chlorpromazine-induced growth hormone release in rats. *Endocrinology*, 95:1608–1613.

Koerker, D. J., Goodner, C. J., and Ruch, W. (1974): Somatostatin action on pancreas. *N. Engl. J. Med.*, 291:262–263.

Kokka, N., and George, R. (1974): Effects of narcotic analgesics, anesthetic and hypothalamic lesions on growth hormone and adrenocorticotropic hormone secretion in rats. In: *Narcotics and the Hypothalamus*, edited by E. Zimmerman and R. George, pp. 137–157. Raven Press, New York.

Kokka, N., Garcia, J. G., Morgan, M., and George, R. (1971): Immunoassay of plasma growth hormone in cats following fasting and administration of insulin, arginine, 2-deoxyglucose and hypothalamic extract. *Endocrinology*, 88:359–360.

Kokka, N., Garcia, J. F., George, R., and Ellioh, H. W. (1972*a*): Growth hormone and ACTH secretion: Evidence for an inverse relationship in rats. *Endocrinology*, 90:735–743.

Kokka, N., Eisenberg, R. M., Garcia, J., and George, R. (1972*b*): Blood glucose, growth hormone, and cortical levels after hypothalamic stimulation. *Am. J. Physiol.*, 222:236–301.

Knobil, E., Meyer, V., and Schally, A. V. (1968): Hypothalamic extracts and the secretion of growth hormone in the rhesus monkey. In: *Growth Hormone*, edited by A. Pecile and E. E. Müller, pp. 226–237. Excerpta Medica, Amsterdam.

Krieger, D. T., and Gewitz, G. P. (1974): Recovery of hypothalamic-pituitary-adrenal function, growth hormone responsiveness and sleep EEG pattern in a patient following removal of an adrenal cortical adenoma. *J. Clin. Endocrinol. Metab.*, 38:1075–1082.

Krieger, D. T., and Glick, S. (1971): Absent sleep peak of growth hormone release in blind subjects: Correlation with sleep EEG stages. *J. Clin. Endocrinol. Metab.*, 33:847–850.

Krieger, D. T., and Glick, S. M. (1974): Sleep EEG stages and plasma growth hormone concentration in states of endogenous and exogenous hypercortisolemia or ACTH elevation. *J. Clin. Endocrinol. Metab.*, 39:986–1000.

Krulich, L., Illner, P., Fawcett, C. P., Quijada, M., and McCann, S. (1972): Dual hypothalamic regulation of growth hormone secretion. In: *Growth and Growth Hormone*, edited by A. Pecile and E. E. Müller, pp. 306–316. Excerpta Medica, Amsterdam.

Lal, S., de la Vega, C., Sourkes, T. L., and Friesen, H. G. (1973): Effect of apomorphine on growth hormone, prolactin, luteinizing hormone and follicle-stimulating hormone levels in human serum. *J. Clin. Endocrinol. Metab.*, 37:719–724.

Lal, S., Ettigi, P., Martin, J. B., Tolis, G., Brown, G. M., Guyda, H., and Friesen, H. G. (1974): Central catecholamine receptor agonists and anterior pituitary secretion. *Clin. Res.*, 22:732A.

Lal, S., Tolis, G., Martin, J. B., Brown, G. M., and Guyda, H. (1975a): Effects of clonidine on growth hormone, prolactin, luteinizing hormone, follicle-stimulating hormone and thyroid-stimulating hormone in the serum of normal men. *J. Clin. Endocrinol. Metab.*, 41:703–708.

Lal, S., Martin, J. B., de la Vaga, C., and Friesen, H. G. (1975b): Comparison of the effect of apomorphine and L-dopa on serum growth hormone levels in man. *Clin. Endocrinol.*, 4:277–278.

Laron, Z., Pertazelan, A., and Karp, M. (1966): Pituitary dwarfism with high serum levels of growth hormone. *Isr. J. Med. Sci.*, 4:883–894.

Liuzzi, A., Chiodini, P. G., Botalla, L., Cremascoli, G., and Silvestrini, F. (1972): Inhibitory effect of L-dopa on GH release in acromegalic patients. *J. Clin. Endocrinol. Metab.*, 35:941–943.

Liuzzi, A., Chiodini, P. G., Botalla, L., Cremascoli, G., Müller, E. E., and Silvestrini, F. (1974a): Decreased plasma growth hormone (GH) levels in acromegalics following CB 154 (2-Br-α-ergocryptine) administration. *J. Clin. Endocrinol. Metab.*, 38:910–912.

Liuzzi, A., Chiodini, P. G., Botalla, L., Silvestrini, F., and Müller, E. E. (1974b): Growth hormone (GH)-releasing activity of TRH and GH-lowering effect of dopaminergic drugs in acromegaly: Homogeneity in the two responses. *J. Clin. Endocrinol. Metab.*, 39:871–876.

Lovinger, R. D., Connors, M. H., Kaplan, S. L., Ganong, W. F., and Grumbach, M. M. (1974a): Effect of L-dihydroxyphenylalanine (L-dopa), anesthesia and surgical stress on the secretion of growth hormone in the dog. *Endocrinology*, 95:1317–1321.

Lovinger, R., Boryczka, A. T., Schackelford, R., Kaplan, S. L., Ganong, W. F., and Grumbach, M. M. (1974b): Effect of synthetic somatotropin release inhibiting factor on the increase in plasma growth hormone elicited by L-dopa in the dog. *Endocrinology*, 95:943–946.

Lovinger, R., Boryczka, A. T., Sackelford, R., Kaplan, S. L., Ganong, W. F., and Grumbach, M. M. (1975): The role of brain amines in the regulation of growth hormone secretion in the dog. *Endocrinology*, 96:A178.

Lucke, C., and Glick, S. M. (1971a): Effect of medroxyprogesterone acetate on the sleep induced peak of growth hormone secretion. *J. Clin. Endocrinol. Metab.*, 33:851–853.

Lucke, C., and Glick, S. M. (1971b): Experimental modification of the sleep-induced peak of growth hormone secretion. *J. Clin. Endocrinol. Metab.*, 32:729–736.

Lucke, C., Adelman, N., and Glick, S. M. (1972): The effect of elevated free fatty acids (FFA) on the sleep-induced human growth hormone (hGH) peak. *J. Clin. Endocrinol. Metab.*, 35:407–412.

Machlin, L. J., Takahashi, T., Horino, M., Hertelendy, F., Gordon, R. S., and Kipnis, D. (1968): Regulation of growth hormone secretion in non-primate species. In: *Growth Hormone*, edited by A. Pecile and E. E. Müller, pp. 292–303. Excerpta Medica, Amsterdam.

Machlin, L. J., Jacobs, L. S., Cirulis, N., Kimes, R., and Miller, R. (1974): An assay for growth hormone and prolactin-releasing activities using a bovine pitutary cell culture system. *Endocrinology, 95*:1350–1358.

Malacara, J. M., Valverde, R., and Reichlin, S. (1972): Elevation of plasma radioimmunoassayable growth hormone in the rat induced by porcine hypothalamic extract. *Endocrinology, 91*:1189–1198.

Malven, P. V. (1974): Altered release of GH, LH and prolactin (PRL) induced by electrical stimulation of the median eminence (ME) in unanesthetized sheep. *Endocrinology, 94*:A127.

Martin, J. B. (1972): Plasma growth hormone (GH) response to hypothalamic or extrahypothalamic electrical stimulation. *Endocrinology, 91*:107–115.

Martin, J. B. (1973): Neural regulation of growth hormone secretion: Medical progress report. *N. Engl. J. Med., 288*:1384–1393.

Martin, J. B. (1973/1974): Studies on the mechanism of pentobarbital-induced GH release in the rat. *Neuroendocrinology, 13*:339–350.

Martin, J. B. (1974a): The role of hypothalamic and extrahypothalamic structures in the control of GH secretion. In: *Advances in Human Growth Hormone Research,* edited by S. Raiti, pp. 223–249. NIH Publication No. 74–612, Washington, D.C.

Martin, J. B. (1974b): Inhibitory effect of somatostatin (SRIF) on the release of growth hormone (GH) induced in the rat by electrical stimulation. *Endocrinology, 94*:497–503.

Martin, J. B., and Jackson, I. (1975): Neural regulation of TSH and GH secretion. In: *Anatomical Neuroendocrinology,* edited by W. Stumpf and L. Grant. Karger, New York (*in press*).

Martin, J. B., and Reichlin, S. (1972): Plasma thyrotropin (TSH) response to hypothalamic electrical stimulation and to injection of synthetic thyrotropin releasing hormone (TRH). *Endocrinology, 90*:1079–1085.

Martin, J. B., and Renaud, L. P. (1974): Hypothalamic and extrahypothalamic regulatory mechanisms for hypothalamic hormone secretion. In: *Neuroendocrine Integration: Basic and Applied Aspects,* edited by L. Fisher. Raven Press, New York (*in press*).

Martin, J. B., Kontor, J., and Mead, P. (1973): Plasma GH responses to hypothalamic, hippocampal and amygdaloid electrical stimulation: Effects of variation in stimulus parameters and treatment with α-methyl-p-tyrosine (α-MT). *Endocrinology, 92*:1354–3161.

Martin, J. B., Renaud, L. P., Brazeau, P. (1974a): Pulsatile growth hormone secretion: Suppression by hypothalamic ventromedial lesions and by long-acting somatostatin. *Science, 186*:538–540.

Martin, J. B., Lal, S., Tolis, G., and Friesen, H. G. (1974b): Inhibition by apomorphine of prolactin secretion in patients with elevated serum prolactin. *J. Clin. Endocrinol. Metab., 39*:180–182.

Martin, J. B., Willoughby, J. O., and Tannenbaum, G. S. (1975a): Evidence for an intrinsic central nervous system rhythm governing episodic GH secretion in the rat. *Endocrinology, 96*:A177.

Martin, J. B., Audet, J., and Saunders, A. (1975b): Effect of somatostatin and hypothalamic ventromedial lesions on GH release induced by morphine. *Endocrinology, 96*:881–889.

Martin, J. B., Tannenbaum, G., Willoughby, J. O., Renaud, L. P., and Brazeau, P. (1975c): Functions of the central nervous system in regulation of pituitary GH secretion. In: *Proceedings, International Conference on Hypothalamic Releasing Factors,* Milan, Italy. Excerpta Medica, Amsterdam (*in press*).

Martin, J. B., Renaud, L. P., and Brazeau, P. (1975d): Hypothalamic peptides: New evidence for "peptidergic" pathways in the C.N.S. *Lancet, 2*:393–395.

McCann, S. M. (1974): Regulation of secretion of follicle-stimulating hormone and luteinizing hormone. In: *Handbook of Physiology-Endocrinology,* Vol. 4, Part 2, edited by E. Knobil and W. H. Sawyer, pp. 489–517. Williams & Wilkins, Baltimore.

McIntyre, H. B., and Odell, W. D. (1974): Physiological control of growth hormone in the rabbit. *Neuroendocrinology, 16*:8–21.

Merimee, T. J., Fineberg, S. E., and Tyson, J. E. (1969): Fluctuations of human growth hormone secretion during menstrual cycle: Response to arginine. *Metabolism,* 18:606–608.

Meyer, V., and Knobil, E. (1966): Stimulation of growth hormone secretion by vasopressin in the rhesus monkey. *Endocrinology,* 70:1016–1018.

Mims, R. B., Scott, C. L., Modebe, O. M., and Bethune, J. E. (1973): Prevention of L-dopa-induced growth hormone stimulation by hyperglycemia. *J. Clin. Endocrinol. Metab.,* 37:660.

Mitchell, J. A., Smyrl, R., Hutchins, M., Schindler, W. J., and Critchlow, V. (1972): Plasma growth hormone levels in rats with increased naso-anal lengths to hypothalamic surgery. *Neuroendocrinology,* 10:31–45.

Mitchell, J. A., Hutchins, M., Schindler, W. J., and Critchlow, V. (1973): Increases in plasma growth hormone concentration and naso-anal length in rats following isolation of the medial basal hypothalamus. *Neuroendocrinology,* 12:161–173.

Mitra, R., and Johnson, H. D. (1972): Growth hormone response to acute thermal exposure in cattle. *Proc. Soc. Exp. Biol. Med.,* 139:1086–1089.

Mogenson, C. J., and Huang, Y. H. (1973): The neurobiology of motivated behavior: In: *Progress in Neurobiology,* edited by G. A. Kerkut and J. H. Phillis, pp. 53–83. Pergamon Press, Oxford.

Motta, M., Fraschini, F., and Martini, L. (1969): "Short" feedback mechanisms in the control of anterior pituitary function. In: *Frontiers in Neuroendocrinology 1969,* edited by W. F. Ganong and L. Martini, pp. 211–254. Oxford University Press, New York.

Müller, E. E. (1973): Nervous control of growth hormone secretion. *Neuroendocrinology,* 11:338–369.

Müller, E. E., Giustina, G., Miedico, D., Cocchi, D., and Pecile, A. (1972): Analogous pattern of bioassayable and radioimmunoassayable growth hormone in some experimental conditions of rat and mouse. In: *Growth and Growth Hormone,* edited by A. Pecile, and E. E. Müller, pp. 283–290. Excerpta Medica, Amsterdam.

Müller, E. E., Brambilla, F., Cavagnini, F., Peracchi, M., and Panerai, A. (1974): Slight effect of L-tryptophan on growth hormone release in normal human subjects. *J. Clin. Endocrinol. Metab.,* 39:1–5.

Murphy, J. T., and Renaud, L. P. (1969): Mechanism of inhibition in the ventromedial nucleus of the hypothalamus. *J. Neurophysiol.,* 32:85–102.

Newman, G., Roberts, W., Frohman, L. A., and Bernardis, L. L. (1967): Plasma GH levels in rats following amygdala pyriform cortex lesions. *Proc. Can. Fed. Biol. Soc.,* 10:41.

Noel, G. L., Suh, H. K., Stone, J. G., and Frantz, A. G. (1972): Human prolactin and growth hormone release during surgery and other conditions of stress. *J. Clin. Endocrinol. Metab.,* 35:840–851.

O'Brien, C. P., and Bach, L. M. N. (1970): Observations concerning hypothalamic control of growth. *Am. J. Physiol.,* 218:226–230.

Ondo, J. G., and Kitay, J. I. (1973): Effects of urethane on pituitary-adrenal function in the rat. *Proc. Soc. Exp. Biol. Med.,* 143:894–898.

Pandos, P., Strauch, G., and Bricaire, H. (1970): Corticotrophin-induced growth-hormone release. *Lancet,* 2:527.

Parker, D. C., and Rossman, L. G. (1971): Human growth hormone release in sleep: Nonsuppression by acute-hyperglycemia. *J. Clin. Endocrinol. Metab.,* 32:65–69.

Parker, D. C., and Rossman, L. G. (1973): Physiology of human growth hormone release in sleep. In: *Endocrinology,* edited by R. O. Scow, pp. 655–660. Excerpta Medica, Amsterdam.

Parker, D. C., and Rossman, L. G. (1974): Sleep-wake cycle and human growth hormone, prolactin, and luteinizing hormone. In: *Advances in Growth Hormone Research,* edited by S. Raiti, pp. 294–320. DHEW Publication No. (NIH) 74–612. Washington, D.C.

Parker, D. C., Morishima, M., Koerker, D. J., Gale, C. C., and Goodner, C. J. (1972): Pilot study of growth hormone release in sleep of the chair-adapted baboon: Potential as model of human sleep release. *Endocrinology,* 91:1462–1467.

Parker, D. C., Rossman, L. G., and Vanderlaan, E. F. (1973): Sleep-related nyctohemeral and briefly episodic variation in human plasma prolactin concentrations. *J. Clin. Endocrinol. Metab.,* 36:1119–1124.

Parker, D. C., Rossman, L. G., Siler, T. M., Rivier, J., Yen, S. S. C., and Guillemin, R. (1974): Inhibition of the sleep-related peak in physiologic human growth hormone release by somatostatin. *J. Clin. Endocrinol. Metab.*, 38:496–499.

Parks, J. S., Amrhein, J. A., Vaidya, V., Moshang, T., Jr., and Bongiovanni, A. M. (1973): Growth hormone responses to propranolol-glucagon stimulation: A comparison with other tests of growth hormone reserve. *J. Clin. Endocrinol. Metab.*, 37:85–92.

Patel, Y. C., Weir, G. C., and Reichlin, S. (1975): Anatomic distribution of somatostatin (SRIF) in brain and pancreatic islets as studied by radioimmunoassay (RIA). *Endocrinology*, 96:A127.

Pawel, M. A., Sassin, J. F., and Weitzman, E. D. (1972): The temporal relation between HGH release and sleep stage changes at nocturnal sleep onset in man. *Life Sci.*, 11:587–593.

Peake, G. T., Wilson, M., Steiner, A. L., and Dhariwal, A. P. S. (1973): Effects of a purified growth hormone releasing factor on growth hormone secretion and pituitary cyclic nucleotide content. *Metabolism*, 22:769–772.

Pelletier, G., Labrie, F., Arimura, A., and Schally, A. V. (1974): Electron microscopic immunohistochemical localization of growth hormone-release inhibiting hormone (somatostatin) in the rat median eminence. *Am. J. Anat.*, 140:445–450.

Plotnikoff, N. P., Kastin, A. J., and Schally, A. V. (1974): Growth hormone release inhibiting hormone: Neuropharmacological studies. *Pharmacol. Biochem. Behav.*, 2:693–696.

Powell, G. F., Hopwood, N. J., and Barratt, E. S. (1973): Growth hormone studies before and during catch-up growth in a child with emotional deprivation and short stature. *J. Clin. Endocrinol. Metab.*, 37:674–679.

Quabbe, H-J., Schilling, E., and Helge, H. (1966): Pattern of growth hormone secretion during a 24-hour fast in normal adults. *J. Clin. Endocrinol. Metab.*, 26:1173–1177.

Raisman, G., and Field, P. M. (1971): Anatomical considerations relevant to the interpretation of neuroendocrine experiments. In: *Frontiers in Neuroendocrinology 1971*, edited by L. Martini and W. F. Ganong, pp. 1–44. Oxford University Press, New York.

Rappaport, R. S., and Grant, N. H. (1973): Growth hormone releasing factor of microbial origin. *Nature (Lond.)*, 248:73–75.

Rayfield, E. J., George, D. T., and Biesel, W. (1974): Altered growth hormone homeostasis during acute bacterial sepsis in the rhesus monkey. *J. Clin. Endocrinol. Metab.*, 38:746–754.

Reichlin, S. (1966). Regulation of somatotrophic hormone secretion. In: *The Pituitary Gland,* edited by G. W. Harris and B. T. Donovan, pp. 270–298. Butterworths, London.

Reichlin, S. (1974): Regulation of somatotrophic hormone secretion. In: *Handbook of Physiology-Endocrinology*, Vol. 4, Part 2, edited by E. Knobil and W. H. Sawyer, pp. 405–447. Williams & Wilkins, Baltimore.

Renaud, L. P., and Martin, J. B. (1975a): Electrophysiological studies of connections of hypothalamic ventromedial nucleus neurons in the rat: Evidence for a role in neuroendocrine regulation. *Brain Res.*, 93:145–151.

Renaud, L. P., and Martin, J. B. (1975b): Thyrotropin releasing hormone (TRH): Depressant action of central neuronal activity. *Brain Res.*, 85:1–5.

Renaud, L. P., Brazeau, P., and Martin, J. B. (1975): Depressant action of TRH, LH-RH and somatostatin on the activity of central neurons. *Nature (Lond.)*, 225:233–235.

Rice, R. W., and Critchlow, V. (1975): Extrahypothalamic control of stress-induced inhibition of growth hormone in the rat. *Fed. Proc.*, 34:273.

Rubin, R. T., Gouin, P. R., Arenander, A. T., and Poland, R. E. (1973a): Human growth hormone release during sleep following prolonged flurazepam administration. *Res. Commun. Chem. Pathol. Pharmacol.*, 6:331–334.

Rubin, A. L., Levin, S. R., Bernstein, R. I., Tyrrell, J. B., Noacco, C., and Forsham, P. H. (1973b): Stimulation of growth hormone by luteinizing hormone-releasing hormone in active acromegaly. *J. Clin. Endocrinol. Metab.*, 37:160.

Ruch, W., Koerker, D. J., Carino, M., Johnson, S. D., Webster, B. R., Ensinck, J. W., Goodner, C. J., and Gale, C. C. (1974): Studies on somatostatin (somatotropin release inhibiting factor) in conscious baboons. In: *Advances in Human Growth Hor-*

mone Research, edited by S. Raiti, pp. 271–293. DHEW Publication No. (NIH) 74–612, Washington, D.C.

Sakuma, M., and Knobil, E. (1970): Inhibition of endogenous growth hormone secretion by exogenous growth hormone infusion in the rhesus monkey. *Endocrinology,* 86:890–894.

Sandow, J., Arimura, A., and Schally, A. V. (1972): Stimulation of growth hormone release by anterior pituitary perfusion in the rat. *Endocrinology,* 90:1315–1319.

Sassin, J. F., Parker, D. C., Johnson, L. C., Rossman, L. G., Mace, J. W., and Gotlin, R. W. (1969): Effects of slow wave sleep deprivation on human growth hormone release in sleep: Preliminary study. *Life Sci.,* 8:1299–1307.

Sassin, J. F., Jacoby, J. H., Finkelstein, J., Fukushima, D., and Weitzman, E. (1971): Episodic release of growth hormone and cortisol in monkeys. *Neurology (Minneap.),* 21:431–432.

Sassin, J. F., Frantz, A. G., Weitzman, E. D., and Kapen, S. (1972): Human prolactin: 24-hour pattern with increased release during sleep. *Science,* 177:1205–1207.

Schalch, D. S., and Reichlin, S. (1968): Stress and growth hormone release. In: *Growth Hormone,* edited by A. Pecile and E. E. Müller, pp. 211–225. Excerpta Medica, Amsterdam.

Schally, A. V., Müller, E. E., and Sawano, S. (1968): Effect of porcine growth hormone releasing factor on the release and synthesis of growth hormone in vitro. *Endocrinology,* 82:271–276.

Schally, A. V., Baby, Y., Nair, R. M. G., and Bennett, C. D. (1971): The amino acid sequence of a peptide with growth hormone releasing activity isolated from porcine hypothalamus. *J. Biol. Chem.,* 246:6647–6650.

Schally, A. V., Arimura, A., and Kastin, A. J. (1973a): Hypothalamic regulatory hormones. *Science,* 179:341–350.

Schally, A. V., Redding, T. W., Takahara, J., Coy, D. H., and Arimura, A. (1973b): Lack of growth hormone-releasing activity of (pyro) Glu-ser-NH$_2$. *Biochem. Biophys. Res. Commun.,* 55:556–562.

Schindler, W. J., Hutchins, M. O., and Septimus, E. J. (1972): Growth hormone secretion and control in the mouse. *Endocrinology,* 91:483–490.

Segal, D. S., and Mandell, A. J. (1974): Differential behavioural effects of hypothalamic polypeptides. In: *The Thyroid Axis Drugs and Behaviour,* edited by A. J. Prange, Jr., pp. 129–134. Raven Press, New York.

Siler, T. M., VanderBerg, G., and Yen, S. S. C. (1973): Inhibition of growth hormone release in humans by somatostatin. *J. Clin. Endocrinol. Metab.,* 37:632–634.

Siler, T. M., Yen, S. S. C., Vale, W., and Guillemin, R. (1974): Inhibition by somatostatin on the release of TSH induced in man by thyrotropin-releasing factor. *J. Clin. Endocrinol. Metab.,* 38:742–745.

Smith, G. P., and Root, A. W. (1971): Dissociation of changes in growth hormone and adrenocortical hormone levels during brain stimulation of monkeys. *Neuroendocrinology,* 8:235–244.

Smythe, G. A., and Lazarus, L. (1974a): Suppression of human growth hormone secretion by melatonin and cyproheptadine. *J. Clin. Invest.,* 54:116–121.

Smythe, G. A., and Lazarus, L. (1974b): Growth hormone responses to melatonin in man. *Science,* 184:1373–1374.

Spitz, I., Gonen, B., and Rabinowitz, D. (1972): Growth hormone release in man revised: Spontaneous vs stimulus-initiated tides. In: *Growth and Growth Hormone,* edited by A. Pecile and E. E. Müller, pp. 371–381. Excerpta Medica, Amsterdam.

Stachura, M. E., Dhariwal, A. P. S., and Frohman, L. A. (1972): Growth hormone synthesis and release in vitro: Effects of partially purified ovine hypothalamic extract. *Endocrinology,* 91:1071–1078.

Takahara, J., Arimura, A., and Schally, A. V. (1974): Effect of catecholamines in the TRH-stimulated release of prolactin and growth hormone from sheep pituitaries in vitro. *Endocrinology,* 95:1490–1494.

Takahashi, Y., Kipnis, D. M., and Daughaday, W. H. (1968): Growth hormone secretion during sleep. *J. Clin. Invest.,* 47:2079–2090.

Tannenbaum, G. S., and Martin, J. B. (1975a): Pulsatile growth hormone (GH) secretion: Dissociation from plasma insulin levels during feeding. *Fed. Proc.,* 34:311.

Tannenbaum, G. S., and Martin, J. B. (1975b): Evidence for an endogenous ultradian rhythm governing growth hormone secretion in the rat. (Submitted to *Endocrinology*)

Toivola, P. T. K., and Gale, C. C. (1972): Stimulation of growth hormone release by microinjection of norepinephrine into hypothalamus of baboons. *Endocrinology*, 90:895–902.

Toivola, P. T. K., Gale, C. C., Goodner, C. J., and Werrbach, J. H. (1972): Central α-adrenergic regulation of growth hormone and insulin. *Hormones*, 3:193–213.

Tolis, G., Kovacs, L., Martin, J. B., and Friesen, H. G. (1975): Dynamic evaluation of growth hormone (GH) and prolactin (hPRL) secretion in active acromegaly with high and low GH output. *Acta Endocrinol. (Kbh.) (in press)*.

Tsushima, T., Friesen, H. G., Chang, T. W., and Raben, M. S. (1974): Studies by radioreceptor assay (RRA) of a factor with growth hormone-like activity in incubation media of spargana of Spirometra mansonoides. *Endocrinology*, 94:A69.

Tyrell, J. B., Lorenzi, M., Forsham, P. H., and Gerich, J. E. (1975): The effect of somatostatin on secretion of adrenocorticotropin in normal subjects and in patients with Nelson's syndrome and Cushing's disease. *Endocrinology*, 96:A350.

Unger, R. H. (1975): The essential role of glucagon in the pathogenesis of diabetes mellitus. *Lancet*, 1:14–16.

Vale, W., Rivier, C., Palkovits, M., Saavedna, J. M., and Brownstein, S. M. (1974a): Ubiquitous brain distribution of inhibitors of adenohypophysial secretion. *Endocrinology*, 94:A145.

Vale, W., Rivier, C., Brazeau, P., and Guillemin, R. (1974b): Effects of somatostatin on the secretion of thyrotropin and prolactin. *Endocrinology*, 95:968–977.

van Haelst, L., Van Cauter, E., Degaute, J. P., and Goldstein, J. (1972): Circadian variations of serum thyrotropin levels in man. *J. Clin. Endocrinol. Metab.*, 35:479–482.

Velasco, M. E., and Taleisnik, S. (1969a): Effect of hippocampal stimulation on the release of gonadotropin. *Endocrinology*, 84:1154–1159.

Velasco, M. E., and Taleisnik, S. (1969b): Release of gonadotropins induced by amygdaloid stimulation in the rat. *Endocrinology*, 84:132–139.

Weitzman, E. D., Fukushima, D., Nogeive, C., Roffwarg, H., Gallagher, T. F., and Hellman, L. (1971): Twenty-four hour pattern of the episodic secretion of cortisol in normal subjects. *J. Clin. Endocrinol. Metab.*, 33:14–22.

Weitzman, E. D., Nogeire, C., Perlow, M., Fukushima, D., Sassin, J., McGregor, P., Gallagher T. F., and Hellman, L. (1974): Effects of a prolonged 3-hour sleep-wake cycle on sleep stages, plasma cortisol, growth hormone and body temperature in man. *J. Clin. Endocrinol. Metab.*, 38:1018–1030.

Werder, K. V., Stevens, W. C., Cromell, T. H., Eger, E. I., and Forsham, P. H. (1970): Growth hormone secretion during long-term anesthesia in man. *Horm. Metab. Res.*, 2:309–310.

Wieland, R. G., Hallberg, M. C., and Zorn, E. M. (1973): Growth hormone response to intramuscular glucagon. *J. Clin. Endocrinol. Metab.*, 37:329–331.

Wilber, J. F., and Porter, J. C. (1970): Thyrotropin and growth hormone releasing activity in hypophysial portal blood. *Endocrinology*, 87:807–811.

Wilber, J. F., Nagel, T., and White, W. F. (1971): Hypothalamic growth hormone releasing activity (GRA): Characterization by the in vitro rat pituitary and radioimmunoassay. *Endocrinology*, 89:1419–1424.

Willoughby, J., Brazeau, P., Renaud, L. P., and Martin, J. B. (1975): Pulsatile GH secretion in the rat: Absent correlation with prolactin surges and sleep-wake cycles. (Submitted to *Endocrinology*).

Yen, S. S. C., Silver, T. M., and De Vane, G. W. (1974): Effect of somatostatin in patients with acromegaly: Suppression of growth hormone, prolactin, insulin and glucose levels. *N. Engl. J. Med.*, 290:935–938.

Youdaev, N. A., and Outecheva, Z. F. (1973): Abstract D.B.7. In: *9th International Congress of Biochemistry*, Stockholm, p. 453.

Zahnd, G. R., Nadeau, A., and von Mulhendahl, K. E. (1969): Effects of corticotrophin on plasma levels of human growth hormone. *Lancet*, 2:1278.

Zimmerman, E. A., Carmel, P. W., Husain, M. K., Ferin, M., Tannenbaum, M., Frantz, A. G., and Robinson, A. G. (1973): Vasopressin and neurophysin: High concentrations in monkey hypophyseal portal blood. *Science*, 182:925–927.

Frontiers in Neuroendocrinology, Vol. 4,
edited by L. Martini and W. F. Ganong.
Raven Press, New York © 1976.

Chapter 6

Regulation of Prolactin Secretion

Robert M. MacLeod

*Department of Internal Medicine, University of Virginia School of Medicine,
Charlottesville, Virginia 22901*

During the past decade there has been a resurgence of interest in the mechanisms regulating the secretion and mode of action of prolactin. The relative lack of investigation of this hormone, as compared with other anterior pituitary hormones, may relate to the fact that it was only recently demonstrated unequivocally that primate prolactin is a distinct chemical entity (Niall et al., 1973). The arduous and insensitive cropsac bioassay also stifled widespread physiological experimentation. Since the introduction of the radioimmunoassay and polyacrylamide electrophoretic methods of analysis, investigation and conclusions concerning this hormone have multiplied manyfold. Many excellent reviews on the biochemical and physiological actions of prolactin have appeared recently (Horrobin, 1974), and no attempt is made here to deal with these aspects. In addition, there are several reviews concerning the regulation of prolactin secretion (Meites and Clemens, 1972; Wolstenholme and Knight, 1972; Pasteels and Robyn, 1973).

This area of research in neuroendocrinology has advanced to the point of identifying several hypothalamic biogenic amines which exert a powerful stimulus on systems regulating prolactin synthesis and release. The main purpose of this chapter is to review these systems and their pharmacological manipulation.

ROLE OF THE HYPOTHALAMUS

The anatomical connection between the median eminence and hypophysis is critical in maintaining the physiological control of prolactin secretion. Everett (1954) reported on the biological effects of hypersecretion of prolactin following transplantation of the pituitary gland beneath the kidney capsule. Isolation of the pituitary from the hypothalamus by stalk section likewise causes an increase in the plasma concentration of prolactin, and placement of electrolytic lesions in the hypophysiotropic area of the median eminence increases both serum prolactin concentration (Chen et al., 1970; Bishop et al., 1971) and production of pituitary prolactin (MacLeod and

Lehmeyer, 1972). Innervation of the medial basal hypothalamus (MBH) is also important in maintaining hormone levels because partial or total deafferentation of the MBH results in lowered circulating levels of prolactin in male rats (Blake et al., 1973). Thus the influence that the hypothalamus exerts on prolactin is profound and complex. In order to comprehend the mechanisms governing prolactin secretion, many investigators have devised techniques to identify the physiologically active components of the hypothalamus.

Inhibitory Influence

The primary action of the hypothalamus on the secretion of mammalian prolactin is inhibitory. Pasteels (1961) and Talwalker et al. (1963) were among the first to demonstrate that an acidic extract of hypothalamic tissue inhibited the *in vitro* secretion of prolactin. The system of Talwalker et al. (1963), however, was refractory to neuropharmacological agents such as acetylcholine, epinephrine, norepinephrine, serotonin, histamine, oxytocin, and vasopressin. They concluded that the hypothalamus contained an unidentified factor(s) that inhibited the *in vitro* synthesis and release of prolactin. The concept that hypothalamic extracts inhibit the secretion of prolactin was extended to other species by the work of Nicoll et al. (1970a). These studies also introduced evidence that hypothalamic extracts may have an additional ability to stimulate the *in vitro* release of prolactin.

The *in vivo* inhibitory effects of hypothalamic extracts on the circulating prolactin concentration are well documented. Amenomori and Meites (1970) reported that crude hypothalamic preparations decreased serum prolactin at 1 and 4 hr after injection into normal but nonlactating rats. Watson et al. (1971) extended these observations by injecting similar extracts into the jugular vein and determining the serum prolactin levels 8 min later. Intact male rats responded with a significant decrease in circulating prolactin, but castrated male rats did not. More recent experiments from this laboratory (Kuhn et al., 1974) show that reconstituted ultrafiltrates of acidic hypothalamic extracts produced a transient decrease in blood prolactin in suckled rats. They suggest that earlier failure of others to observe a decrease in a similar preparation might be explained by an inhibiting factor with a short biological half-life. That these systemically administered extracts probably have their primary effect directly on the pituitary is suggested by the data of Kamberi et al. (1971a), who infused extracts of brain tissue into a portal blood vessel leading to the pituitary. A typical dose-response curve of inhibition was obtained with hypothalamic extracts, and the suppressive effect on plasma prolactin lasted for 90 min following extract infusion. Although Kamberi's data showed that cerebrocortical extracts had no effect on plasma prolactin levels, Arimura et al. (1972) reported that cortical extracts as well as hypothalamic extracts significantly decreased serum prolactin levels in pentobarbital-anesthetized rats. Cortical extracts had no effect in rats with hypothalamic lesions. They suggest that these extracts may decrease prolactin levels not by a direct action on the pituitary but rather by the release of a hypothalamic factor, which in turn inhibits secretion by the pituitary.

Stimulatory Influence

The *in vitro* studies of Nicoll et al. (1970*a*) provide evidence that prolactin secretion may be under stimulatory as well as inhibitory control. During the initial period of pituitary gland incubation, hypothalamic extracts produced an inhibition of prolactin secretion, although a subsequent increase in hormone release was observed during a more prolonged incubation period. Ample physiological data support the concept of a hypothalamic mechanism capable of stimulating prolactin secretion. Abrupt increases in circulating prolactin are known to follow stressful stimuli, ether anesthesia, suckling, or the milking of cows.

Evidence supporting the concept of a hypothalamic prolactin-releasing hormone (PRH) was presented by Valverde-R et al. (1972) using methanol extracts of rat and pig stalk-median eminences. These materials produced a stimulatory response that was log-dose-dependent over a 10-fold range in male rats pretreated with estradiol and progesterone. The authors eliminated thyrotropin-releasing hormone (TRH), oxytocin, and vasopressin as the active prolactin-releasing factor in their extracts. Attempts to demonstrate the presence of a prolactin release-inhibiting hormone (PIH) were unsuccessful. Nevertheless, evidence is accumulating to suggest that prolactin secretion is regulated by a hypothalamic mechanism capable of stimulating as well as inhibiting the secretion of prolactin.

ROLE OF BIOGENIC AMINES IN INHIBITING PROLACTIN SECRETION

It is increasingly evident that biogenic amines have an important function in regulating the secretion of prolactin. A specific function for the hypothalamic catecholamines was suggested by Kanematsu et al. (1963), who produced lactation and a decreased pituitary prolactin concentration in ovariectomized rabbits following reserpine injection. Since lactation could not be produced by this treatment following placement of electrolytic lesions in the hypothalamus, it was concluded that reserpine exerted its action through the hypothalamus. The anatomical data of Hökfelt (1967) showed that the tuberoinfundibular dopaminergic neurons terminate in the median eminence adjacent to the portal blood vessels leading to the anterior pituitary. Other dopaminergic neurons originate in the arcuate nucleus, pass through the median eminence, and terminate in the neurointermediate lobe of the pituitary gland. Although no large quantities of catecholamines can be detected in the anterior pituitary in adult rats, there is suggestive evidence of their presence in this tissue in newborn rats (Baumgarten et al., 1972; Jacobowitz, 1973). Although specific cellular localization has not been accomplished, Hyyppä and Wurtman (1973) reported the presence of serotonin in the pituitary. Catecholamines contained in hypothalamic neurons thus may exert a direct effect on pituitary prolactin secretion after being transported to the pituitary or, alternatively, have an indirect effect on the pituitary by acting on the hypophysiotropic area of the hypothalamus, causing

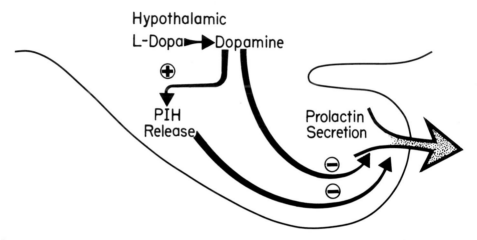

FIG. 6–1. Direct action of dopamine, inhibiting prolactin secretion; and the alternative proposal suggesting that dopamine stimulates the release of PIH, which subsequently inhibits prolactin secretion.

secretion of a second messenger (PIH), which suppresses prolactin secretion (Fig. 6–1).

Direct Inhibition of Prolactin Secretion by Catecholamines

The alternative possibilities of direct or indirect action of catecholamines on the secretion of prolactin were reviewed by van Maanen and Smelik (1968). They observed that placement of reserpine in the basal hypothalamus induced pseudopregnancy, and that treatment with a monamine oxidase inhibitor prevented this disturbance of the estrous cycle. They hypothesized "that the monoaminergic tuberoinfundibular neural system could be responsible for the neurohormonal control of prolactin secretion via the release of the inhibitor neurotransmitter into the portal vessel system."

Evidence supporting the hypothesis that catecholamines directly inhibit the secretion of prolactin was first provided by the work of MacLeod (1969) and Birge et al. (1970), and confirmed by Koch et al. (1970). Incubation of pituitary glands with leucine 4,5-^{3}H results in incorporation of the radioisotope into prolactin, which is largely secreted into the incubation medium. The primary effect of 5×10^{-7} M dopamine is to inhibit the secretion of electrophoretically separated radioactive prolactin; and as a result, isotopically labeled hormone accumulates in the pituitary tissue before its synthesis is inhibited (Table 6–1). The concentration of radioimmunoassayable prolactin secreted into the incubation medium is also decreased in the presence of dopamine; however, the decrease is not proportionally as great as with the newly synthesized prolactin due to the initial uninhibited secretion of preformed prolactin. In collaboration with Dr. Carlo Bruni, we examined pituitary lactotrophs by electron microscopy and found that the rough endoplasmic reticulum is greatly enlarged and filled with secretory material when the pituitary gland is incubated with catecholamines (MacLeod and Lehmeyer, 1972).

TABLE 6–1. *Dopamine-mediated inhibition of the in vitro secretion of prolactin*

	^{3}H-prolactin (cpm/mg pituitary)		Radioimmunoassayable prolactin (μg/mg pituitary)
	Pituitary	Medium	Medium
Control	1,746 ± 362	8,517 ± 1172	13.20 ± 1.36
Dopamine 5×10^{-7} M	2,144 ± 598	369 ± 156	3.92 ± 0.53

Four hemipituitary glands from female rats were incubated in 1 ml tissue culture medium 199 containing 1 μCi ^{3}H-leucine-4,5 for 5 hr in an atmosphere of 95% oxygen/5% carbon dioxide in a Dubnoff shaker at 37°C. Aliquots of pituitary homogenate and incubation medium subjected to polyacrylamide gel electrophoresis as described by MacLeod (1969). There were three or four flasks in each group.

Dopamine at concentrations of 5×10^{-7} M, or 76 ng/ml, always produces a large decrease in prolactin secretion. The use of lower concentrations of dopamine has produced limited success, possibly because the pituitary contains a monamine oxidase capable of metabolizing large quantities of catecholamines (MacLeod et al., 1970). Moreover, there is active oxidation of these agents by atmospheric oxygen. Shaar et al. (1973), however, recently reported that dopamine concentrations as low as 10^{-9} M inhibit *in vitro* secretion of lactogenic hormone. There is thus a growing body of evidence that dopamine may be a physiological inhibitor of prolactin secretion, and because of the *in vitro* action of the catecholamine it may act directly on the pituitary gland *in situ* (Fig. 6–1). Bower et al. (1974) recently presented evidence of a similar mechanism regulating the secretion of melanocyte-stimulating hormone (MSH) from the pituitary.

The concept that catecholamines exert an inhibitory action on prolactin secretion was strengthened by the work of Shaar and Clemens (1974), who examined the catecholamine content of hypothalamic extracts known to inhibit prolactin secretion. They found that the PIH activity in hypothalamic extracts could be totally accounted for by the dopamine and norepinephrine content in the hypothalamus. Enzymatic digestion with monamine oxidase or treatment with alumina rendered the hypothalamic extracts inactive, whereas peptic digests retained their activity and inhibited the secretion of prolactin.

Effect of L-DOPA

The concentration of catecholamines in the brain is increased by administration of L-DOPA following its metabolic conversion to dopamine and norepinephrine. Lu and Meites (1972) showed that L-DOPA, within 30 min of injection into rats, caused a dramatic decrease in serum prolactin and an increase in pituitary prolactin concentration. This effect of L-DOPA is utilized as a clinical assessment of pituitary function in man (Kleinberg and Frantz, 1971; Malarkey et al., 1971; Frantz et al., 1972; Friesen et al., 1972; Turkington, 1972). Oral administration of 500 mg L-DOPA causes a suppression in serum prolactin within 1 to 3 hr, with a return to normal values within approximately 6 hr. Even after chronic administration of the drug, withdrawal of therapy is followed by a prompt rise in serum hormone levels.

The mechanism through which the L-DOPA/dopamine-induced suppression of serum prolactin occurs has been vigorously debated. Lu and Meites (1972) and Donoso et al. (1974) measured serum prolactin in rats bearing pituitary grafts after injecting L-DOPA; the drug decreased the elevated serum prolactin concentrations produced by the pituitary transplant. Donoso et al. (1974) concluded that the dopamine formed in the brain acts directly on the pituitary and not at the hypothalamic level to inhibit prolactin secretion, a view consistent with their earlier findings that L-DOPA decreased serum prolactin levels in rats with lesions in the median eminence (Donoso et al., 1973). Lu and Meites (1972) claimed that L-DOPA increased the synthesis and release of the hypothalamic PIH, and this acted on the pituitary to decrease the secretion of prolactin. In support of this proposal they cited studies of Kamberi et al. (1971b) who found that intraventricular infusion of catecholamines decreased plasma prolactin levels, whereas the direct perfusion of the pituitary gland through one of the portal blood vessels produced no such decrease. These conclusions were recently challenged by Takahara et al. (1974a), who showed that when dopamine dissolved in a glucose solution was infused into a hypophysial portal blood vessel it caused a significant decrease in serum prolactin. Thus the inability of Kamberi et al. (1971b) to alter serum prolactin by introducing dopamine through a portal vessel may be related to oxidation of the catecholamine. Takahara et al. (1974a) also partially purified a PIH fraction prepared from pig hypothalami and showed that this preparation, after repeated chromatography and countercurrent distribution, contained a sufficient amount of dopamine and norepinephrine to account for all of the PIH activity.

The concept proposed by MacLeod (1969; MacLeod et al., 1970) that hypothalamic dopamine inhibits prolactin secretion by direct action is supported by the work of Donoso et al. (1973, 1974). Placement of electrolytic lesions in the median eminence caused serum prolactin levels to increase, and a prompt decrease was produced by L-DOPA injection. Additionally, the inhibition that L-DOPA produced in rats with transplanted pituitary glands was prevented if the rats were given injections of drugs that blocked the decarboxylation of L-DOPA to dopamine in the brain. After reviewing the possible mechanisms for the L-DOPA-induced suppression of serum prolactin, Noel et al. (1973) also suggested that one action of dopamine in humans may be to inhibit directly the secretion at the pituitary.

Effect of Reserpine, Phenothiazines, and Other Agents on Prolactin Secretion

The administration of tranquilizers to some patients has long been known to cause breast enlargement and galactorrhea. Following the pioneering work of Barraclough and Sawyer (1959) and Kanematsu et al. (1963), Coppola et al. (1965) suggested that reserpine-induced pseudopregnancy in rats was due to a depletion of brain norepinephrine. This phenomenon was blocked by L-DOPA but not by α-methyldopa.

These results correlated well with the data of Ratner et al. (1965), which showed that the ability of hypothalami of reserpine-treated rats to inhibit the *in vitro* secretion of prolactin was decreased as compared with hypothalami from normal rats. Although these authors eliminated serotonin and norepinephrine from consideration, it was concluded that reserpine acted on the hypothalamus to suppress secretion of a substance that inhibits prolactin secretion. Subsequent study by this group caused them to modify their concept that catecholamines are not involved in the mechanisms governing prolactin secretion. They suggested that the function of the hypothalamic catecholamine is to promote the release of a hypothalamic PIH (Koch et al., 1970).

Phenothiazine derivatives, especially perphenazine, have long been known to induce mammary development and initiate milk secretion in many species. Injection of perphenazine causes a prompt increase in serum prolactin levels (Ben-David et al., 1970; Lu et al., 1970; MacLeod and Lehmeyer, 1974a) and increases synthesis of the hormone (MacLeod and Lehmeyer, 1972), especially in male rats (MacLeod et al., 1970; MacLeod and Lehmeyer, 1974b). Thus perphenazine acts functionally (although not biochemically) in a manner similar to reserpine and α-methyl-p-tyrosine (MacLeod, 1969; MacLeod et al., 1970). Much effort has been directed toward investigating the mechanism of action of several of these tranquilizers. The data in Table 6–2 show that incubation of pituitary glands from male or female rats in the presence of 5×10^{-7} M dopamine produced a dramatic decrease in the secretion of newly synthesized ^{3}H-prolactin. Other groups of

TABLE 6–2. *Inhibition of the* in vitro *secretion of prolactin and its blockade following perphenazine injection*

	Prolactin (cpm/mg pituitary)	
Group	Pituitary	Medium
Female rats		
Control	675	2,425 ± 425
Dopamine 5 × 10⁻⁷ M	1,500	150 ± 25
Perphenazine	1,490	1,900 ± 405
Perphenazine + dopamine	1,490	1,250 ± 360
Male rats		
Control	210	480 ± 20
Dopamine 5 × 10⁻⁷ M	360	50 ± 10
Perphenazine	700	2,500 ± 50
Perphenazine + dopamine	840	2,510 ± 125

Perphenazine 1 mg was injected daily for 4 days.

rats that received the daily injection of 1 mg perphenazine for 4 days demonstrated an increase in prolactin synthesis, and in male rats the drug caused a fivefold increase in *in vitro* prolactin secretion. When the pituitary glands from perphenazine-treated rats were incubated with dopamine, the usual inhibiting action was not observed. That the onset of this perphenazine effect is very rapid is demonstrated by the data in Fig. 6–2. The longer the interval between the perphenazine injection and the time of sacrifice and

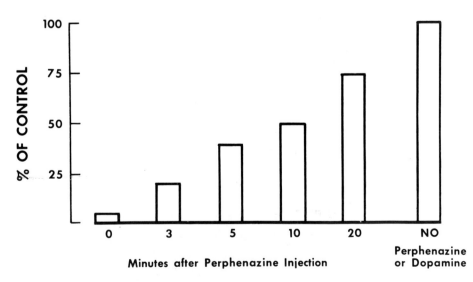

FIG. 6–2. Blockade by perphenazine injection of the dopamine-mediated inhibition of *in vitro* prolactin secretion. Effect of injecting 1 mg perphenazine into rats on the subsequent *in vitro* incubation of their pituitary glands with 5 × 10⁻⁷ M dopamine. (From MacLeod and Lehmeyer, 1974c.)

incubation of the pituitary glands with 5×10^{-7} M dopamine, the less is the effectiveness of the dopamine-mediated inhibition of prolactin secretion. Thus a partial blockade of the dopamine effect on prolactin is seen within 3 min after injection of the tranquilizer.

Perphenazine might conceivably produce this effect by one or a combination of several mechanisms: (1) the drug could act on the hypothalamus to decrease the content of PIH (Ratner et al., 1965; Ben-David et al., 1970; Danon and Sulman, 1970); (2) it could act on the hypothalamus to decrease the catecholamine content and subsequently decrease the content of PIH (Lu et al., 1970; Meites et al., 1972); (3) it could act in the hypothalamus to deplete the catecholamine content, which in time could release the pituitary from inhibitory control; or (4) it could act directly on the pituitary to block the effect of catecholamines and thereby permit prolactin release.

We recently presented evidence for the last of these postulates (MacLeod and Lehmeyer, 1974a). The data presented in Fig. 6–3 show that although perphenazine has no *in vitro* effect of its own, when coincubated with dopamine it blocks the dopamine-mediated inhibition of ³H-prolactin secretion. High specificity of the effectiveness of the tranquilizer is suggested because the dopamine effect is blocked by very small concentrations of the drug.

Another drug, haloperidol, is a competitive antagonist of catecholamines and blocks neurotransmission at dopaminergic receptors (Andén et al., 1966). Dickerman et al. (1972) showed that as little as 10 μg haloperidol per 100 g body weight increased serum prolactin levels within 1 hr of in-

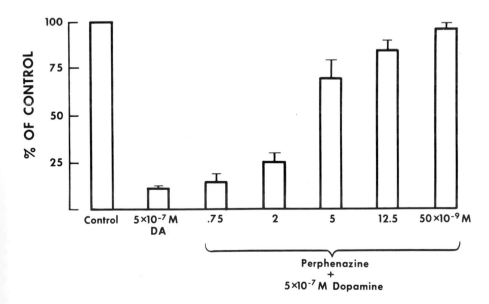

FIG. 6–3. *In vitro* blockade of the dopamine-mediated inhibition of prolactin release with perphenazine. (From MacLeod and Lehmeyer, 1974c.)

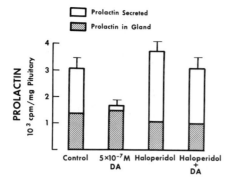

FIG. 6–4. Effect of haloperidol injection on the *in vitro* dopamine-induced suppression of prolactin secretion. Haloperidol (0.1 mg) was administered daily for 4 days. (From MacLeod and Lehmeyer, 1974c.)

jection. Additionally, the ability of hypothalamic extracts to decrease serum prolactin levels was significantly decreased in rats given injections of the drug. In a subsequent article Dickerman et al. (1974) suggested that haloperidol probably decreases the hypothalamic catecholamine content and thus decreases the hypothalamic factors responsible for the control of serum prolactin.

Our interpretation of the mode of action of haloperidol on prolactin secretion varies significantly from the above (MacLeod and Lehmeyer, 1973a). Specifically, we showed that injected haloperidol had an effect on the pituitary gland, producing increased synthesis and release of prolactin and blocking the ability of dopamine to inhibit the *in vitro* secretion of ³H-prolactin (Fig. 6–4). Although there is no reason to doubt that haloperidol may have an effect in the hypothalamus, we believe the drug has an important action directly on the pituitary to block the inhibitory action of hypothalamic catecholamines. Evidence for this postulate is presented in Fig. 6–5. The inhibition produced by dopamine of the *in vitro* secretion of both ³H-prolactin and of radioimmunoassayable prolactin was reversed by coincubation with 5×10^{-9} M haloperidol.

These experimental findings were recently confirmed by Quijada et al.

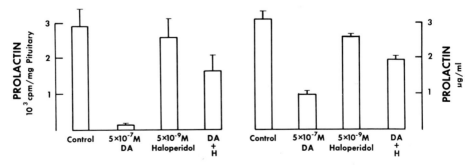

FIG. 6–5. *In vitro* blockade by haloperidol on the dopamine-mediated inhibition of prolactin secretion. *Left*: Prolactin measured by release of ³H-prolactin. *Right*: Prolactin measured by radioimmunoassay. (From MacLeod and Lehmeyer, 1974c.)

(1973). In an additional experiment, however, these authors claim that dopamine caused the release of PIH from rat hypothalami *in vitro,* and that subsequent incubation of pituitary glands in this medium together with haloperidol resulted in decreased prolactin secretion. A concentration of 10 μg haloperidol ($\sim 5 \times 10^{-5}$ M) per incubation caused a slight decrease ($\sim 20\%$) in prolactin release in their studies. We found, however, that this amount of haloperidol caused a much larger decrease ($\sim 80\%$) in prolactin secretion (*unpublished observations*). Dickerman et al. (1972) also found that 10 ng haloperidol decreased the *in vitro* secretion of prolactin. Hence the findings of Quijada et al. (1973) may be interpreted as an effect of haloperidol on the pituitary to inhibit prolactin secretion.

Effect of Pimozide on Prolactin Secretion

The neuroleptic drug pimozide is a specific dopamine receptor-blocking agent (Jansen et al., 1968; Andén et al., 1970) and a potent stimulator of prolactin secretion. Injecting the drug into rats significantly increased the circulating level of prolactin and the *in vitro* capacity of the pituitary to synthesize the labeled hormone (Fig. 6–6); it also rendered the rat pituitary gland refractory to the usual inhibitory *in vitro* action of dopamine (MacLeod and Lehmeyer, 1973a, 1974a) and thus has a biological action similar to perphenazine and haloperidol.

Pimozide also is capable of blocking the action of dopamine *in vitro* (Fig. 6–7). Thus 10^{-8} M pimozide overcame the action of 5×10^{-7} M dopamine; 10^{-9} M of the blocker was partially active in restoring prolactin release. These data once again demonstrate the effectiveness of a dopaminergic blocking agent in inhibiting the action of a hypothalamic catecholamine directly in the pituitary gland. Although Ojeda et al. (1974a) observed that an implant of pimozide in the pituitary gland produced a gradual in-

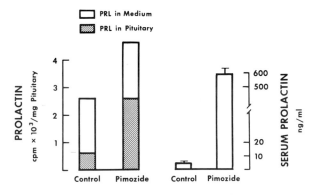

FIG. 6–6. Effect of pimozide injection on serum prolactin levels (*right*) and *in vitro* synthesis and release (*left*) of prolactin. (From MacLeod and Lehmeyer, 1974a.)

crease in serum prolactin, similar results were produced when the drug was implanted in the median eminence-arcuate region. The authors agreed with our thesis that prolactin is under dopaminergic inhibitory control, but they maintain that the pimozide also blocks median eminence-arcuate dopaminergic receptors, thus preventing the tonic stimulation of PIH release. That the dopaminergic inhibitory control of prolactin secretion seems to develop soon after birth was suggested by the observation that pimozide injection produced a rise in plasma prolactin at 3 days of age but not at birth (Ojeda and McCann, 1974).

Lawson and Gala (1975) recently studied the changes produced by neural blocking and stimulating agents on plasma prolactin levels in ovariectomized, estrogen-treated rats. Dopaminergic, α-adrenergic, and serotoninergic blocking agents were much more active than β-adrenergic blocking

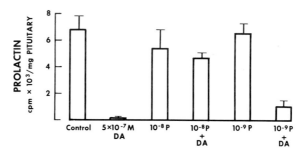

FIG. 6–7. In vitro blockade by pimozide (P) of the dopamine (DA)-mediated inhibition of prolactin release. (From MacLeod and Pace, unpublished observations.)

agents in increasing prolactin levels. Cholinergic blocking agents were without effect.

The aforementioned drugs—reserpine, perphenazine, haloperidol, and pimozide—increase serum prolactin levels following their injection, although their modes of action may vary considerably. Although reserpine increases serum prolactin concentration, the pituitary glands are still responsive to the inhibitory action that catecholamines produce during an in vitro incubation (MacLeod and Lehmeyer, 1972). Additionally, reserpine cannot block the action of catecholamines in vitro; hence it probably acts centrally and not at the pituitary level. The pituitary gland, thus removed from the inhibitory action of the catecholamines, is free to secrete increased amounts of prolactin.

The mode of action of the other drugs is very likely more complex. Each of these agents probably blocks the receptor sites of hypothalamic catecholamines, but their precise biochemical mode of action is unknown. They also have a pronounced action at the pituitary level, blocking the in vivo action of catecholamines; the mechanism of this action is under active investigation.

Based on these studies our conclusion is that hypothalamic catecholamines directly inhibit prolactin secretion. If there is an additional hypothalamic hormone involved in inhibiting this secretion, its acceptance must await positive biochemical identification.

PHARMACOLOGICAL AGENTS THAT MIMIC THE BIOLOGICAL ACTION OF DOPAMINE

Apomorphine

Since apomorphine has some of the pharmacological activities of dopamine and can stimulate dopamine receptors, its effect on prolactin secretion was studied by several groups of investigators. Although originally thought to decrease the amount of circulating prolactin by acting on the hypothalamus, it was demonstrated that this alkaloid can act directly on the pituitary. As shown in Fig. 6–8, 6.4×10^{-8} M apomorphine caused a 60% decrease in labeled prolactin secreted by the pituitary (MacLeod and Lehmeyer, 1973a). In rats given prior injections of perphenazine or whose pituitary glands were incubated with the drug the prolactin-secreting cells were completely protected from the inhibitory action of apomorphine.

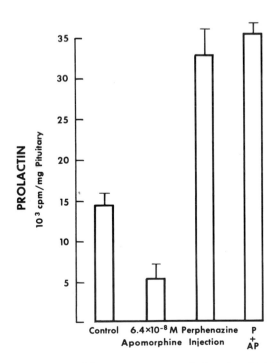

FIG. 6–8. Blockade by perphenazine (P) of the apomorphine (AP)-mediated inhibition of prolactin release. (From MacLeod and Lehmeyer, 1974c.)

Smalstig et al. (1974) observed that administration of apomorphine significantly attenuated the chlorpromazine-induced rise in serum prolactin levels. Additionally, apomorphine prevented the increase in serum prolactin in lactating rats and the rise of serum prolactin at proestrus. As little as 3.2×10^{-8} M apomorphine consistently inhibited prolactin release, and this effect was in turn reversed by concomitant incubation with the specific dopaminergic blocking agent pimozide. These *in vitro* studies confirmed our earlier work (MacLeod and Lehmeyer, 1973a) in which we demonstrated that apomorphine can act directly on the pituitary gland.

More recently Ojeda et al. (1974b) presented evidence that the introduction of apomorphine or dopamine into the third ventricle of ovariectomized, estrogen-treated rats caused a decrease in plasma prolactin. Prior subcutaneous injection of pimozide prevented the dopamine-induced decrease in prolactin levels. The authors feel, however, that the major action of the drugs is on PIH neurons in the brain and not on the pituitary itself. This concept is dependent on their belief that PIH will someday be demonstrated to be something other than a hypothalamic catecholamine.

In two clinical studies (Lal et al., 1973; Martin et al., 1974) apomorphine decreased serum prolactin in four of 12 patients studied. Chlorpromazine blocked the ability of apomorphine to affect serum prolactin levels.

Ergot Alkaloids

Perhaps the best established pharmacological agents used to inhibit prolactin secretion are the ergot alkaloids. Meites and Clemens (1972) reviewed the data demonstrating that a wide variety of ergot derivatives decrease the serum prolactin concentration. In our studies administration of 0.05 or 0.2 mg ergotamine daily for 7 days had no effect on prolactin or growth hormone (GH) synthesis or release (MacLeod and Lehmeyer, 1972, 1973b); ergocornine and ergocryptine significantly decreased prolactin but had no effect on GH release. Wuttke et al. (1971) suggested that ergocornine acts in the hypothalamus to increase PIH and through this mechanism produces a reduction in prolactin secretion; they did not exclude the possibility, however, that the ergot may act directly on the pituitary gland. Several groups have demonstrated that the latter is an important mode of action of the ergot alkaloids (Nicoll et al., 1970b; Lu et al., 1971; Lehmeyer and MacLeod, 1972; MacLeod and Lehmeyer, 1972; Pasteels et al., 1971). Thus as seen in Fig. 6–9, the addition of 3×10^{-7} M ergocryptine caused a 90% decrease in the amount of newly synthesized prolactin secreted by pituitary glands incubated *in vitro*. The ergot acts as a potent analogue to dopamine, and this probably relates to the known α-adrenergic- or dopaminergic-stimulating action of the alkaloids.

The *in vitro* and *in vivo* inhibitory effects of ergocryptine and all the ergots can be systematically blocked by injecting haloperidol, pimozide, or per-

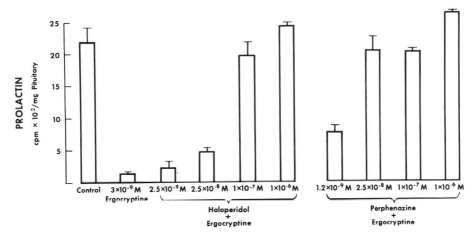

FIG. 6–9. Blockade of the ergocryptine-mediated inhibition of prolactin secretion by various doses of haloperidol and perphenazine. (From MacLeod and Lehmeyer, 1974c.)

phenazine; or by incubating the pituitary with these agents (Fig. 6–9). This is additional evidence that the pituitary gland has α-adrenergic and/or dopaminergic receptors which mediate inhibition of prolactin secretion.

A direct association between serum prolactin concentration and milk yields in the goat was observed by Hart (1973) and McMurtry and Malven (1974). They noted that injection of 2-Br-α-ergocryptine or ergocryptine lowered the amount of milk produced and decreased normal or elevated circulating prolactin concentrations.

The usefulness of the ergot derivatives in suppressing the prolactin-induced stimulation of experimental mammary tumor growth has been demonstrated by many investigators (Nagasawa and Meites, 1970; Cassell et al., 1971; Quadri and Meites, 1971; Arai et al., 1972; Yanai and Nagasawa, 1972; Sinha et al., 1974). Treatment of nonpuerperal galactorrhea with 2-Br-α-ergocryptine has been very successful. The prompt cessation of milk secretion accompanied by restoration of regular menses is probably secondary to the dramatic fall in serum prolactin levels. Hyperprolactinemia and galactorrhea tends to recur after therapy is discontinued (Lutterbeck et al., 1971; Besser et al., 1972; del Pozo et al., 1974). Although most investigators report that ergot derivatives do not affect the secretion of other hormones, Miyai et al. (1974) showed that 2-Br-α-ergocryptine caused a transient decrease in serum TSH levels in hypothyroid patients.

PROLACTIN-SECRETING PITUITARY TUMORS

A large number of experimental, transplantable pituitary tumors synthesize and secrete large quantities of prolactin and other pituitary hormones. These tumor hormones have biological and neuroendocrine effects that are similar to those of pituitary gland hormones. Thus the hypothalamus and other higher centers in rats bearing these tumors detect the excessively high serum concentration of the tumor hormones and, presumably through the feedback mechanisms, activate the release of specific inhibitor hypophysiotropic hormones. This decreases the capability of the pituitary gland to synthesize and release the appropriate hormones. Several groups have demonstrated that animals bearing these tumors have atropic pituitary glands and synthesize decreased quantities of hormones (MacLeod et al., 1966, 1968; Chen et al., 1967; MacLeod and Abad, 1968). Surgical removal of the tumors results in prompt restoration of pituitary function.

We previously speculated that a causal relationship may exist between the increased serum prolactin concentration in rats bearing pituitary tumors and the dopamine-mediated decrease in prolactin secretion by the host's

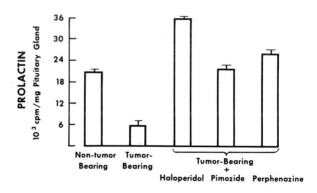

FIG. 6–10. Suppression of pituitary gland prolactin release by pituitary tumors and restoration by dopaminergic blocking agents (From MacLeod and Lehmeyer, 1974c.)

pituitary gland. Such a hypothesis is compatible with Hökfelt and Fuxe's (1972) observation that prolactin injection caused marked activation of the tuberoinfundibular dopamine neurons of rats. This activation was also observed in pregnant and lactating rats. A prompt decrease in dopamine turnover in the neurons accompanied the injection of ergocornine and 2-Br-α-ergocryptine. No such effect was noted in the norepinephrine neurons terminating in the hypothalamus.

The data presented in Fig. 6–10 show that the prolactin secreted by pituitary tumor MtTW15 caused a 65% decrease in the ability of the host's pituitary gland to secrete newly synthesized prolactin into the incubation medium (MacLeod and Lehmeyer, 1974c). Experiments were designed to block the accumulation of dopamine in the neurons of tumor-bearing rats via administration of haloperidol, pimozide, or perphenazine. The drugs caused a restoration of prolactin secretion. Therefore the serum prolactin probably increased the activity of the tuberoinfundibular dopamine neurons, with increased secretion of the catecholamine into the portal blood supply and a consequent reduction in prolactin secretion.

Voogt and Carr (1974) recently studied the effect of suckling on plasma prolactin and the synthesis rates of hypothalamic catecholamines. This stimulus brought about an increase in circulating prolactin after 4 min, but the rate of dopamine synthesis did not increase until 15 min after exposure of the mother to the pups. They conclude, in agreement with Hökfelt and Fuxe (1972), that the increased blood prolactin may trigger a short-loop negative feedback, increasing the activity of the dopaminergic neurons, which in turn decreases prolactin secretion.

ROLE OF ESTROGENS

Estrogens have long been known to cause hypertrophy of the pituitary gland and increase prolactin secretion (Ratner et al., 1963). It has also been demonstrated that ovariectomy is accompanied by a decrease in prolactin production, which is reversed by injecting estrogens or testosterone (Catt and Moffat, 1967; MacLeod et al., 1969). The increment in serum prolactin in those experiments was proportional to the amount of estradiol administered. Very large doses of estradiol caused a slight decrease from peak response, but even 500 μg estradiol produced a significant increase in pituitary and serum prolactin levels (Chen and Meites, 1970). The circulating level of prolactin was greatly increased in androgenized female rats, but further increases were not observed when large amounts of estrogens were administered (Mallampati and Johnson, 1973). However, ovariectomy in these rats or in spontaneously constant-estrous rats decreased the serum prolactin concentration (Ratner and Peake, 1974).

Prolactin release during the estrous cycle is a rhythmic, internally controlled phenomenon, with a large increase on the afternoon of proestrus (Kwa and Verhofstad, 1967; Sar and Meites, 1967; Niswender et al., 1969; Amenomori et al., 1970; Neill, 1970). Estrogens are essential for this surge of prolactin release because the injection of antiserum to estrogen on the second day of diestrus abolished the expected increase in serum prolactin (Neill et al., 1971). This inhibition could be neutralized by the concomitant injection of diethylstilbestrol. Hökfelt and Fuxe (1972) and Ahrén et al. (1971) subsequently correlated the nadir of serum prolactin levels during diestrus with increased dopamine turnover in the tuberoinfundibular neurons during diestrus and the elevated serum prolactin levels at proestrus with a decrease in hypothalamic dopamine turnover.

Other studies also show that estrogens exert specific effects on hypothalamic catecholamines. Dopamine turnover in the tuberoinfundibular neurons was decreased in ovariectomized rats and was restored by administering estrogens or testosterone (Fuxe et al., 1969). Stefano and Donoso

(1967), reported that ovariectomy decreased hypothalamic dopamine content. In contrast, the turnover of hypothalamic norepinephrine was increased following ovariectomy (Stefano and Donoso, 1967), and its rate of synthesis was increased (Anton-Tay et al., 1969). However, Bapna et al. (1971) reported a decrease in synthesis. These data support the hypothesis that estrogens stimulate prolactin secretion by altering the effective physiological concentration of dopamine that is delivered to or perceived by the pituitary gland.

PROLACTIN-RELEASING HORMONES AND TRH

To date there has been no identification of a hypothalamic hormone or factor that possesses exclusive ability to stimulate prolactin secretion. However, it is abundantly evident that TRH functions well in this regard.

Although there is no evidence that TRH increases plasma GH levels in humans or sheep (Debeljuk et al., 1973), administration of the tripeptide increases plasma somatotropin concentrations in rats (Takahara et al., 1974b). Prior treatment of sheep with triiodothyronine blunted the increase in serum prolactin and thyrotropin-stimulating hormone (TSH) concentrations produced by TRH. This correlates well with the finding that hypothyroid patients are more responsive than hyperthyroid patients to the prolactin-releasing activity of TRH (Snyder et al., 1973; Noel et al., 1974). Administration of thyroid hormones to a group of hypothyroid patients caused a significant decrease in prolactin release in response to TRH. Conversely, in patients with hyperthyroidism, the response to TRH increased following antithyroid treatment. Noel et al. (1974) showed that the smallest amounts of TRH capable of producing an increase in plasma TSH concentration also increased plasma prolactin, an observation which supports the concept that TRH has a physiological role in the control of prolactin secretion. That TRH acts directly on the pituitary gland and not through a hypothalamic factor is suggested by the finding that TRH stimulated prolactin secretion by ectopic pituitary transplants in rats with bilateral median eminence lesions (Porteus and Malven, 1974) and by pituitary tumor cells *in vitro* (Tashjian et al., 1971).

Stimulation of the *in vitro* secretion of prolactin by the normal pituitary gland is dependent on the *in vivo* hormonal environment of the host. Although Lu et al. (1972) were unable to demonstrate an *in vitro* effect of TRH on pituitary glands from male rats, a subsequent report showed that estrogenization of rats caused them to respond to 0.2 to 5.0 μg TRH (Mueller et al., 1973). Vale et al. (1973) showed that pituitary glands from euthyroid rats were minimally responsive to TRH, but prior treatment of the rats with propylthiouracil increased the *in vitro* sensitivity of prolactin release in response to TRH.

We recently conducted a study of the *in vitro* effect of TRH (Hill-Samli

TABLE 6–3. *TRH blockade of the inhibitory effects of dopamine, apomorphine, and ergocryptine on prolactin secretion*

Inhibitor	^{3}H-prolactin released into medium (cpm/mg pituitary)	Radioimmunoassayable prolactin released into medium (μg/mg pituitary)
Experiment I		
Control	8,079 ± 619	2.85 ± 0.15
TRH 25 ng/ml	8,665 ± 1,060	—
Dopamine 2 × 10^{-7} M	651 ± 87	1.33 ± 0.15
Dopamine 2 × 10^{-7} M + TRH 5 ng/ml	1,750 ± 856	1.52 ± 0.22
Dopamine 2 × 10^{-7} M + TRH 25 ng/ml	4,217 ± 808[a]	2.18 ± 0.24[a]
Experiment II		
Control	7,615 ± 838	5.85 ± 0.58
Ergocryptine 4 × 10^{-4} M	462 ± 109	2.61 ± 0.39
Ergocryptine 4 × 10^{-4} M + TRH 5 ng/ml	2,745 ± 415[a]	4.32 ± 0.21[a]
Apomorphine 5 × 10^{-8} M	2,614 ± 582	2.75 ± 0.25
Apomorphine 5 × 10^{-8} M + TRH 5 ng/ml	6,017 ± 692[a]	4.57 ± 0.40[a]

[a] Value significantly greater than value for inhibitor alone ($p < 0.02$).

and MacLeod, 1974, 1975). The data presented in Table 6–3 show that, although TRH had no effect on the secretion of prolactin, adding the tripeptide partially overcame the inhibitory action of dopamine. Additional data demonstrate that the potent dopaminergic agents ergocryptine and apomorphine inhibit prolactin secretion when added in low concentrations *in vitro,* and the concomitant incubation with TRH reversed the inhibitory action of these substances. No effect of either treatment was noted on GH secretion. Takahara et al. (1974*c*) conducted similar experiments in sheep pituitary preparations. In their study dopamine inhibited the secretion of prolactin and GH, and the presence of TRH reversed the inhibitory action of the catecholamine. All of these findings are consonant with those of Noel et al. (1973), who demonstrated that the TRH-mediated increase in human plasma prolactin was suppressed by prior administration of L-DOPA. These data suggest that dopamine and TRH have, respectively, properties of prolactin-inhibiting and prolactin-releasing hormones. This concept is also discussed by Rivier and Vale (1974).

An interesting contrary view was recently reported by Gautvik et al. (1974), who noted that suckling elevated serum prolactin levels but did not increase circulating TSH, thyroxine, or triiodothyronine. The subjects' thyroid function responded normally to exogenous TRH. They suggest that although TRH can cause prolactin secretion the action of the tripeptide alone does not explain the prolactin release that occurs with suckling. Further investigation is required before these data can be correlated with those of Grimm and Reichlin (1973), who reported that the *in vitro* release of TRH from hypothalamic fragments is stimulated by dopamine and norepinephrine, and inhibited by serotonin.

SUMMARY AND CONCLUSIONS

Prolactin secretion has been observed to decrease following the L-DOPA-induced increase in hypothalamic catecholamines. Conversely, agents which decrease brain catecholamine concentration increase prolactin secretion. These results can be explained in at least two ways: (1) L-DOPA, after decarboxylation to dopamine, may act directly on the pituitary gland to inhibit the secretion of prolactin; and (2) dopamine may act in the hypothalamus to release "PIH." There is strong evidence that the hypothalamic catecholamines dopamine and norepinephrine are potent inhibitors of the

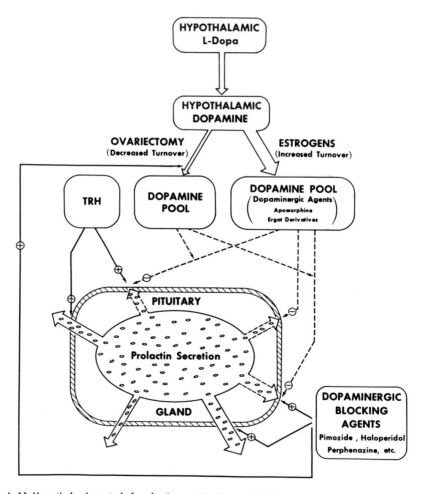

FIG. 6–11. Hypothalamic control of prolactin secretion. As noted in the text, estrogens influence the turnover of the hypothalamic dopamine pool and thereby influence prolactin secretion. Dopaminergic agents such as apomorphine and ergot derivatives mimic the effects of dopamine, and dopaminergic blocking agents are antagonistic at the pituitary and hypothalamic levels.

in vitro secretion of prolactin and that their effect is blocked by several dopaminergic blocking agents at very low concentrations (Fig. 6–11). Apomorphine and the ergot alkaloids, which are known as dopaminergic stimulators, inhibit prolactin secretion following their injection or addition to the pituitary *in vitro*. Their action is blocked *in vivo* and *in vitro* by dopaminergic blocking agents. Likewise, the action of TRH on the pituitary gland is probably direct and can partially overcome the inhibitory action of dopamine. The hypothesis that dopamine releases a "PIH" must be considered unproved until a hypothalamic hormone that inhibits prolactin secretion is isolated and identified. Conversely, the hypothesis that hypothalamic dopamine functions as a neurohormone to inhibit the secretion of prolactin directly has a strong experimental foundation.

REFERENCES

Ahrén, K., Fuxe, K., Hamberger, L., and Hökfelt, T. (1971): Turnover changes in the tubero-infundibular dopamine neurons during the ovarian cycle of the rat. *Endocrinology*, 88:1415–1424.

Amenomori, Y., and Meites, J. (1970): Effect of a hypothalamic extract on serum prolactin levels during the estrous cycle and lactation. *Proc. Soc. Exp. Biol. Med.*, 134:492–495.

Amenomori, Y., Chen, C. L., and Meites, J. (1970): Serum prolactin levels in rats during different reproductive states. *Endocrinology*, 86:506–510.

Andén, N. E., Dahlstrom, A., Fuxe, K., and Hökfelt, T. (1966): The effect of haloperidol and chlorpromazine on the amine levels of central monoamine neurons. *Acta Physiol. Scand.*, 68:419–420.

Andén, N. E., Butcher, S. G., Corrodi, H., Fuxe, K., and Ungerstedt, U. (1970): Receptor activity and turnover of dopamine and noradrenaline after neuroleptics. *Eur. J. Pharmacol.*, 11:303:314.

Anton-Tay, F., Pelham, R. W., and Wurtman, R. J. (1969): Increased turnover of ³H-norepinephrine in rat brain following castration or treatment with ovine follicle-stimulating hormone. *Endocrinology*, 84:1489–1492.

Arai, Y., Suzuki, Y., and Masuda, S. (1972): Effects of ergocornine on reserpine-induced lactogenic response of male rat mammary glands. *Endocrinol. Jap.*, 19:111–114.

Arimura, A., Dunn, J. D., and Schally, A. V. (1972): Effect of infusion of hypothalamic extracts on serum prolactin levels in rats treated with Nembutal, CNS depressants, or bearing hypothalamic lesions. *Endocrinology*, 90:378–383.

Bapna, J., Neff, N. H., and Costa, E. (1971): A method for studying norepinephrine and serotonin metabolism in small regions of rat brain: Effect of ovariectomy on amine metabolism in anterior and posterior hypothalamus. *Endocrinology*, 89:1345–1349.

Barraclough, C. A., and Sawyer, C. H. (1959): Induction of pseudopregnancy in the rat by reserpine and chlorpromazine. *Endocrinology*, 65:563–571.

Baumgarten, H. G., Björklund, A., Holstein, A. F., and Nobin, A. (1972): Organization and ultrastructural identification of the catecholamine nerve terminals in the neural lobe and pars intermedia of the rat pituitary. *Z. Zellforsch.*, 126:483–517.

Ben-David, M., Danon, A., and Sulman, F. G. (1970): Acute changes in blood and pituitary prolactin after a single injection of perphenazine. *Neuroendocrinology*, 6:336–342.

Besser, G. M., Parke, L., Edwards, C. R. W., Forsyth, I. A., and McNeilly, A. S. (1972): Galactorrhea: Successful treatment with reduction of plasma prolactin by brom-ergocryptine. *Br. Med. J.*, 3:669–672.

Birge, C. A., Jacobs, L. S., Hammer, C. T., and Daughaday, W. H. (1970): Cathecholamine inhibition of prolactin secretion by isolated rat adenohypophyses. *Endocrinology,* 86:120–130.

Bishop, W., Krulich, L., Fawcett, C. P., and McCann, S. M. (1971): The effect of median eminence (ME) lesions on plasma levels of FSH, LH and prolactin in the rat. *Proc. Soc. Exp. Biol. Med.,* 136:925–927.

Blake, C. A., Scaramuzzi, R. J., Norman, R. L., Hilliard, J., and Sawyer, C. H. (1973): Effects of hypothalamic deafferentation on circulating levels of LH, FSH, prolactin and testosterone in the male rat. *Endocrinology,* 92:1419–1425.

Bower, A., Hadley, M. E., and Hruby, V. J. (1974): Biogenic amines and control of melanophore stimulating hormone-release. *Science,* 184:70–72.

Cassell, E. E., Meites, J., and Welsch, C. W. (1971): Effects of ergocornine and ergocryptine on growth of 7,12-dimethylbenzanthracene-induced mammary tumors in rats. *Cancer Res.,* 31:1051–1053.

Catt, K., and Moffat, B. (1967): Isolation of internally labeled rat prolactin by preparative disc electrophoresis. *Endocrinology,* 80:324–328.

Chen, C. L., and Meites, J. (1970): Effects of estrogen and progesterone on serum and pituitary prolactin levels in ovariectomized rats. *Endocrinology,* 86:503–505.

Chen, C. L., Minaguchi, H., and Meites, J. (1967): Effects of transplanted pituitary tumors on host pituitary secretion. *Proc. Soc. Exp. Biol. Med.,* 126:317–325.

Chen, C. L., Amenomori, Y., Lu, K. H., Voogt, J. L., and Meites, J. (1970): Serum prolactin levels in rats with pituitary transplants or hypothalamic lesions. *Neuroendocrinology,* 6:220–227.

Coppola, J. A., Leonardi, R. G., Lippman, W., Perrine, J. W., and Ringler, I. (1965): Induction of pseudopregnancy in rats by depletors of endogenous catecholamines. *Endocrinology,* 77:485–490.

Danon, A., and Sulman, F. G. (1970): Storage of prolactin-inhibiting factor in the hypothalamus of perphenazine-treated rats. *Neuroendocrinology,* 6:295–300.

Debeljuk, A., Arimura, A., Redding, T., and Schally, A. V. (1973): Effect of TRH and triiodothyronine on prolactin release in sheep. *Proc. Soc. Exp. Biol. Med.,* 142:421–423.

del Pozo, E., Varga, L., Wyss, H., Tolis, G., Friesen, H., Wenner, R., Vetter, L., and Uettwiler, A. (1974): Clinical and hormonal response to bromocriptin (CB-154) in the galactorrhea syndromes. *J. Clin. Endocrinol. Metab.,* 39:18–26.

Dickerman, S., Clark, J., Dickerman, E., and Meites, J. (1972): Effects of haloperidol on serum and pituitary prolactin and on hypothalamic PIF in rats. *Neuroendocrinology,* 9:332–340.

Dickerman, S., Kledzik, G., Gelato, M., Chen, H. J., and Meites, J. (1974): Effects of haloperidol on serum and pituitary prolactin, LH and FSH, and hypothalamic PIF and LRF. *Neuroendocrinology,* 15:10–20.

Donoso, A. O., Bishop, W., and McCann, S. M. (1973): The effects of drugs which modify catecholamine synthesis on serum prolactin in rats with median eminence lesions. *Proc. Soc. Exp. Biol. Med.,* 143:360–363.

Donoso, A. O., Banzán, A. M., and Barcaglioni, J. C. (1974): Further evidence on the direct action of L-dopa on prolactin release. *Neuroendocrinology,* 15:236–239.

Everett, J. W. (1954): Luteotrophic function of autografts of the rat hypophysis. *Endocrinology,* 54:685–690.

Frantz, A. G., Habif, D. U., Hyman, G. A., and Suh, K. H. (1972): Remission of metastatic breast cancer after reduction of circulating prolactin in patients treated with L-dopa. *Clin. Res.,* 20:234–241.

Friesen, H., Gudya, H., Hwang, P., Tyson, J. E., and Barbeau, A. (1972): Functional evaluation of prolactin secretion: A guide to therapy. *J. Clin. Invest.,* 51:706–709.

Fuxe, K., Hökfelt, T., and Nilsson, O. (1969): Castration, sex hormones and tuberoinfundibular dopamine neurons. *Neuroendocrinology,* 5:107–120.

Gautvik, K. M., Tashjian, A. H., Jr., Kourides, I. A., Weintraub, B. D., Graeber, C. T., Maloof, F., Suzuki, K., and Zuckerman, J. E. (1974): Thyrotropin-releasing hormone is not the sole physiologic mediator of prolactin release during suckling. *N. Engl. J. Med.,* 290:1162–1165.

Grimm, Y., and Reichlin, S. (1973): Thyrotropin-releasing hormone (TRH): Neurotransmitter regulation of secretion by mouse hypothalamic tissue in vitro. *Endocrinology,* 93:626–631.

Hart, I. C. (1973): Effect of 2-bromo-α-ergocryptine on milk yield and the level of prolactin and growth hormone in the blood of the goat at milking. *J. Endocrinol.,* 57:179–180.

Hill-Samli, M., and MacLeod, R. M. (1974): Interaction of thyrotropin-releasing hormone and dopamine on the release of prolactin from the rat interior pituitary in vitro. *Endocrinology,* 95:1189–1192.

Hill-Samli, M., and MacLeod, R. M. (1975): TRH blockade of the ergocryptine and apomorphine inhibition of prolactin release in vitro. *Proc. Soc. Exp. Biol. Med.,* 149: 511–514.

Hökfelt, T. (1967): The possible ultrastructural identification of tuberoinfundibular dopamine-containing nerve endings in the median eminence of the rat. *Brain Res.,* 5:121–123.

Hökfelt, T., and Fuxe, K. (1972): Effects of prolactin and ergot alkaloids on the tubero-infundibular dopamine (DA) neurons. *Neuroendocrinology,* 9:100–122.

Horrobin, D. F. (1974): *Prolactin 1974.* Medical and Technical Publishing, London.

Hyyppä, M., and Wurtman, R. J. (1973): Biogenic amines in the pituitary gland: What is their origin and function? Pituitary indoleamines. In: *Drug Effects on Neuroendocrine Regulation,* edited by E. Zimmerman, W. H. Gispen, B. H. Marks, and D. De Wied, pp. 211–215. Elsevier, New York.

Jacobowitz, D. M. (1973): Distribution of biogenic amines in the pituitary gland. In: *Drug Effects on Neuroendocrine Regulation,* edited by E. Zimmerman, W. H. Gispen, B. H. Marks, and D. De Wied, pp. 199–209. Elsevier, New York.

Jansen, A. J., Niemegeers, C. J. E., Schellekens, K. H. L., Dresse, A., Lenaerts, F. M., Pinchard, A., Schaper, W. K. A., Van Neuten, J. M., and Verbruggen, F. J. (1968): Pimozide, a chemically novel, highly potent and orally long-acting neuroleptic drug. *Arzneim. Forsch.,* 18:261–279.

Kamberi, I. A., Mical, R. S., and Porter, J. C. (1971a): Pituitary portal vessel infusion of hypothalamic extract and release of LH, FSH, and prolactin. *Endocrinology,* 88:1294–1299.

Kamberi, I. A., Mical, R. S., and Porter, J. C. (1971b): Effect of anterior pituitary perfusion and intraventricular injection of catecholamines on prolactin release. *Endocrinology,* 88:1012–1020.

Kanematsu, S., Hilliard, J., and Sawyer, C. H. (1963): Effect of reserpine on pituitary prolactin content and its hypothalamic site of action in the rabbit. *Acta Endocrinol. (Kbh.),* 44:467–474.

Kleinberg, D. L., and Frantz, A. G. (1971): Human prolactin: Measurement in plasma by in vitro bioassay. *J. Clin. Invest.,* 50:1557–1568.

Koch, Y., Lu, K. H., and Meites, J. (1970): Biphasic effects of catecholamines on pituitary prolactin release in vitro. *Endocrinology,* 87:673–675.

Kuhn, E., Krulich, L., Fawcett, C. P., and McCann, S. M. (1974): The ability of hypothalamic extracts to lower blood prolactin levels in lactating rats. *Proc. Soc. Exp. Biol. Med.,* 146:104–108.

Kwa, H. G., and Verhofstad, F. (1967): Radioimmunoassay of rat prolactin. *Biochim. Biophys. Acta,* 133:186–188.

Lal, S., de la Vega, C. E., Sourkes, T. L., and Friesen, H. G. (1973): Effect of apomorphine on growth hormone, prolactin, luteinizing hormone and follicle-stimulating hormone levels in human serum. *J. Clin. Endocrinol. Metab.,* 37:719–724.

Lawson, D. M., and Gala, R. R. (1975): The influence of adrenergic, dopaminergic, cholinergic, and serotoninergic drugs on plasma prolactin levels in ovariectomized, estrogen-treated rats. *Endocrinology,* 90:313–318.

Lehmeyer, J. E., and MacLeod, R. M. (1972): Suppression of pituitary tumor function by alkaloids. *Proc. Am. Assoc. Cancer Res.,* 13:90 (abstract).

Lu, K. H., and Meites, J. (1972): Effects of L-dopa on serum prolactin and PIF in intact and hypophysectomized, pituitary-grafted rats. *Endocrinology,* 91:868–872.

Lu, K. H., Amenomori, Y., Chen, C. L., and Meites, J. (1970): Effects of central acting drugs on serum and pituitary prolactin levels in rats. *Endocrinology,* 87:667–670.

Lu, K. H., Koch, Y., and Meites, J. (1971): Direct inhibition by ergocornine of pituitary prolactin release. *Endocrinology*, 89:229–233.

Lu, K. H., Shaar, C. J., Kortright, K. H., and Meites, J. (1972): Effects of synthetic TRH on in vitro and in vivo prolactin release in the rat. *Endocrinology*, 91:1540–1545.

Lutterbeck, P. M., Pryor, J. S., Varga, L., and Wenner, R. (1971): Treatment of non-puerperal galactorrhea with an ergot alkaloid. *Br. Med. J.*, 3:228–229.

MacLeod, R. M. (1969): Influence of norepinephrine and catecholamine-depleting agents on the synthesis and release of prolactin and growth hormone. *Endocrinology*, 85:916–923.

MacLeod, R. M., and Abad, A. (1968): On the control of prolactin and growth hormone synthesis in rat pituitary glands. *Endocrinology*, 83:799–806.

MacLeod, R. M., and Lehmeyer, J. E. (1972): Regulation of the synthesis and release of prolactin. In: *Lactogenic Hormones,* edited by G. E. W. Wolstenholme and J. Knight, pp. 53–82. Churchill Livingstone, London.

MacLeod, R. M., and Lehmeyer, J. E. (1973a): Pituitary gland alpha-adrenergic receptors and their function in prolactin secretion. *Endocrinology*, 92:A-50 (abstract).

MacLeod, R. M., and Lehmeyer, J. E. (1973b): Suppression of pituitary tumor growth and function by ergot alkaloids. *Cancer Res.*, 33:849–855.

MacLeod, R. M., and Lehmeyer, J. E. (1974a): Studies on the mechanism of the dopamine-mediated inhibition of prolactin secretion. *Endocrinology*, 94:1077–1085.

MacLeod, R. M., and Lehmeyer, J. E. (1974b): Reciprocal relationship between the in vitro synthesis and secretion of prolactin and growth hormone. *Proc. Soc. Exp. Biol. Med.*, 145:1128–1131.

MacLeod, R. M., and Lehmeyer, J. E. (1974c): Restoration of prolactin synthesis and release by administration of monoaminergic blocking agents to pituitary tumor-bearing rats. *Cancer Res.*, 34:345–350.

MacLeod, R. M., Smith, M. C., and DeWitt, G. W. (1966): Hormonal properties of transplanted tumors and their relation to the pituitary gland. *Endocrinology*, 79:1149–1156.

MacLeod, R. M., DeWitt, G. W., and Smith, M. C. (1968): Suppression of pituitary gland hormone content by pituitary tumor hormones. *Endocrinology*, 82:889–894.

MacLeod, R. M., Abad, A., and Eidson, L. L. (1969): In vivo effect of sex hormones on the in vitro synthesis of prolactin and growth hormone in normal and pituitary tumor-bearing rats. *Endocrinology*, 84:1475–1483.

MacLeod, R. M., Fontham, E. H., and Lehmeyer, J. E. (1970): Prolactin and growth hormone production as influenced by catecholamines and agents that affect brain catecholamines. *Neuroendocrinology*, 6:283–294.

Malarkey, W. B., Jacobs, L. S., and Daughaday, W. H. (1971): Levodopa suppression of prolactin in nonpuerperal galactorrhea. *N. Engl. J. Med.*, 285:1160–1163.

Mallampati, R. S., and Johnson, D. C. (1973): Serum and pituitary prolactin, LH, and FSH in androgenized female and normal rats treated with various doses of estradiol benzoate. *Neuroendocrinology*, 11:46–56.

Martin, J. B., Lal, S., Tolis, G., and Friesen, H. G. (1974): Inhibition by apomorphine of prolactin secretion in patients with elevated serum prolactin. *J. Clin. Endocrinol. Metab.*, 39:180–182.

McMurtry, J. P., and Malven, P. V. (1974): Experimental alterations of prolactin levels in goat milk and blood plasma. *Endocrinology*, 95:559–564.

Meites, J., and Clemens, J. (1972): Hypothalamic control of prolactin secretion. *Vitam. Horm.*, 30:165–221.

Meites, J., Lu, K. H., Wuttke, W., Welsch, C. W., Nagasawa, H., and Quadri, S. K. (1972): Recent studies on functions and control of prolactin secretion in rats. *Recent Prog. Horm. Res.*, 28:471–526.

Miyai, K., Onishi, T., Hosokawa, M., Ishibashi, K., and Kumahara, Y. (1974): In-hibition of thyrotropin and prolactin secretions in primary hypothyroidism by 2-Br-α-ergocryptine. *J. Clin. Endocrinol. Metab.*, 39:391–394.

Mueller, G. P., Chen, H. J., and Meites, J. (1973): In vivo stimulation of prolactin release in the rat by synthetic TRH. *Proc. Soc. Exp. Biol. Med.*, 144:613–615.

Nagasawa, H., and Meites, J. (1970): Suppression by ergocornine and iproniazid of carcinogen-induced mammary tumors in rats; effects on serum and pituitary prolactin levels. *Proc. Soc. Exp. Biol. Med.,* 135:469–472.

Neill, J. D. (1970): Effect of "stress" on serum prolactin and luteinizing hormone levels during the estrous cycle of the rat. *Endocrinology,* 87:1192–1197.

Neill, J. D., Freeman, M. E., and Tillson, S. A. (1971): Control of the proestrus surge of prolactin and LH secretion by estrogens in the rat. *Endocrinology,* 89:1448–1453.

Niall, H. D., Hogen, M. L., Tregear, G. W., Segre, G. V., Hwang, P., and Friesen, H. (1973): The chemistry of growth hormone and the lactogenic hormones. *Recent Prog. Horm. Res.,* 29:387–416.

Nicoll, C. S., Fiorindo, R. P., McKennee, C. T., and Parsons, J. A. (1970a): Assay of hypothalamic factors which regulate prolactin secretion. In: *Hypophysiotropic Hormones of the Hypothalamus: Assay and Chemistry,* edited by J. Meites, pp. 115–150. Williams & Wilkins, Baltimore.

Nicoll, C. S., Yaron, Z., Nutt, N., and Daniels, E. (1970b): Effects of ergotamine tartrate on prolactin and growth hormone secretion by rat adenohypophysis in vitro. *Biol. Reprod.,* 5:59–66.

Niswender, G. D., Chen, C. L., Midgley, A. R., Jr., Meites, J., and Ellis, S. (1969): Radioimmunoassay for rat prolactin. *Proc. Soc. Exp. Biol. Med.,* 130:793–797.

Noel, G. L., Suh, H. K., and Frantz, A. G. (1973): L-Dopa suppression of TRH-stimulated prolactin release in man. *J. Clin. Endocrinol. Metab.,* 36:1255–1258.

Noel, G. L., Dimond, R. C., Wartofsky, L., Earll, J. M., and Frantz, A. G. (1974): Studies of prolactin and TSH secretion by continuous infusion of small amounts of thyrotropin-releasing hormone (TRH). *J. Clin. Endocrinol. Metab.,* 39:6–17.

Ojeda, S. R., and McCann, S. M. (1974): Development of dopaminergic and estrogenic control of prolactin release in the female rat. *Endocrinology,* 95:1499–1505.

Ojeda, S. R., Harms, P. G., and McCann, S. M. (1974a): Effect of blockade of dopaminergic receptors on prolactin and LH release: Median eminence and pituitary sites of action. *Endocrinology,* 94:1650–1657.

Ojeda, S. R., Harms, P. G., and McCann, S. M. (1974b): Possible role of cyclic AMP and prostaglandin E₁ in the dopaminergic control of prolactin release. *Endocrinology,* 95:1694–1703.

Pasteels, J. L. (1961): Sécrétion de prolactine par l'hypophyse en culture de tissus. *C. R. Acad. Sci. [D] (Paris),* 253:2140.

Pasteels, J. L., and Robyn, C., editors (1973): *Human Prolactin.* Excerpta Medica, Amsterdam.

Pasteels, J. L., Danguy, A., Frerotte, M., and Ectors, F. (1971): Inhibition de la sécrétion de prolactine par l'ergocornine et la 2-Br-α-ergocryptine: Action direct sur l'hypophyse en culture. *Ann. Endocrinol. (Paris),* 32:188–192.

Porteus, S. F., and Malven, P. V. (1974): Stimulation of prolactin release in vivo by thyrotropin-releasing hormone (TRH) through direct action on the ectopic rat pituitary. *Endocrinology,* 94:1699–1703.

Quadri, S. K., and Meites, J. (1971): Regression of spontaneous mammary tumors in rats by ergot drugs. *Proc. Soc. Exp. Biol. Med.,* 138:999–1001.

Quijada, M., Illner, P., Krulich, L., and McCann, S. M. (1973): The effect of catecholamines on hormone release from anterior pituitaries and ventral hypothalami incubated in vitro. *Neuroendocrinology,* 13:151–163.

Ratner, A., and Peake, G. T. (1974): Maintenance of hyperprolactinemia by gonadal steroids in androgen-sterilized and spontaneously constant-estrus rats. *Proc. Soc. Exp. Biol. Med.,* 146:680–683.

Ratner, A., Talwalker, P. K., and Meites, J. (1963): Effect of estrogen administration in vivo on prolactin release by rat pituitary in vitro. *Proc. Soc. Exp. Biol. Med.,* 112:12–15.

Ratner, A., Talwalker, P. K., and Meites, J. (1965): Effect of reserpine on prolactin-inhibiting activity of rat hypothalamus. *Endocrinology,* 77:315–319.

Rivier, C., and Vale, W. (1974): In vivo stimulation of prolactin secretion in the rat by thyrotropin releasing factor, related peptides, and hypothalamic extracts. *Endocrinology,* 95:978–983.

Sar, M., and Meites, J. (1967): Changes in pituitary prolactin release and hypothalamic PIF content during the estrous cycle of rats. *Proc. Soc. Exp. Biol. Med.*, 125:1018–1021.

Shaar, C. J., and Clemens, J. A. (1974): The role of catecholamines in the release of anterior pituitary prolactin in vitro. *Endocrinology*, 95:1202–1212.

Shaar, C. J., Smalstig, E. B., and Clemens, J. A. (1973): The effect of catecholamines, apomorphine and monoamine oxidase on rat anterior pituitary prolactin release in vitro. *Pharmacologist*, 15:256 (abstract).

Sinha, Y. N., Selby, F. W., and VanderLaan, W. P. (1974): Effects of ergot drugs on prolactin and growth hormone secretion, and on mammary nucleic acid content in C3H/Bi mice. *J. Natl. Cancer Inst.*, 52:189–191.

Smalstig, E. B., Sawyer, B. D., and Clemens, J. A. (1974): Inhibition of rat prolactin release by apomorphine in vivo and in vitro. *Endocrinology*, 95:123–129.

Snyder, P. J., Jacobs, L. S., Utiger, R. D., and Daughaday, W. H. (1973): Thyroid hormone inhibition of prolactin response to thyrotropin-releasing hormone. *J. Clin. Invest.*, 52:2324–2329.

Stefano, F. J., and Donoso, A. O. (1967): Norepinephrine levels in the rat hypothalamus during the estrous cycle. *Endocrinology*, 81:1405–1406.

Takahara, J., Arimura, A., and Schally, A. V. (1974a): Suppression of prolactin release by a purified porcine PIF preparation and catecholamines infused into a rat hypophysial portal vessel. *Endocrinology*, 95:462–465.

Takahara, J., Arimura, A., and Schally, A. V. (1974b): Stimulation of prolactin and growth hormone release by TRH infused into a hypophysial portal vessel. *Proc. Soc. Exp. Biol. Med.*, 146:831–835.

Takahara, J., Arimura, A., and Schally, A. V. (1974c): Effect of catecholamines on the TRH-stimulated release of prolactin and growth hormone from sheep pituitaries in vitro. *Endocrinology*, 95:1490–1494.

Talwalker, P. K., Ratner, A., and Meites, J. (1963): In vitro inhibition of pituitary prolactin synthesis and release by hypothalamic extracts. *Am. J. Physiol.*, 205:213–218.

Tashjian, A. H., Jr., Barowsky, N. J., and Jensen, D. K. (1971): Thyrotropin-releasing hormone: Direct evidence for stimulation of prolactin production by pituitary cells in culture. *Biochem. Biophys. Res. Commun.*, 43:516–523.

Turkington, R. W. (1972): Inhibition of prolactin secretion and successful therapy of the Forbes-Albright syndrome with L-dopa. *J. Clin. Endocrinol. Metab.*, 34:306–311.

Vale, W., Blackwell, R., Grant, G., and Guillemin, R. (1973): TRF and thyroid hormones on prolactin secretion by rat anterior pituitary cells in vitro. *Endocrinology*, 93:26–33.

Valverde-R, C., Chieffo, V., and Reichlin, S. (1972): Prolactin-releasing factor in porcine and rat hypothalamic tissue. *Endocrinology*, 91:982–993.

Van Maanen, J. H., and Smelik, P. G. (1968): Induction of pseudopregnancy in rats following local depletion of monoamines in the median eminence of the hypothalamus. *Neuroendocrinology*, 3:177–186.

Voogt, J. L., and Carr, L. A. (1974): Plasma prolactin levels and hypothalamic catecholamine synthesis during suckling. *Neuroendocrinology*, 16:108–118.

Watson, J. T., Krulich, L., and McCann, S. M. (1971): Effect of crude rat hypothalamic extract on serum gonadotropin and prolactin levels in normal and orchidectomized male rats. *Endocrinology*, 89:1412–1418.

Wolstenholme, G. E. W., and Knight, J., editors (1972): *Lactogenic Hormones.* Churchill Livingstone, London.

Wuttke, W., Cassell, E., and Meites, J. (1971): Effects of ergocornine on serum prolactin and LH, and on hypothalamic content of PIF and LRF. *Endocrinology*, 88:737–741.

Yanai, R., and Nagasawa, H. (1972): Inhibition of mammary tumorigenesis by ergot alkaloids and promotion of mammary tumorigenesis by pituitary isografts in adreno-ovariectomized mice. *J. Natl. Cancer Inst.*, 48:715–719.

Frontiers in Neuroendocrinology, Vol. 4,
edited by L. Martini and W. F. Ganong.
Raven Press, New York © 1976.

Chapter 7

Secretion of Corticotropin-Releasing Hormone In Vitro

Mortyn T. Jones, Edward Hillhouse, and Janet Burden

Sherrington School of Physiology, St. Thomas's Hospital Medical School, London, SE1, England

The secretion of corticotropin-releasing hormone (CRH) is a complex phenomenon that involves the interaction of a large number of control factors, including stress, circadian rhythm, and feedback mechanisms. Thus the activity of the CRH neuron is dependent on both excitatory and inhibitory inputs integrated at the hypothalamic level. The role of neurotransmitters and corticosteroids in CRH regulation *in vivo* has been investigated by a number of workers (Kendall, 1971; Yates et al., 1971; Krieger, 1973; Van Loon, 1973), but it is difficult to determine the exact site of action of these substances. Halàsz (1969) showed that the isolated hypothalamus exhibits a high degree of functional ability *in vivo,* and this preparation has been widely used to study hypothalamic control of anterior pituitary function. The rat hypothalamus is small and remains viable over at least a 2-hr incubation. We have therefore used it initially to investigate factors controlling CRH secretion (Bradbury et al., 1973). The functional integrity of the hypothalamus *in vitro* has been demonstrated by its ability to synthesize and secrete CRH (Hillhouse et al., 1975), luteinizing hormone-releasing hormone (LRH), thyrotropin-releasing hormone (TRH; S. Jeffcoate, D. Holland, E. Hillhouse, J. Burden, and M. Jones, *unpublished observations*), and the neurohypophyseal hormones (Bridges et al., 1975).

HYPOTHALAMUS IN VITRO

Advantages to using the hypothalamus in *in vitro* CRH experiments include:

1. The preparation enables CRH secretion to be measured directly.

2. It enables a variety of hormones and drugs to be tested for an effect at the hypothalamic level. This can be accomplished either by pretreatment and removal of the tissue or by addition of the substance *in vitro.*

3. No anesthetic is required.

4. The environment is constant.

5. Since the preparation is used only for a maximum of 2 hr after removal from the animal, it is unlikely that dedifferentiation of neurons occurs, as

seems to happen in the cultured hypothalamus *in vitro* (Sachs et al., 1973).
Disadvantages to its use include the following:

1. One of the greatest problems with *in vitro* preparations of cerebral tissues is that they display an abnormal electrolyte balance characterized by the retention of sodium and chloride ions and the loss of potassium ions (Keesey et al., 1965). In addition, the tissue invariably accumulates fluid (Hökfelt, 1968) and both extra- and intracellular edema become apparent. The hypothalamus *in vitro* does not differ from other preparations of nervous tissue in this respect (Bradbury et al., 1973) and thus is in an abnormal state, which might lead to the malfunction of various neuronal networks.

2. Once the hypothalamus has been isolated from the rest of the brain, it is devoid of all its neuronal and feedback inputs. Thus in its response to a neurotransmitter *in vitro* the preparation might differ from the tissue *in vivo*.

3. It was suggested by Oota et al (1974) and Hökfelt (1973) that one means of neuroendocrine control could be by anatomical diffusion barriers. *In vitro,* these would probably not be present.

4. Enzymes released from hypothalamic tissue *in vitro* can cause degradation of some of the hypothalamic hormones, e.g., TRH (S. Jeffcoate, *unpublished observations*).

METHODS

Preparation of Hypothalamic Tissue

Male rats weighing 100 to 175 g are housed in an air-conditioned room with a controlled light cycle (07:00 to 21:00 hr; 7 A.M. to 9 P.M.). Rat chow and water, or in the case of adrenalectomized rats 0.9% saline, are available *ad libitum*. Experiments are performed between 07:00 and 10:00 hr (7 A.M. and 10 A.M.) to minimize variation in the CRH content of the tissue (Hiroshige, 1973). The animals are removed from their cages with a minimum of stress and decapitated. The skull is removed, the frontal lobes lifted, the optic nerves cut, and the whole brain deflected backward. The pituitary stalk severs at the level of the diaphragma sellae. The brain is placed on a Petri dish and the hypothalamus dissected out using a pair of iris scissors. The hypothalamus is lifted by gripping the cut ends of the optic nerves with a pair of fine forceps. The tissue to be removed is bordered rostrally by the optic chiasm, laterally by the hypothalamic fissures, and caudally by the mamillary bodies. The dorsal extent of the cut is approximately 2 mm. Once the hypothalamus has been dissected, it is transferred to an incubation flask. The whole procedure from time of sacrifice to commencement of incubation takes less than 1 min. Hypothalami are incubated singly for studies on the effect of electrical stimulation and in groups of three for all other experiments. The Teflon incubation flasks are held in a Dubnoff metabolic shaker which carries the distributors for both electrical stimuli and the gas mixture. In some experiments the median eminence was removed and incubated alone either with or without the presence of putative neurotransmitters.

The composition of the incubating medium is similar to that of cerebrospinal fluid (CSF) except that the K^+ level is raised to twice the normal value in an attempt to maintain the intracellular K^+ concentration. The chemical composition is as follows: NaCl 126 mM, KCl 6 mM, Na_2HPO_4 1 mM, $MgSO_4 \cdot 7H_2O$ 0.877 mM, $NaHCO_3$ 22mM, $CaCl_2$ 1.45 mM, glucose 200mg%. The solution is made with deionized water and gassed with 95% O_2/5% CO_2; the pH is 7.4, the osmolarity 298 mmole/liter, and the temperature 36.6° C.

Histological Examination of the Hypothalamus

To determine the consistency of block size, 50 hypothalami from an actual experiment were subjected to histological sectioning (Fig. 7–1). Each block consisted of all the major hypothalamic nuclei, the proximal pituitary stalk, and the mamillary bodies. A few sections also included a small rim of thalamic tissue. No pyknotic nuclei were seen. Recently in collaborative experiments with W. Wittkowski, we demonstrated good preservation of the fine structure of the median eminence of the incubated hypothalamus (Fig. 7–2).

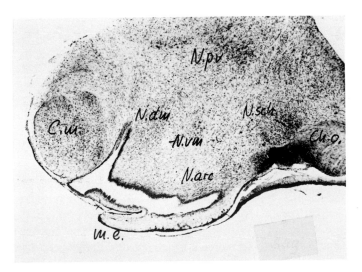

FIG. 7–1. Incubated hypothalamus. C.m., mamillary body. Ch.O, optic chiasm. N.pv, nucleus paraventricularis. N.dm, nucleus dorsomedialis. N.vm, nucleus ventromedialis. N.sch, nucleus suprachiasmaticus. N.arc, arcuate nucleus. m.e., median eminence. Bouin-fixed sagittal paraffin section stained with chromalume hematoxylin phloxine. ×25.

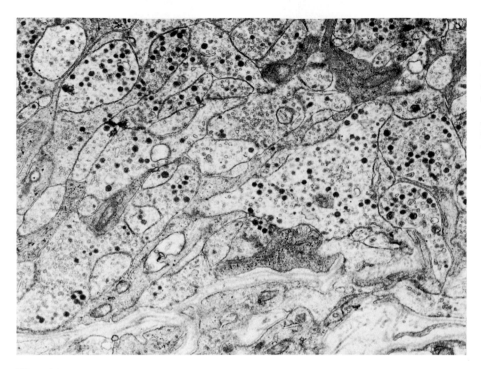

FIG. 7–2. Electron micrograph of the median eminence from a hypothalamus incubated *in vitro* for 40 min (30 min preincubation, 10 min incubation). The tissue was fixed according to the method of Peters (1970). The picture shows part of the palisade layer limited by the basement membrane of the perivascular space with numerous nerve endings with dense-core vesicles and some glial processes. × 16,000. (From W. Wittkowski, *unpublished observations.*)

Viability Studies

The oxygen consumption of the hypothalamus *in vitro* is linear over a 3-hr period, and the amount of oxygen consumed by the tissue varies from 68.8 to 120 μmoles/g/hr (Bradbury et al., 1973). These results on the oxygen consumption are comparable to those reported by McIlwain (1956) for mammalian brain slices and compare favorably with data for oxygen consumption *in vivo* based on arteriovenous oxygen differences in the monkey (McIlwain, 1956). Observations on the electrolyte balance of the tissue have shown that the hypothalamus *in vitro* behaves in a manner similar to slices of cerebral cortex (Keesey et al., 1965; Bradbury et al., 1973). Thus the tissue gains sodium, chloride, and fluid, and loses potassium. Much of this redistribution of the electrolytes takes place within the first few minutes of incubation. This may represent mechanical damage to cells on the cut surfaces leading to potassium loss (Pappius and Elliot, 1956). Another possibility is an exchange of tissue potassium for sodium and a net uptake of fluid (Bachelard et al., 1962).

Rat brain slices increase in weight during incubation, and the rat hypothalamus does not differ from other brain slices in this respect (Bradbury et al., 1973). Thus the swelling and apparent extracellular space increase fairly steadily. At 1 hr the swelling is 9.6% and the ^{51}Cr-ethylenediaminetetraacetic acid (EDTA) space 25.1% of the wet weight. This degree of swelling is considerably lower than that obtained by some investigators with brain slices (Bachelard et al., 1962) and compares favorably with that obtained by Keesey et al. (1965) who incubated slices of guinea pig cerebral cortex and obtained 13.5% swelling. Pappius et al. (1962) suggested that the degree of trauma is responsible for the swelling of brain slices, and that the water is taken up mainly by the extracellular space. The hypothalamus has an undamaged ventral surface, which may explain the low degree of swelling. Electronmicroscopic studies on cerebral slices *in vitro* revealed mainly astroglial swelling (Thorack et al., 1965; Hökfelt, 1968), which may account for most of the ionic changes observed.

Since excitation of neural tissue is brought about by changes in the permeability to sodium and potassium ions, some idea as to the function of the tissue *in vitro* can be obtained from the response of these ions during electrical stimulation. When the hypothalamus is stimulated electrically *in vitro* for a period of 10 min, the tissue gains sodium and loses potassium ions, but the normal electrolyte balance is restored following a 10-min recovery period. These results agree with those reported by Keesey et al. (1965) in their experiments on slices of guinea pig cerebral cortex *in vitro*.

The results presented in this section suggest that some of the features of both resting and stimulated neural tissue are well maintained by the rat hypothalamus *in vitro*. Thus the tissue used in these experiments, although by no means normal, does show considerable metabolic activity and is able to maintain a reasonable electrolyte balance. The speed with which the tissue is removed appears to be important, as Lowry et al (1964) showed that the levels of adenosine triphosphate (ATP) and creatinine phosphate fall to almost zero by 2 min.

Assay of CRH

The assay used for most of the experiments was *in vivo-in vitro* assay using 48-hr basal hypothalamus-lesioned animals (Bradbury et al., 1973; Jones et al., 1975). Recently we measured plasma ACTH in basal hypothalamus-lesioned animals using the cytochemical assay for ACTH described by Daly et al. (1974) as well as primed hemisected pituitary *in vitro* (Buckingham et al., 1975). Figure 7–3 shows the log dose-response relationships of different volumes of CRH obtained from hypothalami stimulated with serotonin (5-hydroxytryptamine; 5-HT). In many of the experiments the samples were also assayed for vasopressin (Bisset et al., 1967a,b). These

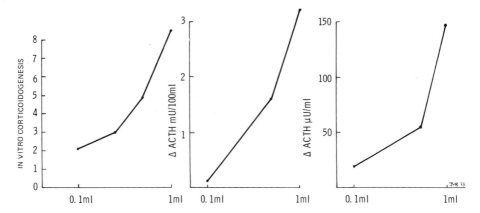

FIG. 7–3. Effect of diluting CRH from the 5-HT-stimulated hypothalamus *in vitro* on various CRH assays. The units of corticoidogenesis are micrograms per 100 mg/hr. A: *In vitro* corticoidogenesis of 48-hr ME-lesioned rat. B: Plasma ACTH (cytochemical assay) of the 48-hr ME-lesioned rat. C: ACTH (cytochemical assay) from hemisected primed pituitaries *in vitro*. (From Gillham et al., 1975a,b.)

experiments enabled us to determine the specificity of the *in vitro* response of the hypothalamus to various neurotransmitters. Thus 5-HT released CRH but had no effect on the release of neurohypophyseal hormones. Dopamine, on the other hand, caused the release of vasopressin and oxytocin but had no effect on CRH release (Bridges et al., 1975).

FUNCTIONAL ABILITY OF THE RAT HYPOTHALAMUS IN VITRO

Neurotransmitter Regulation of CRH Secretion In Vitro

Acetylcholine

Acetylcholine has been implicated in the central control of CRH secretion by a number of investigators (Hedge and Smelik, 1968; Steiner et al., 1969; Krieger and Krieger, 1970; Marks et al., 1970; Hedge and De Wied, 1971). We investigated the effect of acetylcholine on the *in vitro* secretion of CRH from both the isolated hypothalamus (Burden et al., 1974a; Hillhouse et al., 1974a, 1975) and the median eminence (Bradbury et al., 1973). Acetylcholine in doses of 1 to 5 pg/ml causes a dose-dependent release of CRH from the hypothalamus *in vitro* (Fig. 7–4) but is ineffective when tested on the median eminence *in vitro* even in doses of up to 10 ng/ml. Estimations of the amount of acetylcholine present in the hypothalamus of the rat range from 2.9 μg/g (Krieger, 1973) to 7 μg/g (Kobayashi and Matsui, 1969). It can be calculated that the hypothalamic blocks used in these experiments contain approximately 150 ng acetylcholine, so the acetylcholine concentrations required to effect CRH secretion are well within the physiological range. The amount of acetylcholine present in the median

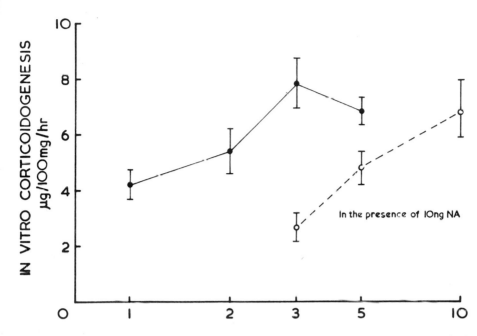

FIG. 7–4. Log dose-response curve for acetylcholine (left curve), and the effect of norepinephrine (NA) on the response. Acetylcholine concentrations in picograms per milliliter of medium are shown on the horizontal axis. (From Hillhouse et al., 1975.)

eminence of the rat is reported to be 0.8 μg/g (Clementi et al., 1971). Assuming that the weight of each incubated median eminence is 5 mg, each piece of tissue contains approximately 4 ng acetylcholine. The amount of acetylcholine used in the experiments on the median eminence—and found to be ineffective—is therefore greater than the actual amount present in the tissue. These experiments suggest that acetylcholine stimulates CRH secretion by acting at the dendritic or somal level of the CRH neuron.

A recent report showed that the release of CRH from isolated sheep synaptosomes can be caused by direct application of acetylcholine in concentrations of nanograms per milliliter (Edwardson and Bennett, 1974). This suggests that, in sheep at least, there are cholinergic excitatory synapses with neurosecretory neurons in the median eminence. Other investigations have shown that activation of the pituitary-adrenal axis follows implantation of carbachol in the median eminence of cats (Krieger and Krieger, 1970). However, in the same experiments the implantation of norepinephrine, 5-HT, and γ-aminobutyric acid (GABA) also caused an increase in corticosteroid secretion; these effects may have been due to high local concentrations of these substances causing nonspecific release of CRH.

We have now extended our observations on the site of action of acetylcholine and demonstrated that it has no effect on CRH secretion from blocks containing the ventromedial and dorsomedial nuclei, the periventricular nucleus, the arcuate nucleus, and the median eminence (R. Bock, M. Jones, and E. Hillhouse, *unpublished observations*). This suggests that the CRH cell bodies lie outside these areas.

Experiments on the pharmacology of the acetylcholine-induced release of CRH *in vitro* reveal that the effect is mediated via a mixed receptor system which is predominantly nicotinic (Burden et al., 1974a; Hillhouse et al., 1975). The pure muscarinic agent bethanacol, in doses of 3 to 100 ng, does not significantly alter the release of CRH above basal levels. Hexamethonium antagonizes the acetylcholine-stimulated release *in vitro,* but atropine only partially antagonizes the effect (Fig. 7–5). Atropine has been shown by several investigators (Hedge and Smelik, 1968; Krieger et al., 1968; Hedge

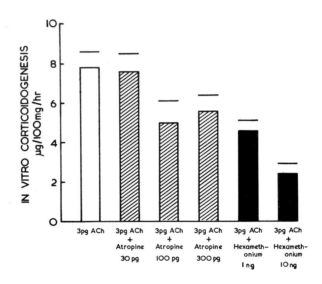

FIG. 7–5. Response to acetylcholine in the presence of atropine and hexamethonium. (From Hillhouse et al., 1975.)

and De Weid, 1971) to modify ACTH secretion, but atropine in high concentrations is known to have a local anesthetic effect. The systemic or intraventricular administration of atropine to dogs does not alter ACTH release (Ganong, 1972, 1973). Our results indicate that acetylcholine acts directly at the hypothalamic level to release CRH via a mixed receptor system that is predominantly nicotinic.

5-Hydroxytryptamine

5-Hydroxytryptamine (5-HT) has been implicated in the central control of ACTH secretion for a long time, but there has been uncertainty whether its role is excitatory or inhibitory (Naumenko, 1967; Telegdy and Vermes, 1973). In view of these divergent reports we decided to investigate the effect of 5-HT since there is good evidence that it acts as a neurotransmitter in the hypothalamus (Hökfelt, 1970; Moss et al., 1972; Kuhar and Agajanian, 1973).

In our experiments the addition of 5-HT to the incubation medium caused an increase in CRH secretion (Burden et al., 1974b; Jones et al., 1975). The results are illustrated in Fig. 7–6 and show a dose-dependent release of CRH over a range of 100 pg/ml to 10 ng/ml. The amounts of 5-HT present in the hypothalamus of the rat ranges from 1.28 to 2.31 μg/g

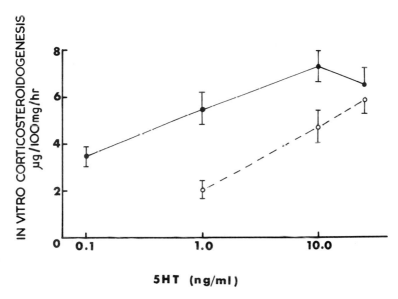

FIG. 7–6. Log dose-response curve to 5-HT (*solid curve*) and the effect of 10 ng norepinephrine on the response (*broken curve*).

(Stoner and Elson, 1971; Vermes et al., 1973) giving a total tissue content of 40 to 60 ng. Thus the amounts of 5-HT required to effect the secretion of CRH are well within the physiological range, especially if one takes into account the presence of diffusion barriers and reuptake mechanisms. The effect of 5-HT on CRH secretion *in vitro* appears to be mediated by specific serotonergic receptors because methysergide antagonizes the action of 5-HT *in vitro* (Jones et al., 1975).

The implantation of 5-HT into various regions of the CNS results in activation of the pituitary-adrenal system in both the cat (Krieger and Krieger, 1970) and the guinea pig (Naumenko, 1967). In the rat, however, 5-HT implantation into various hypothalamic areas resulted in inhibition of the ether stress-induced response (Telegdy and Vermes, 1973). Administration of 5-HT into the lateral ventricle has been shown to block the ether and surgical stress-induced response in both the dog (Van Loon,

1973) and the rat (Vermes et al., 1973). In experiments on conscious rats with chronically implanted intraventricular cannulas, the administration of 5-HT into the lateral ventricle activates the adrenocortical system; the effect is not affected by prior reserpinization but is abolished by Nembutal anesthesia (Abe and Hiroshige, 1974). The experiments of Van Loon (1973) and Vermes et al. (1972) were performed on anesthetized animals, which may account for the discrepancy in the results obtained. Other investigators have shown that the administration of 5-HT into the ventricular system of rats neither stimulates nor inhibits ACTH secretion consistently in normal or reserpine-treated rats (Hall and Marks, *unpublished observations,* cited by Marks et al., 1970). In guinea pigs injection of 5-HT into the lateral ventricles causes an increase in plasma corticosteroids both in intact and midbrain-sectioned guinea pigs (Naumenko, 1968). This suggests that the stimulatory action of 5-HT on the pituitary-adrenal system is due to a central, not a peripheral, action. However, in all these experiments the doses of 5-HT used were extremely high, and as with all intraventricular injection studies the precise site of action of the indoleamine remained undetermined.

Vermes et al. (1972) showed that when hypothalamic extracts are added to the pituitary together with 5-HT the release of ACTH is inhibited. However, this probably is just a pharmacological effect at the pituitary level. A number of reports have appeared in the literature implicating 5-HT in the control of the circadian periodicity of the hypothalamopituitary-adrenal axis (Krieger and Rizzo, 1969; Scapagnini et al., 1970). Of particular interest, in view of our findings on the serotonergic and cholinergic control of CRH secretion, are two studies by Krieger's group on the participation of the central nervous system (CNS) in controlling the circadian periodicity of plasma 17-hydroxycorticosteroid levels in the cat (Krieger et al., 1968; Krieger and Rizzo, 1969). The administration of anticholinergic agents was shown to block the afternoon peak in plasma corticosteroid levels in the cat (Krieger et al., 1968), which suggests the participation of central cholinergic structures in the circadian rhythm of ACTH secretion. Further studies then revealed that drugs which are able to affect the metabolism of 5-HT or its action were also capable of preventing the daily rise in plasma corticosteroid levels (Krieger and Rizzo, 1969). Drugs that deplete brain norepinephrine levels had no effect on the circadian periodicity of ACTH secretion, and none of the drugs used had any effect on the stress response to insulin hypoglycemia or to *Pseudomonas* polysaccharide. This suggests that central cholinergic and serotonergic pathways are involved in the circadian rhythm of ACTH release and are different from those which mediate certain types of stress responses.

We investigated the effect of an experimentally induced cholinergic blockade on the secretion of CRH in response to 5-HT (Burden et al., 1974*b;* Hillhouse et al., 1974*a;* Jones et al., 1975). Both hexamethonium and atropine reduced the response to 5-HT so that it was not significantly different from the basal values. This suggests that the 5-HT acts via a cholinergic interneuron that contains specific serotonergic receptors since the effect is blocked by methysergide. In the rat the cell bodies of the acetylcholine-containing neurons must be situated within the hypothalamus. This partly agrees with the conclusions reached by Naumenko (Naumenko, 1968; Popova et al., 1972) who suggested that 5-HT acted directly on the hypothalamus although it was thought that other neurotransmitters might be involved.

Other Monoamines

One of the most confusing fields of study at the moment is the role of brain monoamines in the control of ACTH secretion (Ganong, 1972, 1973; Van Loon, 1973; Abe and Hiroshige, 1974). The effect of norepinephrine, dopamine, and histamine on the *in vitro* release of CRH from the isolated rat hypothalamus was tested (Hillhouse et al., 1975). None of these monoamines caused a significant alteration in the basal secretion of CRH when administered in doses up to 10 ng/ml. The rat hypothalamus contains 1.57 to 2 μg norepinephrine per gram and 0.2 to 0.4 μg dopamine per gram (Stoner and Elson, 1971; Scapagnini and Preziosi, 1972). A calculation similar to that performed for acetylcholine and 5-HT shows that the blocks of hypothalamic tissue used in the experiments contain approximately 48 to 60 ng norepinephrine and 6 to 12 ng dopamine. Thus at concentrations near those present in the tissue the two catecholamines did not affect CRH secretion. Norepinephrine did appear to depress the basal secretion of CRH, although this was not a significant effect. A norepinephrine dose of 100 ng/ml, which is in excess of the amount present in the tissue, did not further depress the basal secretion. Histamine, which has been shown to be present in the hypothalamus in concentrations approximately one-half those of norepinephrine (Chapter 1), had no effect on the basal secretion of CRH in doses up to 10 ng/ml.

Many reports have appeared in the literature supporting a central noradrenergic neuroinhibitory pathway to CRH release (Ganong, 1972; Fuxe et al., 1973; Van Loon, 1973). We used the rat hypothalamus *in vitro* to test this hypothesis by examining the effect of norepinephrine and the other monoamines on both the acetylcholine and 5-HT-induced release of CRH (Hillhouse et al., 1975). Table 7–1 shows that norepinephrine in a concentration of 10 ng/ml abolished the stimulatory effect of acetylcholine (3 pg/ml) on CRH release. Neither dopamine nor histamine at the same concentration exhibited any inhibitory effect. Norepinephrine caused the log dose-response curves for both acetylcholine and 5-HT to shift to the right. The results are illustrated in Figs. 7–4 and 7–6. The minimum effective dose of norepinephrine was found to be 3 ng/ml, which is considerably less than the amount present in the blocks of tissue. These results support the hypothesis that there may be a central noradrenergic pathway that inhibits CRH release.

Pharmacological experiments using drugs known to affect catecholamine synthesis and metabolism have suggested a role for hypothalamic catecholamines in the control of ACTH secretion (Ganong, 1972; Scapagnini and Preziosi, 1972; Van Loon, 1973). Using data compiled from experiments with his co-workers Ganong (1972) plotted a graph which shows an inverse relationship between plasma corticosterone concentrations in the rat and hypothalamic norepinephrine levels. However, not all reports have supported this hypothesis (Kaplanski et al., 1972; Lippa et al., 1973; Ulrich and Yuwiler, 1973). The interpretation of some of these experiments may be com-

TABLE 7–1. Effect of phentolamine and norepinephrine on acetylcholine-induced CRH release

Substances added	In vitro corticosterone (μg/100 mg/hr)
ACh (3 pg)	8.0 ± 0.5
ACh (3 pg) + NE (3 ng)	6.0 ± 0.6
ACh (3 pg) + NE (10 ng)	2.3 ± 0.3[a]
ACh (3 pg) + NE (10 ng) + phentolamine (100 ng)	6.0 ± 0.5

ACh, acetylcholine. NE, norepinephrine.
[a] Significantly different from phentolamine: $p < 0.005$.

plicated by the possible development of denervation hypersensitivity, which is a well-documented phenomenon in the peripheral nervous system. Thus small amounts of catecholamines might be able to maintain normal function in the presence of increased sensitivity. Experiments are now in progress to allow this possibility to be investigated using the preparation of the rat hypothalamus in vitro. Another possibility is that other neuroinhibitory pathways that are not catecholaminergic might be able to take over the role of the noradrenergic pathways and help to maintain the functional integrity of the system. This seems to be a distinct possibility, as our experiments have shown that both GABA and melatonin can inhibit CRH release from the rat hypothalamus in vitro (Burden et al., 1974c; Jones et al., 1975).

Probably the most convincing evidence in favor of a central noradrenergic neuroinhibitory control of ACTH secretion is that of Fuxe and his co-workers (Fuxe et al., 1973). The 6-hydroxydopamine-induced degeneration of the dorsal noradrenergic pathways of the brain had no effect on either the hypothalamic catecholamine fluorescence or on normal activity of the pituitary-adrenal axis. However, when the ventral noradrenergic pathway was destroyed, there was a considerable loss of hypothalamic norepinephrine terminals, which resulted in an enhanced ether stress response at 1 day after the lesion but not at 1 week. Again this suggests that either denervation hypersensitivity is taking place or that other neuroinhibitory pathways can compensate for loss of the noradrenergic pathways.

We also examined the effect of phentolamine, an α-adrenergic blocking agent, on the inhibitory action of norepinephrine (Burden et al., 1974b; Hillhouse et al., 1975). Table 7-1 shows that norepinephrine in doses of 3 to 10 ng/ml causes a dose-dependent reduction in the release of CRH in response to acetylcholine, and that this inhibitory action of norepinephrine is antagonized by phentolamine in doses of 100 ng/ml to 1 μg/ml. This is in agreement with the results of Scapagnini and Preziosi (1973) who investigated the effect of α- and β-blocking agents on the noradrenergic inhibition of ACTH secretion in the rat. Systemic administration of phentolamine produced an increase in plasma corticosteroid levels, and intraventricular administration of a systemically ineffective dose had a similar effect. Propranolol had no effect on the plasma corticosterone levels. Dallman and Yates (1969) showed that iproniazid potentiates the inhibitory effect of dexamethasone following stress, and that prior administration of phentolamine reduced this effect (Scapagnini and Preziosi, 1973). The present results are in accord with the hypothesis of Ganong (1972) that there is a central noradrenergic neuroinhibitory pathway to CRH release mediated via an α-adrenergic receptor mechanism.

Putative Amino Acid Neurotransmitters

Although the role of certain amino acids as neurotransmitters in the CNS is rapidly becoming established, their role as potential modulators of CRH secretion has received little attention. Therefore we examined the effect of several of these agents on CRH secretion (Burden et al., 1974c; Jones et al., 1975). The basal release of CRH was not significantly altered by adding the putative amino acid neurotransmitters aspartate, glutamate, glycine, or GABA to the incubating medium in concentrations up to 10 ng/ml. As none of the amino acids stimulated the release of CRH, it was decided to determine if they inhibited secretion of the releasing hormone. It was found that only GABA reduced the stimulatory action of acetylcholine on CRH release (Table 7-2). GABA in doses of 100 pg to 10 ng/ml caused a dose-dependent reduction in the release of CRH in response to acetylcholine (3 pg/ml), and the inhibitory action of GABA could also be demonstrated using 5-HT as a stimulus to CRH release. GABA is highly concentrated in the lateral preoptic region of the rat hypothalamus and is present in concentrations up to 380 μg/g. Thus the amounts of GABA needed to inhibit CRH release is only a minute fraction of the tissue content and suggests that it may play a role in CRH secretion. Glycine did not reduce the stimulatory action of either acetylcholine or 5-HT. In order to determine if the effect of the GABA was mediated via an action on a specific GABA receptor, the effect of picro-

TABLE 7-2. *Effect of GABA and melatonin on ACh-stimulated CRH release*

Substances added[a]	No. of exp. observ.	In vitro corticosterone (μg/100 ng/hr)
ACh	12	7.8 ± 0.9
ACh + GABA (100 pg)	8	5.5 ± 0.6[b]
ACh + GABA (1 ng)	10	3.1 ± 0.4[c]
ACh + GABA (10 ng)	8	2.3 ± 0.3[c]
ACh + melatonin (10 ng)	9	3.8 ± 0.4[c]
ACh + melatonin (100 ng)	14	3.6 ± 0.5[c]

[a] In each case 3 pg ACh was used.
[b] Significantly different from ACh (3 pg): $p < 0.05$.
[c] Significantly different from ACh (3 pg): $p < 0.005$.

toxin, a GABA antagonist, was investigated. Table 7–3 shows that picrotoxin in doses of 10 to 100 ng/ml significantly reduced the inhibitory action of GABA (10 ng/ml) on the release of CRH in response to 5-HT (10 ng/ml).

It has been proposed that the amino acids glutamate and aspartate have an excitatory action on neurons, but our results suggest that they have no functional significance in the control of CRH release. The presence of GABA in the hypothalamus together with neurons sensitive to the microiontophoretic application of GABA has been reported by a number of investigators (Pruntek and Philippu, 1973; Robinson and Wells, 1973). Our results implicate these neurons in the control of CRH release. It is noteworthy that GABA is a more potent inhibitory neurotransmitter than norepinephrine in our test system. Since the response to both 5-HT and acetylcholine is inhibited by GABA, it is suggested that GABA acts directly on the CRH neurons, which must contain specific GABA receptors as the effect is abolished by picro-

TABLE 7-3. *Effect of GABA and melatonin on 5-HT-stimulated CRH release*

Substances added[a]	No. of exp. observ.	In vitro corticosterone (μg . 100 mg/hr)
5-HT	15	7.2 ± 0.7
5-HT + GABA (100 pg)		6.3 ± 0.89
5-HT + GABA (1 ng)	10	3.4 ± 0.5[b]
5-HT + GABA (10 ng)	7	1.6 ± 0.2[b]
5-HT + GABA (10 ng) + picrotoxin (1 ng)	9	3.0 ± 0.5[c]
5-HT + GABA (10 ng) + picrotoxin (10 ng)	10	5.1 ± 0.5[c]
5-HT + GABA (10 ng) + picrotoxin (100 ng)	10	4.7 ± 0.5[c]
5-HT + melatonin (10 ng)	18	3.4 ± 0.35[b]
5-HT + melatonin (100 ng)	7	3.5 ± 0.65[b]
5-HT + melatonin (1 μg)	7	2.7 ± 0.7[b]

[a] In each case 10 ng 5-HT was used.
[b] Significantly different from 5-HT (10 ng): $p < 0.005$.
[c] Significantly different from 5-HT (10 ng) + GABA (10 ng): $p < 0.01$.

toxin. Recently this work was confirmed *in vivo* by using intraventricular administration of both GABA and picrotoxin (Makara and Stark, 1974).

Yagi and Sawaki (1975) showed that collaterals from parvicellular cells synapse with GABA inhibitory neurons. It is therefore possible that the effect seen with GABA may represent the mechanism of autofeedback whereby CRH regulates its own release.

Effect of Melatonin

Since melatonin is a metabolite of 5-HT, it is possible that it might influence CRH secretion. Several reports have already appeared to this effect (Wurtman and Anton-Tay, 1969; Motta et al., 1971). We investigated the effect of melatonin on the secretion of CRH *in vitro* (Burden et al., 1974c; Jones et al., 1975). Melatonin, in concentrations up to 10 ng/ml, did not significantly alter the basal secretion of CRH. However, doses of 10 ng/ml to 1 μg/ml significantly reduced the CRH-releasing effect of 5-HT (10 ng/ml). The results are illustrated in Tables 7-2 and 7-3, which also show that a 10 ng/ml dose of melatonin significantly reduced the CRH response to acetylcholine (3 pg/ml). This indicates that the inhibitory action of melatonin must be directly on the CRH neuron.

That the pineal gland is important in the control of the neuroendocrine system was suggested by Wurtman and Anton-Tay (1969); moreover, that melatonin inhibits the release of CRH in response to both 5-HT and acetylcholine may reflect a physiological role. Studies in which the pineal was removed or where melatonin was implanted or injected intraventricularly support our conclusion that melatonin inhibits CRH release. It has been suggested that melatonin acts as an antagonist on the 5-HT receptor; however, our data place the effect distal to the receptor, since melatonin inhibits the action of acetylcholine as well as that of 5-HT. The finding that melatonin and 5-HT have opposing effects on CRH release is significant with respect to experiments in which parachlorophenylalanine (pCPA) has been used to study the role of 5-HT in the central control of CRH secretion (Bhattacharya and Marks, 1970; Scapagnini et al., 1971; Van Delft et al., 1973; Vernikos-Danellis and Berger, 1973). Pretreatment of animals with pCPA interferes with melatonin as well as 5-HT synthesis, and the results of such experiments must be interpreted with caution. It is possible that variations in the levels of these two indoleamines may be important in the control of the circadian rhythm of CRH release.

Interactions Between the Inhibitory Actions of Norepinephrine, GABA, and Melatonin

Since norepinephrine was previously shown to inhibit CRH secretion, it occurred to us that the effect of GABA might be due to the release of

endogenous norepinephrine. We tested for this possibility by adding phentolamine (100 ng/ml and 1 μg/ml) to the hypothalamic incubating medium
containing 5-HT (10 ng/ml) and GABA (1 ng/ml). The phentolamine did
not antagonize the inhibitory action of GABA on CRH release. As it was also
possible that the inhibition seen with norepinephrine was mediated via a
GABA neuron, picrotoxin (100 ng/ml) was added to the hypothalamic

TABLE 7–4. Effects of various antagonists on the ability of GABA, norepinephrine, and melatonin to inhibit 5-HT-stimulated CRH release

Substances added[a]	No. of exp. observ.	In vitro corticosterone (μg/100 mg/hr)
5-HT + melatonin (10 ng)	18	3.4 ± 0.35
5-HT + melatonin (10 ng) + phentolamine (100 ng)	19	3.5 ± 0.5
5-HT + melatonin (10 ng) + phentolamine (1 μg)	19	4.1 ± 0.5
5-HT + melatonin (10 ng) + picrotoxin (100 ng)	8	2.8 ± 0.6
5-HT + norepinephrine (10 ng)	10	1.5 ± 0.43
5-HT + norepinephrine (10 ng) + phentolamine (100 ng)	8	4.1 ± 0.9[b]
5-HT + norepinephrine (10 ng) + picrotoxin (100 ng)	8	1.6 ± 0.2
5-HT + GABA (10 ng)	7	1.6 ± 0.2
5-HT + GABA (10 ng) + picrotoxin (100 ng)	14	3.9 ± 0.45[c]
5-HT + GABA (10 ng) + phentolamine (100 ng)	10	2.7 ± 0.3

[a] In each case 10 ng 5-HT was used.
[b] Significantly different from 5-HT + norepinephrine (10 ng): $p < 0.01$.
[c] Significantly different from 5-HT + GABA (10 ng): $p < 0.005$.

medium containing 5-HT (10 ng/ml) and norepinephrine (10 ng/ml). The
picrotoxin did not alter the inhibitory action of norepinephrine on CRH release. The results are summarized in Table 7–4, which also shows that neither
picrotoxin nor phentolamine had any effect on the inhibitory action of melatonin. The three inhibitory substances thus exert their effects through independent mechanisms.

Model of the Neurotransmitters Involved in CRH Release

Our experiments on the rat hypothalamus *in vitro* enabled us to formulate
a model of the neurotransmitters involved in the control of the CRH secretion at the hypothalamic level (Burden et al., 1974c; Jones et al., 1975). The
model (Fig. 7–7) is a highly tentative one based on our *in vitro* data and
those selected from *in vivo* experiments by other workers. Since the anatomical site of the CRH cells is unknown, their location in the model is un-
specified.

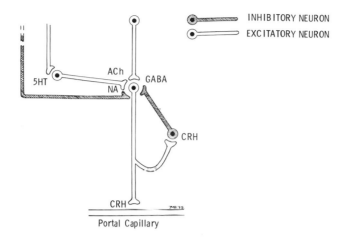

FIG. 7–7. Proposed model of the neurotransmitters involved in the release of CRH from the hypothalamus. The model shows: (1) The CRH neuron with its axon terminating at a portal capillary. A collateral from the CRH neuron synapses with a GABA (inhibitory) Interneuron. (2) Activity in the CRH neuron causes a negative feedback action via excitation of the GABA interneuron (as has been suggested for the tuberoinfundibular neurons by Yagi and Sawaki, 1975). (3) A 5-HT pathway which releases CRH after excitation of a cholinergic interneuron. (4) The final common pathway to CRH release is cholinergic. Two cholinergic neurons are shown. One is the interneuron placed between the 5-HT pathway and the CRH cell (? for control of the circadian rhythm). The other cholinergic neuron does not have a 5-HT synapse and may control the stress-induced release of CRH. (5) A noradrenergic pathway (NA) which is inhibitory to CRH secretion. It should be pointed out that in the case of the GABA neuron another model can be postulated (Jones et al., 1975) in which the neuron originates in the lateral preoptic area and terminates at the CRH axon (i.e., presynaptically).

Negative Feedback Control of CRH Secretion

Long-Loop Feedback

ACTH secretion in the rat is believed to be regulated by two temporally and dynamically distinct corticosteroid feedback mechanisms: a rate-sensitive fast feedback (Dallman and Yates, 1969; Dallman et al., 1972; Jones et al., 1972) and a proportional delayed feedback (Dallman and Yates, 1969; Yates and Maran, 1974). Several sites of feedback have been suggested, ranging from the midbrain to the adrenal (Dallman and Yates, 1968). We used the preparation of the rat hypothalamus *in vitro* to investigate the effects of either adrenalectomy or corticosteroid treatment on CRH secretion *in vitro* (Bradbury et al., 1973; Hillhouse et al., 1974b; 1975; Burden et al., 1975).

Delayed Feedback

Hypothalami were removed from male rats at different time intervals following adrenalectomy, and their function *in vitro* was investigated. The basal secretion of CRH begins to increase between the fourth to the 24th hour following adrenalectomy, reaches a peak at 7 days after the operation, and maintains that level indefinitely (Fig. 7–8). Thus corticosteroids play a role in the maintenance of basal adrenocorticotropic activity, as postulated by Davidson et al. (1968) who reported that the implantation of cortisol in the median eminence of rats results in inhibition of basal corticotropic activity. Adrenalectomy also results in an increase in both the acetylcholine-induced and the electrically stimulated secretion of CRH *in vitro*. This increased CRH secretion develops 1 day after operation and reaches a maximum at 14 days postoperatively. The results (Fig. 7–9) are in agreement with morphological data on the effect of adrenalectomy on granules in the median eminence (Brinkman and Bock, 1973). It is interesting that in the 2-hr adrenalectomized rat no detectable CRH was released from the hypothalamus in response to a standard dose of acetylcholine (3 pg/ml). This agrees with several reports that the CRH content of the median eminence, as well as the ACTH content of the pituitary, of the rat undergo a substantial decrease 1 to 3 hr after adrenalectomy (Vernikos-Danellis, 1956a,b; Dallman et al., 1972; Buckingham and Hodges, 1974). Replacement therapy with corticosterone (5 mg/kg) prevented hypersecretion of CRH induced by adrenalectomy (Bradbury et al., 1973).

Adrenalectomy has long been known to result in high resting levels and hypersecretion after stress, but it has only recently been shown that this hypersecretion after stress occurs within 10 min (Dallman et al., 1972). Hodges and Vernikos (1960) suggested that the exaggerated response was

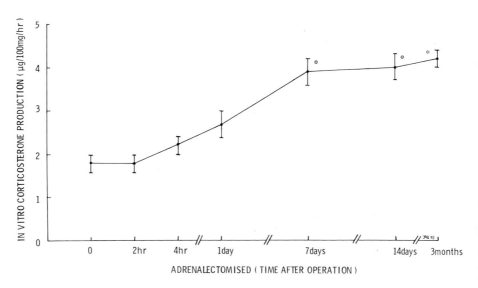

FIG. 7–8. Effect of adrenalectomy on the basal secretion of CRH from the hypothalamus *in vitro*. Asterisks identify values that are significantly elevated over the control ($p < 0.01$).

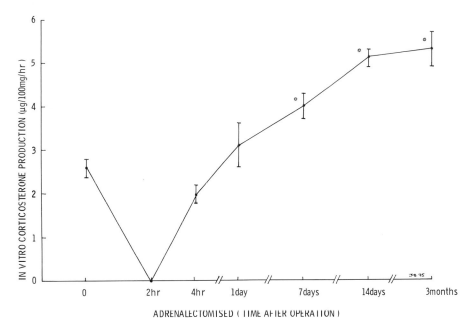

FIG. 7–9. Effect of adrenalectomy on the acetylcholine-induced release of CRH in the hypothalamus *in vitro*. See legend for Fig. 7–8.

due to enhanced ACTH synthesis, which suggests that the adenohypophysis is the main site of corticoid negative feedback. It was previously shown that CRH synthesis occurred in the rat hypothalamus *in vitro* as shown by the output of the neurohormone in response to electrical stimulation (Bradbury et al., 1973). The present experiments show that CRH synthesis is increased by adrenalectomy since its output is greater in response to 5-HT or acetylcholine stimulation of hypothalami taken from adrenalectomized animals than those from intact animals. This increased output takes place without any concomitant decrease in content (Table 7–5). It appears therefore that hypersecretion of ACTH in adrenalectomized animals is the result of a primary increase in CRH synthesis and release followed by increased elaboration of ACTH.

A wide variety of steroids were tested for an effect at the hypothalamic level (Fig. 7–10). Rats adrenalectomized 7 to 14 days previously were treated 4 and 24 hr before the hypothalami were removed from these animals and incubated with acetylcholine (3 pg/ml) to stimulate CRH release. The control histogram represents the amount of CRH activity after acetylcholine stimulation; it can be seen that pretreatment with steroids caused a significant reduction in the amount of CRH released in response in acetylcholine stimulation ($p < 0.01$ or less). Thus corticosterone, cortisol, 11-deoxycorticosterone, and 11-deoxycortisol all exhibit a significant delayed feedback effect

TABLE 7–5. *CRH content of hypothalami before and after incubation with either acetylcholine or 5-hydroxytryptamine*

Treatment[a]	Content (mU ACTH/ hypothalamus)	Release into medium (mU ACTH/ hypothalamus)	Total amount: content + release (mU ACTH/ hypothalamus)
No incubation	8	—	8
Two-hour incubation with ACh (3 pg/ml)	8	10	18
Two-hour incubation with 5-HT (10 ng/ml)	10	20	30

CRH activity was assayed in the ME-lesioned rat and is expressed in terms of standard ACTH (Acthar).

[a] ACh, acetylcholine. 5-HT, 5-hydroxytryptamine.

at both 4 and 24 hr following subcutaneous administration. This confirms previous reports from this and other laboratories (Tiptaft and Jones, 1975). Three steroids—dexamethasone, progesterone, and 11β-17α-dihydroxyprogesterone—showed no delayed feedback effect at 4 hr but did exhibit considerable efficacy at 24 hr. Prednisolone, which is a potent suppressor of

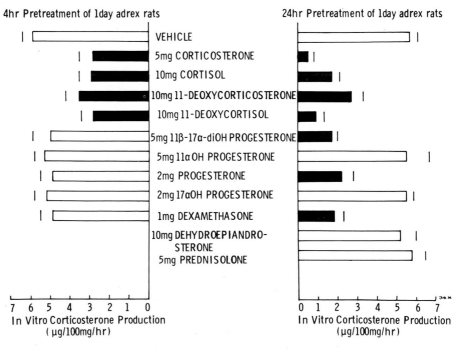

FIG. 7–10. Delayed feedback of various steroids on the hypothalamus. The steroids were administered 4 or 24 hr before testing, as indicated. Adrex, adrenalectomized.

pituitary adrenocorticotropic activity, showed no delayed feedback at 24 hr. However, further experiments using different time intervals and dosages are needed before any firm conclusions can be drawn concerning this steroid.

Experiments have also been performed to determine delayed feedback effects at the pituitary level. Steroids were administered to hypothalamus-lesioned animals at different time intervals prior to intravenous injection of CRH obtained from the rat hypothalamus *in vitro* (Burden et al., 1975). Preliminary results (Table 7–6) show that a wide variety of steroids exert a delayed feedback effect at the pituitary level. These results are interesting because they show that dexamethasone has a delayed feedback effect at the pituitary at 4 hr which by 24 hr has disappeared, whereas the delayed feedback at the hypothalamus is not apparent until 24 hr. Prednisolone, which

TABLE 7–6. Delayed feedback at the pituitary

Treatment	Pretreatment of ME-lesioned rat for 4 hr	Pretreatment of ME-lesioned rat for 24 hr
Vehicle	6.3 ± 0.5	6.2 ± 0.4
Corticosterone (2 mg)	1.7 ± 0.3	0.8 ± 0.2
Cortisol (2 mg)	1.2 ± 0.2	0.4 ± 0.2
11-Deoxycorticosterone (2 mg)	2.4 ± 0.6	2.6 ± 0.3
11-Deoxycortisol (2 mg)	2.3 ± 0.4	—
Dexamethasone (1 mg)	1.5 ± 0.3	5.3 ± 0.7[a]
Progesterone (2 mg)	—	2.8 ± 0.5
Prednisolone (5 mg)	—	1.8 ± 0.2
Aldadiene (10 mg)	—	2.3 ± 0.3
Beclomethasone diproprionate (10 mg)	—	2.8 ± 0.2

ME, median eminence.
[a] Not significantly different from vehicle.

has no effect at the hypothalamus at 24 hr, shows considerable suppression at the pituitary level. Probably the most perplexing result in these experiments is that progesterone shows considerable delayed feedback activity at both the hypothalamus and pituitary, an observation that has not been confirmed *in vivo* (Tiptaft and Jones, 1975). As the effects may be due to conversion of progesterone into a more active steroid *in vivo*, experiments are now in progress to allow examination of the delayed feedback effect of the steroid added directly to the hypothalamus *in vitro*.

Delayed corticosteroid feedback at the hypothalamus is probably due to its influence on the rate of CRH synthesis, since the CRH output in response to both electrical and acetylcholine stimulation is greater than that originally found in the tissue, and the output is reduced compared to that seen in intact animals after pretreatment with the corticosterone (Bradbury et al., 1973). At the pituitary level corticosteroids are thought to exert their delayed feedback effect mainly by suppressing ACTH release rather than synthesis

(Fleischer and Rawls, 1968, 1970), or by inhibiting ACTH synthesis (Hodges and Vernikos, 1960). A protein synthesis step is believed to be involved (Arimura et al., 1969), which presumably explains why there is a delay between administration of corticoids and the appearance of delayed feedback.

The delayed feedback mechanism at the hypothalamic level is remarkable for its nonspecificity since a wide variety of steroids have significant activity. Neither the 11β- nor the 21β-OH groups are essential since even progesterone has significant delayed feedback activity (Fig. 7–11). Thus the fast and the delayed feedback receptors in the hypothalamus differ in both their dynamics and specificity. It is possible that steroids undergo metabolism in the body

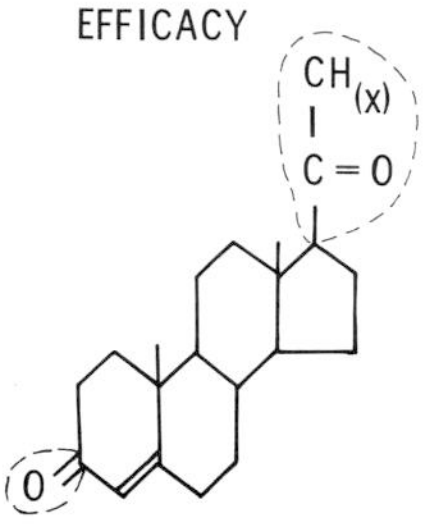

EFFICACY

FIG. 7–11. Delayed feedback. Groups essential for the efficacy of the steroid molecule on the delayed feedback receptor.

during the interval before removal of the hypothalamus for testing *in vitro*. If such changes occur, they are likely to be subtle and not involve a conversion to cortisol or corticosterone.

Fast feedback

Preparation of the rat hypothalamus presented us with an opportunity to investigate the effect of steroids added directly to the tissue *in vitro*. We used this to investigate the fast feedback action of various steroids on CRH secretion (Jones et al., 1974; Burden et al., 1975; Hillhouse et al., 1975). Fast feedback is studied by adding the steroid simultaneously with acetylcholine and measuring the amount of CRH secreted into the incubation medium during the next 10 min. Figure 7–12 shows that corticosterone in concentrations of 1 pg/ml to 10 ng/ml inhibits the release of CRH induced by acetylcholine (3 pg/ml). Control experiments show that these corticosterone doses do not reduce the responsiveness of the animals to exogenous CRH. From these experiments we conclude that the primary site of the fast feedback action of corticosterone is at the hypothalamus, and that CRH output is reduced by doses well within the free steroid concentration range found in the plasma. This laboratory previously showed that the stress response in the intact animal can be reduced by immediate pretreatment with physiological doses of corticosterone (Jones et al., 1974; Tiptaft and Jones, 1975). Thus

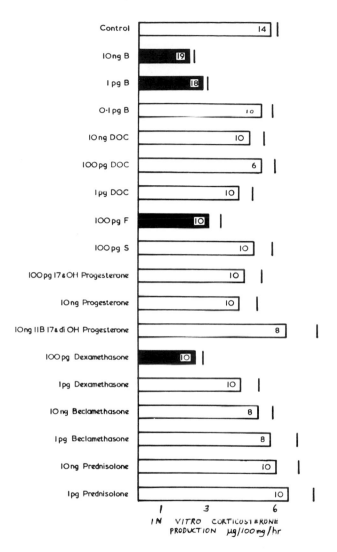

FIG. 7–12. Fast feedback action of various steroids added simultaneously with 3 pg acetylcholine to the hypothalamus *in vitro*. The release of CRH during the succeeding 10 min is shown. Bars, ± SEM.

the corticotropic response to the surgical stress of bilateral sham adrenalectomy is reduced when the rate of rise in plasma corticosterone exceeds 1.3 μg/100 ml/min (Jones et al., 1972); this corresponds to a 1.3 ng/ml/min rate of rise in free steroid in the plasma. The present results demonstrate that such levels reduce CRH output from the hypothalamus *in vitro* and may be responsible for modulation of the stress response *in vivo*.

Figure 7–12 shows the effect of various other steroids on the release of CRH induced by acetylcholine (3 pg/ml). Of all the steroids tested, only corticosterone, cortisol, and dexamethasone were fast feedback agonists. Fast

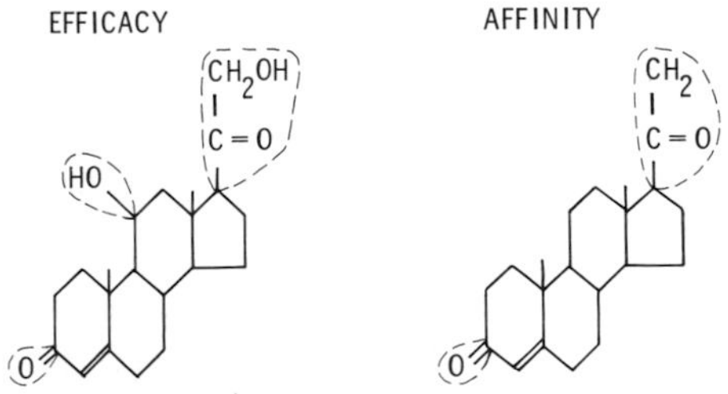

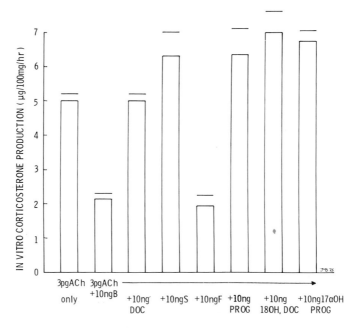

FIG. 7–13. Fast feedback. *Left:* Groups essential for the efficacy of the steroid molecule on the fast feedback receptor. *Right:* Groups essential for the affinity of the steroid molecule on the fast feedback receptor.

feedback to the hypothalamus therefore requires an 11β-OH group and a 21-OH group in the corticosteroid molecule (Fig. 7–13). An additional double bond in the Δ1 position weakens this fast feedback action, but the further addition of a 9-halogen counteracts the weakening effect of dehydrogenation (e.g., dexamethasone and prednisolone). Blocking of the C21β-OH group also abolishes the fast feedback propensity of the steroid at the hypothalamic level (e.g., beclomethasone dipropionate).

FIG. 7–14. Effect of various steroids on the fast feedback action of corticosterone on acetylcholine-stimulated CRH release. These steroids being tested as antagonists were added 5 min before the addition of 3 pg acetylcholine and 10 ng corticosterone. DOC, deoxycorticosterone. S, 11-deoxycortisol. F, cortisol. PROG, progesterone. 18OH,DOC, 18-hydroxydeoxycorticosterone. 17αOH, PROG, 17α-hydroxyprogesterone.

The protocol was changed in the experiment depicted in Fig. 7–14. Five minutes before the stimulation period the hypothalamic fluid was replaced by a solution containing an additional steroid under investigation for antagonistic properties. Therefore during the stimulation period, acetylcholine, corticosterone, and the putative antagonist were present. Figure 7–14 shows that 1 ng/ml of deoxycorticosterone (DOC) antagonized the inhibitory action of corticosterone (100 pg/ml). 11-Deoxycortisol (compound S), progesterone, and 18-OH-DOC in a dose of 10 ng/ml were able to antagonize the inhibitory effect of corticosterone (10 ng/ml). Compound S (10 ng/ml) also antagonized the inhibitory effect of cortisol (10 ng/ml). As the degree of inhibition with cortisol is not as great as that seen with corticosterone, it was decided to determine if cortisol acts as a partial agonist. However, cortisol does not antagonize the effect of 10 ng corticosterone at a dose of 10 ng/ml (Fig. 7–14), and it is unlikely that cortisol is a partial agonist. The antagonism between DOC, compound S, and corticosterone and cortisol (respectively) has been observed in vivo (Tiptaft and Jones, 1975), and the current work confirms previous reports from this and another laboratory (Edwardson and Bennett, 1974; Hillhouse et al., 1975) that this antagonism is hypothalamic in origin. The ability of 18-OH-DOC to antagonize the fast feedback action of corticosterone in vitro confirms a previous report that 18-OH-DOC causes exaggeration of the stress response when administered 10 min prior to an ether stress (Tiptaft and Jones, 1975).

TABLE 7–7. Mechanism of the fast feedback inhibition of acetylcholine-stimulated CRH release

Treatment	In vitro corticosteroid production (μg/100 mg/1 hr)	No. of animals
Experiment I[a]		
Basal	2.7 ± 0.3^b	15
ACh (3 pg)	5.9 ± 0.6	18
ACh (3 pg) + B (1 ng)	2.4 ± 0.3^b	15
ACh (3 pg) + B (1 ng) + phentolamine (100 ng)	3.4 ± 0.3^b	10
ACh (3 pg) + B (1 ng) + picrotoxin (100 ng)	2.8 ± 0.3	10
Experiment II[c]		
Basal	2.7 ± 0.3	15
Basal + B (10 ng)	1.6 ± 0.5	5
K$^+$ (48 mM) injected into the assay animal	2.1 ± 0.7	7
K$^+$ (12 mM)	4.6 ± 0.6	10
K$^+$ (12 mM) + B (10 ng)	$4.5 \pm 0.6^{b,d}$	8
K$^+$ (48 mM)	4.2 ± 0.5	12
K$^+$ (48 mM) + B (10 ng)	$3.1 \pm 0.1^{b,e}$	7

[a] Experiment I: Effect of the putative inhibitory transmitters on CRH release.

[b] $p < 0.01$ compared to ACh (3 pg).

[c] Experiment II: Effect of the simultaneous addition of corticosterone on potassium (K$^+$)-induced CRH release.

[d] Not significant from K$^+$ (12mM) alone.

[e] Not significant from K$^+$ (48 mM) alone.

We found that ACh-stimulated CRH release can be inhibited by norepinephrine and by GABA (Jones et al., 1975). It was therefore decided to test if corticosterone acts via one of these inhibitory pathways. Table 7–7 shows the effect of picrotoxin (100 ng/ml), a GABA antagonist, and phentolamine (100 ng/ml), an α-blocker, on the fast feedback action of corticosterone. The action of corticosterone on acetylcholine-induced release was unaffected, and it can be concluded that corticosterone does not act via a neuroinhibitory pathway. We then tested if the action of corticosterone was mediated by stabilization of the cell membrane. CRH release was induced with 12 or 48 mM K^+; this is not inhibited by corticosterone (10 ng/ml), suggesting that membrane stabilization may be the mechanism of action of the steroid.

Short-Loop Feedback

Several groups have suggested that ACTH exerts a negative feedback effect on the corticotropic response to stress, and it has been shown that intrahypothalamic implants of ACTH inhibit the corticotropic response to stress (Motta et al., 1965). To test the existence of such a short-loop feedback, ACTH was added simultaneously with 5-HT (10 ng/ml) to hypothalami incubated in vitro. The results (Fig. 7–15) show that ACTH, in doses of 100 nU/ml and above, inhibits CRH secretion and support the concept that ACTH exerts a modulating effect on CRH release. Therefore the inhibitory effect of ACTH on the corticotropic response to stress appears to be mediated via suppression of CRH output from the hypothalamus.

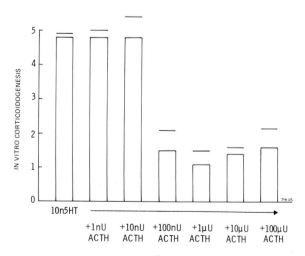

FIG. 7–15. Effect of various doses of ACTH (Acthar®) on 5-HT-stimulated CRH release from the hypothalamus in vitro.

NATURE OF CRH

We have begun to investigate the chemical nature of CRH obtained using the stimulated hypothalamus *in vitro*. This approach has advantages over previous methods of CRH extraction in that the tissue effects a considerable purification of the hormone because stimulation with 5-HT causes CRH to be released specifically; the amount released over 2 hr is greater than that normally found in the tissue (Table 7–5). The preliminary results are described by Gillham et al. (1975*a,b*). Figure 7–16 shows the CRH activity of fractions collected from a column of Sephadex G-25.

There are two peaks of CRH activity corresponding to substances whose molecular weights are approximately 2,500 and 1,300. These peaks do not contain ACTH (cytochemical assay). They themselves are not active on the adrenal *in vitro,* nor do they potentiate the effect of ACTH in this assay. There is also no detectable LRH, TRH, antidiuretic hormone, or oxytocin activity. Studies are now in progress to determine the amino acid sequence of the materials.

SUMMARY

The rat hypothalamus *in vitro* shows a considerable degree of metabolic activity, releases CRH in response to neurotransmitters, and has the ability

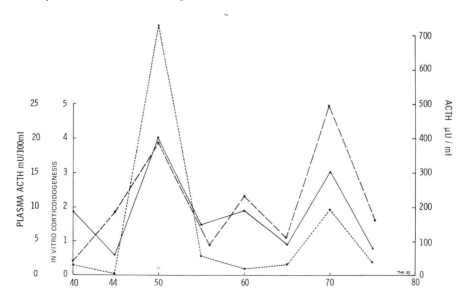

FIG. 7–16. Fractions of fluid collected from 50 hypothalami stimulated with 5-HT and passed through a Sephadex G25 column. The fraction numbers are indicated along the horizontal axis. Three different CRH assays were used: (—), *in vitro* corticoidogenesis of 48-hr ME-lesioned rat. (— —), plasma ACTH (cytochemical assay) of the 48-hr ME-lesioned rat. (------), ACTH (cytochemical assay) from hemisected primed pituitaries *in vitro*.

to synthesize the releasing hormone. CRH secretion is stimulated by acetyl-choline acting predominantly via a nicotinic receptor mechanism. 5-HT also releases CRH and does so by stimulating a cholinergic interneuron since its activity is blocked by hexamethonium as well as methysergide. Thus the final common pathway to CRH release is cholinergic.

Norepinephrine (via an α-receptor mechanism), melatonin, and GABA inhibit CRH secretion. These three agents produce the inhibition via inde-pendent receptor mechanisms. Two separate pathways may be postulated for the GABA neuroinhibitory mechanism. In the first postulate GABA is re-leased from an interneuron whose activity is excited by a collateral from the CRH neuron. In the second postulate a GABA neuronal pathway terminates on the axons of the CRH neurons, i.e., presynaptically. The noradrenergic system is regarded as the neuroinhibitory pathway to CRH release.

CRH release is inhibited by both fast and delayed corticosteroid (long-loop) feedback as well as ACTH (short-loop) feedback. Structure-activity relationships of different steroids suggest that 11β-OH and 21β-OH groups are essential for the fast but not the delayed feedback mechanism.

ACKNOWLEDGMENTS

We express our thanks to the Wellcome Trust and to Smith Kline & French for financial support (to M. T. Jones). We are grateful to the following people who collaborated in this work: Dr. B. Gillham, Dr. S. Jeffcoate, Professor R. Bock, Professor W. Wittkowski, Professor J. R. Hodges, Dr. Julia Buck-ingham, and Dr. T. E. Bridges. R. Bock performed the histological sectioning.

REFERENCES

Abe, K., and Hiroshige, T. (1974): Changes in plasma corticosterone and hypothalamic CRF levels following intraventricular injection or drug-induced changes of brain biogenic amines in the rat. *Neuroendocrinology,* 14:195–211.

Arimura, A., Bowers, C. V., Schally, A. V., Saito, M., and Miller, M. C. (1969): Effect of corticotropin-releasing factor, dexamethasone and actinomycin D on the release of ACTH from rat pituitaries in vitro and in vivo. *Endocrinology,* 85:300–311.

Bachelard, H. S., Campbell, W. J., and McIlwain, H. (1962): The sodium and other ions of mammalian cerebral tissues maintained and electrically stimulated in vitro. *Biochem. J.,* 84:225–236.

Bhattacharya, A. N., and Marks, B. H. (1970): Effects of α-methyltyrosine and p-chlorophenylalanine on the regulation of ACTH secretion. *Neuroendocrinology,* 6:49–55.

Bissett, G. W., Hilton, S. M., and Poissner, A. M. (1967a): Hypothalamic pathways for independent release of vasopressin and oxytocin. *Proc. R. Soc. Lond. [Biol.],* 166: 422–442.

Bissett, G. W., Clark, B. J., Haldar, J., Harris, M. N., Lewis, G. P., and Rocha e Silva, M., Jr. (1967b): The assay of milk-ejecting activity in the lactating rat. *Br. J. Pharmacol. Chemother.,* 31:537–549.

Bradbury, M. W. B., Burden, J., Dicker, A., Hillhouse, E. W., Jones, M. T., and Philbrick, D. (1973): Stimulation of rat hypothalamus in vitro. *J. Physiol. (Lond.),* 234:74P.

Bridges, T. E., Hillhouse, E. W., and Jones, M. T. (1975): The effect of dopamine on neurohypophyseal hormone secretion in vivo and in vitro. *J. Physiol. (Lond.)*, 247: 107P.

Brinkman, H., and Bock, R. (1973): Influence of various corticoids on the augmentation of Gomori positive granules in the median eminence of the rat following adrenalectomy. *Naunyn Schmiedebergs Arch. Pharmacol.*, 280:49–62.

Buckingham, J. L., and Hodges, J. R. (1974): Inter-relationships of pituitary and plasma corticotrophin and plasma corticosterone in adrenalectomised and stressed adrenalectomised rats. *J. Endocrinol.*, 63:213–222.

Buckingham, J. L., Burden, J. L., Hillhouse, E. W., Hodges, J. R., and Jones, M. T. (1975): A sensitive assay for corticotrophin-releasing hormone. *J. Endocrinol. (in press)*.

Burden, J. L., Hillhouse, E. W., and Jones, M. T. (1974a): The effect of various putative neurotransmitters on the release of CRH from the hypophysiotrophic hypothalamus in vitro. *J. Physiol. (Lond.)*, 239:51–52.

Burden, J. L., Hillhouse, E. W., and Jones, M. T. (1974b): The inhibitory action of GABA and melatonin on the release of corticotrophin-releasing hormone from the rat hypophysiotrophic area in vitro. *J. Physiol. (Lond.)*, 239:116–117.

Burden, J. L., Hillhouse, E. W., and Jones, M. T. (1974c): A proposed model of the transmitters involved in the control of corticotrophin-releasing hormone. *J. Endocrinol.*, 63:20–21.

Burden, J. L., Hillhouse, E. W., and Jones, M. T. (1975): Structure-activity relationship of various steroids and the sites of their fast and delayed feedback mechanisms. *J. Endocrinol. (in press)*.

Clementi, F., Ceccarelli, B., Cerati, E., Demonte, M. L., and Pecile, A. (1971): Subcellular organisation of the median-eminence. *Adv. Cytopharmacol.*, 1:331–342.

Dallman, M., and Yates, F. E. (1968): Anatomical and functional mapping of central neuronal input and feedback pathways of the adrenocortical system. *Mem. Soc. Endocrinol.*, 17:39–72.

Dallman, M. F., and Yates, F. E. (1969): Dynamic asymmetries in the corticosteroid feedback path and distribution-metabolism-binding elements in the adrenocortical system. *Ann. N.Y. Acad. Sci.*, 156:696–721.

Dallman, M. F., Jones, M. T., Vernikos-Danellis, J., and Ganong, W. F. (1972): Corticosteroid feedback control of ACTH secretion: Rapid effects of bilateral adrenalectomy on plasma ACTH in the rat. *Endocrinology*, 91:961–968.

Daly, J. R., Loveridge, N., Bitensky, L., and Chayen, J. (1974): The cytochemical bioassay of corticotrophin. *Clin. Endocrinol.*, 3:311–318.

Davidson, J. M., Jones, L. E., and Levine, S. (1968): Feedback regulation of adrenocorticotrophin secretion in "basal" and "stress" conditions: Acute and chronic effects of intrahypothalamic corticoid implantation. *Endocrinology*, 82:655–663.

Edwardson, J. A., and Bennett, G. W. (1974): Modulation of corticotrophin-releasing factor release from hypothalamic synaptosomes. *Nature (Lond.)*, 251:425–427.

Fleischer, N., and Rawls, W. (1968): Inhibition of vasopressin-induced ACTH release from the pituitary by glucocorticoids in vitro. *Endocrinology*, 83:1232–1236.

Fleischer, N., and Rawls, W. (1970): Adrenocorticotrophin (ACTH) synthesis and release in pituitary monolayer culture; the effect of dexamethasone. *Am. J. Physiol.*, 219:445–448.

Fuxe, K., Hökfelt, T., Jonsson, G., Levine, S., Lidbrink, P., and Löfström, A. (1973): Brain and pituitary-adrenal interactions—studies on central monamine neurones. In: *Brain-Pituitary-Adrenal Interrelationships*, edited by A. Brodish and E. S. Redgate, pp. 239–269. Karger, Basel.

Ganong, W. F. (1972): Evidence for a central noradrenergic system that inhibits ACTH secretion. In: *Brain-Endocrine Interaction, Median Eminence: Structure and Function*, pp. 254–266. Karger, Basel.

Ganong, W. F. (1973): Pharmacological aspects of neuroendocrine integration. *Prog. Brain Res.*, 38:41–59.

Gillham, B., Jones, M. T., Hillhouse, E. W., and Burden, J. L. (1975a): Preliminary observations on the nature of corticotrophin-releasing hormone from the rat hypothalamus in vitro. *J. Endocrinol. (in press)*.

Gillham, B., Burden, J. L., Hillhouse, E. W., and Jones, M. T. (1975b): The preparation of the rat hypothalamus in vitro as a source of CRH. *J. Endocrinol. (in press).*

Halász, B. (1969): The endocrine effects of isolation of the hypothalamus from the rest of the brain. In: *Frontiers in Neuroendocrinology,* edited by W. F. Ganong and L. Martini, pp. 307–342. Oxford University Press, New York.

Hedge, G. A., and Smelik, P. G. (1968): Corticotrophin release: Inhibition by intra-hypothalamic implantation of atropine. *Science,* 159:891–892.

Hedge, G. A., and De Weid, D. (1971): Corticotrophin and vasopressin secretion after hypothalamic implantation of atropine. *Endocrinology,* 88:257–259.

Hillhouse, E. W., Burden, J. L., and Jones, M. T. (1974a): The control of CRF release at the hypothalamic level: In: *Neurosecretion: The Final Neuroendocrine Pathway,* edited by F. Knowles and L. Vollrath, p. 308. Springer-Verlag, New York.

Hillhouse, E. W., Burden, J. L., and Jones, M. T. (1974b): Structure-activity relationships of various steroids on the feedback control of corticotrophin-releasing hormone. *J. Endocrinol.,* 63:22.

Hillhouse, E. W., Burden, J. L., and Jones, M. T. (1975): The effect of various putative neurotransmitters on the release of corticotrophin-releasing hormone from the hypothalamus of the rat in vitro. I. The effect of acetylcholine and noradrenaline. *Neuroendocrinology,* 17:1–11.

Hiroshige, T. (1973): CRF assay by intrapituitary injection through the parapharyngeal approach and its physiological validity. In: *Brain-Pituitary-Adrenal Interrelationships,* edited by A. Brodish and E. S. Redgate, pp. 57–58. Karger, Basel.

Hodges, J. R., and Vernikos, J. (1960): The effects of hydrocortisone on the level of corticotrophin in the blood and pituitary glands of adrenalectomized and stressed adrenalectomized rats. *J. Endocrinol.,* 55:489–497.

Hökfelt, T. (1968): In vitro studies on central and peripheral monoamine neurones at the ultrastructural level. *Z. Zellforsch.,* 91:1–74.

Hökfelt, T. (1970): Electron microscopic studies on peripheral and central monoamine neurones. *Aspects of Neuroendocrinology,* edited by W. Bargmann and B. Scharrer, pp. 79–94. Springer-Verlag, Berlin.

Hökfelt, T. (1973): Possible site of action of dopamine in the hypothalamic pituitary control. *Acta Physiol. Scand.,* 89:606–608.

Jones, M. T., Brush, F. R., and Neame, R. L. B. (1972): Characteristics of fast feedback control of corticotrophin release by corticosteroids. *J. Endocrinol.,* 55:489–497.

Jones, M. T., Tiptaft, E. M., Brush, F. R., Fergusson, D. A. N., and Neame, R. L. B. (1974): Evidence for dual corticotrophin-receptor mechanisms in the feedback control of ACTH secretion. *J. Endocrinol.,* 60:223–233.

Jones, M. T., Hillhouse, E. W., and Burden, J. L. (1975): A proposed model of the neurotransmitters involved in the release of corticotrophin-releasing hormone. *J. Endocrinol. (in press).*

Kaplanski, J., Dorst, W., and Smelik, P. G. (1972): Pituitary-adrenal activity and depletion of brain catecholamines after α-methyl-p-tyrosine administration. *Eur. J. Pharmacol.,* 20:238–240.

Keesey, J. C., Wallgren, H., and McIlwain, H. (1965): The sodium, potassium and chloride of cerebral tissues; maintenance, change on stimulation and subsequent recovery. *Biochem. J.,* 95:289–300.

Kendall, J. W. (1971): Feedback control of adrenocorticotrophic hormone secretion. In: *Frontiers in Neuroendocrinology 1971,* edited by L. Martini and W. F. Ganong, pp. 177–207. Oxford University Press, New York.

Kobayashi, H., and Matsui, T. (1969): Fine structure of the median eminence and its functional significance. In: *Frontiers in Neuroendocrinology 1969,* edited by W. F. Ganong and L. Martini, pp. 1–32. Oxford University Press, New York.

Krieger, D. T. (1973): Neurotransmitter regulation of ACTH release. *Mt. Sinai J. Med.,* 40:302–314.

Krieger, D. T., and Rizzo, F. (1969): Serotonin mediation of circadian periodicity of plasma 17-hydroxycorticosteroids. *Am. J. Physiol.,* 217:1703–1707.

Krieger, D. T., Silverberg, A. I., Rizzo, F., and Krieger, H. P. (1968): Abolition of circadian periodicity of plasma 17-OH CS levels in the cat. *Am. J. Physiol.,* 215:959–962.

Krieger, H. P., and Krieger, D. T. (1970): Chemical stimulation of the brain: Effect on adrenal corticoid release. *Am. J. Physiol.*, 218:1632–1641.

Kuhar, M. J., and Aghajanian, G. K. (1973): Selective accumulation of ^{3}H-serotonin by nerve terminals of raphe neurones: An autoradiographic study. *Nature (Lond.)*, 241:187–188.

Lippa, A. S., Antelman, S. M., Fahringer, E. E., and Redgate, E. S. (1973): Relationship between catecholamines and ACTH: Effects of 6-hydroxydopamine. *Nature (Lond.)*, 241:24–25.

Lowry, O. H., Passonneau, J. V., Hesselberger, F. X., and Schulz, D. W. (1964): Effect of Ischaemia on known substrates and co-factors of the glycolytic pathway in brain. *J. Biol. Chem.*, 239:18–30.

Makara, G. B., and Stark, E. (1974): Effect of gamma-aminobutyric acid (GABA) and GABA antagonist drugs on ACTH release. *Neuroendocrinology*, 16:178–190.

Marks, B. H., Hall, M. M., and Bhattacharya, A. N. (1970): Psychopharmacological effects and pituitary-adrenal activity. *Prog. Brain Res.*, 32:57–70.

McIlwain, H. (1956): Electrical influences and speed of chemical change in the brain. *Physiol. Rev.*, 36:355–375.

Moss, R. L., Urban, I., and Cross, B. A. (1972): Microelectrophoresis of cholinergic and aminergic drugs on paraventricular neurones. *Am. J. Physiol.*, 223:310–318.

Motta, M., Mangili, G., and Martini, L. (1965): A short loop feedback in the control of ACTH secretion. *Endocrinology*, 77:392–395.

Motta, M., Schiaffini, O., Piva, F., and Martini, L. (1971): Pineal principles and the control of adrenocorticotrophin secretion. In: *The Pineal Gland*, edited by G. Wolstenholme and P. Knight, pp. 279–291. Churchill Livingstone, London.

Naumenko, E. V. (1967): Role of adrenergic and cholinergic structures in the control of the pituitary-adrenal system. *Endocrinology*, 80:69–76.

Naumenko, E. V. (1968): Hypothalamic chemoreactive structures and the regulation of pituitary-adrenal function: Effects of local injections of norepinephrine, carbachol and serotonin into the brain of guinea pigs with intact brains and after mesencephalic transection. *Brain Res.*, 11:1–10.

Oota, Y., Kobayashi, H., Nishioka, R. S., and Bern, H. A. (1974): Relationship between neurosecretory axon and ependymal terminals on capillary walls in the median eminence of several vertebrates. *Neuroendocrinology*, 16:127–136.

Pappius, H. M., and Elliott, K. A. C. (1956): Water distribution in incubated slices of brain and other tissues. *Can. J. Biochem. Physiol.*, 34:1007–1022.

Pappius, H. M., Klatzo, I., and Elliott, K. A. C. (1962): Further studies on swelling of brain slices. *Can. J. Biochem. Physiol.*, 40:885–898.

Peters, A. (1970): The fixation of central nervous tissue and the analysis of electron micrographs of the neutropil with special reference to the cerebral cortex. In: *Contemporary Research Methods in Neuro-anatomy*, edited by W. J. H. Nauta and S. O. E. Elber, pp. 56–76. Springer-Verlag, Berlin.

Popova, N. K., Maslova, L. N., and Naumenko, E. V. (1972): Serotonin and the regulation of the pituitary-adrenal axis after deafferentation of the hypothalamus. *Brain Res.*, 47:61–67.

Pruntek, S. S., and Phillipu, A. (1973): Superinfusion of the hypothalamus with GABA: The effect on the release of noradrenaline and blood pressure. *Naunyn Schmeidebergs Arch. Pharmacol.*, 276:103–118.

Robinson, N., and Wells, F. (1973): Distribution and localisation of sites of GABA metabolism in the adult rat brain. *J. Anat.*, 114:365–378.

Sachs, H., Pearson, D., Shainberg, A., Shin, S., Bryce, G., Malamed, S., and Mowles, T. (1973): Studies on the hypothalamo-neurohypophyseal complex in organ culture. In: *Recent Studies of Hypothalamic Function*, pp. 50–66. Karger, Basel.

Scapagnini, U., and Preziosi, P. (1972): Role of brain norepinephrine and serotonin in the tonic and phasic regulation of hypothalamic hypophyseal adrenal axis. *Arch. Int. Pharmacodyn. Ther. (Suppl.)*, 196:205–220.

Scapagnini, U., and Preziosi, P. (1973): Receptor involvement in the control of ACTH secretion. *Neuropharmacology*, 12:32–38.

Scapagnini, U., Van Loon, G. R., Moberg, G. P., and Ganong, W. F. (1970): Effect of α-methyl-p-tyrosine on the circadian variation of plasma corticosterone in rats. *Eur. J. Pharmacol.,* 11:266–268.

Scapagnini, U., Moberg, G. P., Van Loon, G. R., DeGroot, J., and Ganong, W. F. (1971): Relation of brain 5-hydroxytryptamine content to the diurnal variation in plasma corticosterone in the rat. *Neuroendocrinology,* 7:90–96.

Steiner, K. A., Ruf, K., and Akert, K. (1969): Steroid sensitive neurons in the rat brain: Anatomical localization and responses to neurohumours and ACTH. *Brain Res.,* 12:74–85.

Stoner, H. B., and Elson, P. M. (1971): The effect of injury on monoamine concentrations in the rat hypothalamus. *J. Neurochem.,* 18:1837–1846.

Telegdy, G., and Vermes, I. (1973): The role of serotonin in the regulation of the hypophysis-adrenal system. In: *Brain-Pituitary-Adrenal Interrelationships,* edited by A. Brodish and E. S. Redgate, pp. 332–333. Karger, Basel.

Thorack, R. M., Dufty, M. L., and Haynes, J. M. (1965): The effect of anisotonic media upon cellular ultrastructure in fresh and fixed rat brain. *Z. Zellforsch.,* 66: 690–700.

Tiptaft, E., and Jones, M. T. (1975): Structure activity relationships of various steroids upon ACTH secretion. *J. Endocrinol. (in press).*

Ulrich, R. S., and Yuwiler, A. (1973): Failure of 6-hydroxydopamine to abolish the circadian rhythm of serum corticosterone. *Endocrinology,* 92:611–614.

Van Delft, A., Kaplanski, M. L., and Smelik, P. G. (1973): Circadian periodicity of pituitary adrenal function after p-chlorophenylalanine administration in the rat. *J. Endocrinol.,* 59:465–474.

Van Loon, G. R. (1973): Brain catecholamines and ACTH secretion. In: *Frontiers in Neuroendocrinology, 1973,* edited by W. F. Ganong and L. Martini, pp. 209–247. Oxford University Press, New York.

Vermes, I., Telegdy, G., and Lissák, K. (1972): Inhibitory action of serotonin on the hypothalamus-induced ACTH release. *Acta Physiol. Acad. Sci. Hung.,* 41:95–98.

Vermes, I., Telegdy, G., and Lissák, K. (1973): Correlation between hypothalamic serotonin content and adrenal function during acute stress: Effect of adrenal corticosteroids on hypothalamic serotonin content. *Acta Physiol. Acad. Sci. Hung.,* 43:33–42.

Vernikos-Danellis, J. (1956a): Effect of stress, adrenalectomy, hypophysectomy and hydrocortisone on the corticotrophin-releasing activity of the rat median eminence. *Endocrinology,* 76:122–126.

Vernikos-Danellis, J. (1956b): Effect of rat median eminence extracts on pituitary ACTH content in normal and adrenalectomised rats. *Endocrinology,* 76:240–245.

Vernikos-Danellis, J., and Berger, L. (1973): Brain serotonin and the pituitary-adrenal system. In: *Serotonin and Behaviour,* edited by J. Barchas and E. Usdin. Academic Press, New York.

Wurtman, R. J., and Anton-Tay, F. (1969): The mammalian pineal as a neuroendocrine transducer. *Recent Prog. Horm. Res.,* 25:499–522.

Yagi, J., and Sawaki, Y. (1975): Recurrent inhibition and facilitation demonstration in the tuberoinfundibular system and effects of strychnine and picrotoxin. *Brain Res.,* 84:155–160.

Yates, F. E., and Maran, J. W. (1974): Stimulation and inhibition of adrenocorticotrophin release. In: *Handbook of Physiology, Section 7: Endocrinology,* Vol. 4, pp. 367–404. American Physiological Society, Washington, D.C.

Yates, F. E., Russel, S. M., and Maran, J. W. (1971): Brain-adenohypophyseal communication in mammals. *Ann. Rev. Physiol.,* 33:393–445.

Frontiers in Neuroendocrinology, Vol. 4,
edited by L. Martini and W. F. Ganong.
Raven Press, New York © 1976.

Chapter 8

Clinical Neuroendocrinology

G. M. Besser and C. H. Mortimer

The Medical Professorial Unit, St. Bartholomew's Hospital, London EC1A 7BE, England

Prior to the introduction of synthetic thyrotropin-releasing hormone (TRH) and gonadotropin-releasing hormone (GnRH) during the period 1969 to 1971 (Folkers et al., 1969; Burgus et al., 1970; Schally et al., 1971) clinical neuroendocrinology did not exist as a separate discipline although several dynamic tests of endocrine function linking centrally mediated mechanisms were in use to augment clinical evaluation. These included insulin-induced hypoglycemia to test ACTH and growth hormone (GH) reserve and the use of centrally acting drugs (James and Landon, 1968; Rees et al., 1971). The value of these techniques was restricted, however, and they had no intrinsic therapeutic potential.

In contrast, when the hypothalamic regulatory hormones became available in a purified synthetic form, they allowed pituitary function to be evaluated directly for the first time. It was then possible to assess the available stores of a pituitary hormone within the gland, as well as the mechanisms involved in integrating the hypothalamic influences on the pituitary with those involving higher centers and the feedback effects of the target gland secretions. An attempt could now be made in clinical practice to evaluate the changes in pituitary hormone synthesis and secretion and to try to distinguish accurately between diseases of the pituitary and hypothalamus as causes of apparent hypopituitarism. In addition, primary target gland dysfunction could be more clearly assessed. More recently it has become clear that in addition to their diagnostic usefulness hypothalamic regulatory substances may be used to treat hypothalamic and pituitary disease.

THYROTROPIN-RELEASING HORMONE

Normal Subjects

In normal subjects intravenous injection of the tripeptide TRH results in a rapid rise in serum thyrotropin (TSH) with a peak at 15 to 30 min (Fig. 8–1). There is a dose-related response in the range of 15 to 500 μg with no additional response after this. TRH is also active if given by mouth,

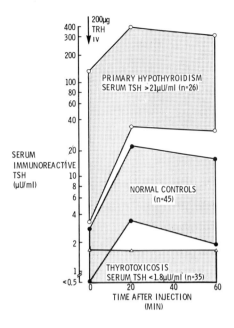

FIG. 8–1. Ranges for serum TSH levels following TRH 200 μg i.v. in normal controls and patients with thyrotoxicosis or primary hypothyroidism. (From Hall et al., 1974.)

but much larger amounts are required (Hall et al., 1970; Haigler et al., 1972; Ormston, 1972; Snyder and Utiger, 1972). Higher TSH responses are seen in women compared with men, although the administration of estrogen to males enhances pituitary responsiveness (Faglia et al., 1973a; Mortimer et al., 1974a). Increasing age in males has been reported to result in a blunting of the TSH response, although this may not be the case in females (Snyder and Utiger, 1972). Circadian variation in pituitary responsiveness to the releasing hormone alters in accordance with the evening rise in basal TSH levels, the greatest response being seen at 11 P.M. (Weeke, 1974). Following TRH there is a rise in serum triiodothyronine (T_3) levels peaking at 2 to 4 hr and serum thyroxine (T_4) at 8 hr (Lawton, 1972). Continuous intravenous infusions or repeated daily administration blunt pituitary responsiveness, probably owing to exhaustion of pituitary stores and to an increase in circulating thyroid hormone levels (Haigler et al., 1971; Gual et al., 1972; Fairclough et al., 1973). Exogenous administration of either T_3 or T_4 suppresses the TSH response in a dose-related manner (Evered et al., 1973; Shenkman et al., 1973). Since the stimulating effect of TRH is blocked by an increase in circulating thyroid hormone level acting at the pituitary, it seems likely that this negative feedback is the principal regulatory mechanism for TSH secretion. It is not yet clear if the secretion of TRH by the hypothalamus itself is altered in humans by varying the concentrations of circulating T_3 and T_4.

Analogues of TRH have been synthesized, including a proline methyl derivative with enhanced biological action. This enhancement may be due to increased binding avidity at the receptor site (Burgus et al., 1973).

Primary Thyroid Disease

A standard clinical intravenous TRH test has been developed which differentiates both hyper- and hypothyroidism from the euthyroid state (Ormston et al., 1971). TRH (200 μg) is given intravenously, and blood is sampled for immunoreactive TSH at 0, 20, and 60 min. TSH rather than T_3 or T_4 must be measured (Fig. 8–1) since only very small changes in the latter hormones occur and such changes are difficult to evaluate in a routine clinical assay (Lawton, 1972). The test is devoid of important side effects, although many patients experience transient flushing and nausea with a deep urethral sensation described as a desire to micturate; this is thought to be due to smooth-muscle spasm.

In *hyperthyroidism,* whether due to Graves' disease or a nodular goiter, the high circulating T_3 and T_4 levels block the action of TRH and there is an insignificant rise in TSH. However, a small response may be obtained by giving larger doses. The response may be suppressed for many weeks after the return of clinical euthyroidism and normal circulating levels of thyroid hormones (Von zur Mühlen et al., 1971). The standard 200 μg TRH test has proved extremely reliable in differential diagnosis of clinically occult or borderline T_4 or T_3 thyrotoxicosis since a normal response excludes this diagnosis. Before the introduction of this test the only equivalent procedure was the T_3 suppression test, which involved a radioactive iodine uptake study before and after 7 days of treatment with a supraphysiological dose of T_3 (80 to 120 μg/day). Not only was this test time-consuming, it was potentially dangerous since it could exacerbate the clinical manifestations of thyrotoxicosis, precipitating heart failure, angina, or atrial fibrillation.

The TSH response to TRH in Graves' disease may be variable. If it is associated with hyperthyroidism the TSH response is uniformly suppressed, but some 60% of patients with Graves' disease who are clinically euthyroid may also fail to respond normally. These patients usually also fail to suppress their thyroidal ^{131}I uptake after T_3 administration, although some discrepancies between the tests have been recognized (Ormston et al., 1973). Presumably this suppression of pituitary TSH secretion in the euthyroid patient with Graves' disease results from a significant proportion of the thyroid hormone production being dependent on nonpituitary thyroid-stimulating immunoglobulins. Similarly euthyroid patients on replacement therapy may not respond to TRH (Evered et al., 1973). Patients with nodular goiters may also be clinically euthyroid but fail to respond to TRH.

The TRH test may be useful in the diagnosis of primary *hypothyroidism,* since although basal serum TSH levels are often elevated there may be overlap with the normal range in mild cases. The TSH response to the releasing hormone is excessive in patients with primary hypothyroidism (Fig. 8–1). This test has now replaced the TSH stimulation test for confirming the presence of mild hypothyroidism. However, it has become apparent that some patients may have normal or mildly elevated basal TSH levels, show an excessive response to TRH, and yet be clinically euthyroid. It is thought that these individuals have a reduced thyroid reserve secretory capacity; the term "subclinical hypothyroidism" has been linked with this condition. It is typically seen in euthyroid patients with thyroiditis or following partial thyroidectomy. However, this appears to be a misnomer since there is no clinical evidence of thyroid insufficiency and circulating thyroid hormone levels are normal. It seems more logical to conclude that these patients are in a compensated state in which the thyroid gland has a reduced reserve capacity for hormone production, but normal T_3 and T_4 levels are maintained by the increased drive of higher TSH levels. Data suggesting that these patients are at a disadvantage have not yet been presented, and for the time being there is no clear indication that they should be treated with thyroxine although prolonged follow-up is essential.

Pituitary and Hypothalamic Disease

In *secondary* (*pituitary*) *hypothyroidism* the TSH response may be normal but is often impaired 20 min after 200 μg TRH i.v. is given (Fleischer et al., 1972; Hall et al., 1972). In patients with *tertiary* (*hypothalamic*) *hypothyroidism,* TSH secretion usually reaches normal levels, although the 60-min value is frequently higher than that at 20 min and may be excessive. This is called the delayed type of response and is never seen in normal subjects. This pattern is characteristic of patients with predominantly hypothalamic disease but an intact pituitary. Occasionally it may draw attention to an otherwise unsuspected hypothalamic lesion. A group of children with hypothalamic hypothyroidism and short stature have been described in whom repeated administration of TRH resulted in a return of normal thyroid function (Costom et al., 1971; Snyder and Utiger, 1973). Exceptions to the classic types of response in pituitary and hypothalamic disease often occur, and the delayed pattern must not be considered of significant diagnostic importance without further corroborative studies (Patel and Burger, 1973).

Other Diseases

In Cushing's syndrome and corticosteroid-treated patients, the TSH response to TRH may be impaired or absent, the response returning when the circulating corticosteroid levels return to normal (Hall et al., 1972; Faglia et al., 1973*b*). Conversely, we have also seen clinically euthyroid patients with Addison's disease (primary adrenocortical failure) who show excessive TSH responses to TRH before treatment. When these patients were retested after replacement therapy comprised of physiological doses of cortisol and fludrocortisone, their TSH responses were normal. The TSH response to TRH is also greater in patients with liver disease and renal failure; since a successful renal transplant results in a return to normal, the effect is thought to be due to impaired blood clearance of TSH and/or TRH (Pokroy et al., 1974).

TRH and Prolactin

Although it was assumed that each hypothalamic regulatory hormone controlled only one pituitary hormone, this has not proved to be the case. TRH releases prolactin in humans as well as in animals (Jacobs et al., 1971). This is a dose-related response when TRH is given intravenously in increasing doses from 6 to 100 μg, the latter dose causing the maximal response (Jacobs et al., 1971). However, it is clear that there are different pituitary cell mechanisms controlling TSH and prolactin secretion since the effects can be dissociated. Thus in thyrotoxicosis the TSH response is suppressed more than the prolactin response (Sachson et al., 1972); and the TSH but not the prolactin response is inhibited by GH release inhibiting hormone (GIH; Hall et al., 1973).

The time course and character of hormone release during TRH infusions are also different, marked pulsatility of prolactin release being seen in contrast to the smoother TSH response (Mortimer et al., 1974a). However, there are similarities since L-DOPA reduces both the prolactin and TSH responses to TRH (Spaulding et al., 1972; Noel et al., 1973). Although TRH is probably not the physiological prolactin-releasing hormone, it may be used to assess pituitary prolactin reserve in normal subjects and patients with pituitary or hypothalamic disease. Responses are absent in Sheehan's syndrome, whereas prolactin levels may rise excessively in the galactorrhea-amenorrhea syndrome and in some patients with pituitary tumors.

TRH and Other Hormones

In normal males there is a small rise in serum FSH levels following bolus injections or infusions of TRH (Mortimer et al., 1973a, 1974a). This response is suppressed by estrogen administration. A similar rise in FSH has not been recorded in normal, hypothyroid, or postmenopausal females, although stimulation of LH secretion by TRH at midcycle has been described in some normal women (Franchimont, 1972). TRH may also cause GH release in some patients with acromegaly (Irie and Tsushima, 1972; Faglia et al., 1973b). This may be the result of the lack of receptor specificity on the membranes of the tumor cells and does not necessarily indicate that TRH has a structural similarity to GH-releasing hormone (GRH). The response is suppressed by GIH (Carr et al., 1975).

Despite the multiplicity of actions of TRH, in clinical practice a combined test with GnRH and insulin-induced hypoglycemia can be used for evaluating pituitary hormonal reserve. Plasma TSH, prolactin, cortisol (for ACTH), LH, FSH, and GH are measured over 2 hr. The response to each stimulus is the same whether it is given alone or in combination (Mortimer et al., 1973a). This indicates that there is no competition between the mechanisms controlling the release of hormones at the pituitary level in man although this has been suggested in rats (Guillemin, 1968).

Therapeutic Value of TRH

TRH has been used in the treatment of carcinoma of the thyroid (Fairclough et al., 1973); the patients received infusions or ingested tablets of TRH. Both regimens were effective in increasing serum TSH levels, although the agent was at least 50 times more active when given intravenously than when administered orally (Haigler et al., 1972). TRH therapy caused the TSH level to rise into the range normally found in primary hypothyroidism without the patient being clinically hypothyroid, and it was hoped that this would result in an increased uptake of ^{131}I by the malignant tumor and its metastases.

The tripeptide has also been found to have central stimulating effects in hypophysectomized animals and was reported to produce transient improvement in mental depression in humans (Kastin et al., 1972; Prange et al., 1972). However, in a double-blind crossover trial, TRH was found to be ineffective when an oral dose of 40 mg/day for 7 days was compared to placebo (Mountjoy et al., 1974). Its use has also been suggested for enhancing milk production in cows and possibly in mothers with large families in developing countries.

Assays

Recent work has been directed to the development of a radioimmunoassay for TRH. Although antisera have been raised, the sensitivity of the assays has not been great enough to allow measurement of circulating levels (Jeffcoate and White, 1974). It is hoped that more sensitive assays will be developed so that further advances may be made in our understanding of the physiological control of pituitary function. It is pertinent in this regard to note the work of Gilbert and her associates (1975) in the development of an ultrasensitive cytochemical bioassay that can measure TRH in femtogram per milliliter amounts.

GONADOTROPIN-RELEASING HORMONE

The classic experiments of Harris (1950), Harris and Johnson (1950), McCann (1962), and McCann and Dhariwal (1966) in animals led to the concept that the hypothalamus regulated the release of LH and FSH by means of two releasing hormones, LRH and FRH, which were carried to the anterior pituitary by the hypothalamic portal circulation. However, Schally et al. (1971) were able to isolate only a single GnRH—the decapeptide commonly called LRH—from extracts of porcine hypothalami. Further work showed that this hormone was capable of stimulating the release of both LH and FSH from the pituitary, although under most circumstances more LH than FSH was released. The question remains open as to the identity of a separate FRH. Preliminary evidence was provided by Bowers et al. (1973) who isolated a fraction which produced FSH release *in vitro* although it was inactive *in vivo*. The weight of evidence at present suggests that although there may be a second GnRH with predominant FRH activity the single decapeptide is capable of producing differential changes in gonadotropins by interacting with the feedback effects of gonadal steroids. We feel that there are no conceptual reasons which necessitate a separate FRH, and consequently we have used the term gonadotropin-releasing hormone (GnRH) in this chapter.

Normal Subjects

Following the initial isolation and description of its structure, GnRH was synthesized by many laboratories and is available for physiological evaluation (Geiger et al., 1971; Sievertsson et al., 1971). In normal adult human subjects, as in animals, GnRH causes an increase in both LH and FSH in a dose-related manner when 25 to 500 μg is given as an intravenous bolus. However, less FSH is secreted than LH (Besser et al., 1972a). Following bolus injections the rapid rise in both gonadotropins appears to be simultaneous. However, if the decapeptide is infused continuously in normal males, the rise in FSH occurs first (within 3 to 10 min) and the rise in LH later (9 to 20 min). The LH levels continue to rise after the FSH has reached a plateau at 20 to 30 min. In addition, secretion of the gonadotropins occurs in pulsatile patterns which are asynchronous for the two hormones despite continuous infusion of the releasing hormone. The time course of release is clearly different for each gonadotropin. It seems likely that there are periods when the pituitary gonadotrop is refractory to the action of the releasing hormone, and this refractory period differs for each hormone (Mortimer et al., 1973b). Further work has shown that when GnRH is administered immunoreactive GnRH levels may reach 249 to 580 pg/ml in the systemic circulation before any rise in LH is seen; the FSH response occurs when GnRH levels are much lower (30 to 221 pg/ml). It appears therefore that the threshold for FSH secretion is lower than that for LH, and there is a clear lag period between the rise in circulating levels of GnRH and pituitary secretion of the gonadotropins.

Treatment with small doses of ethinyl estradiol (30 μg/day for 3 days) suppresses the gonadotropin responses in males, and FSH is more highly suppressed than LH (Mortimer et al., 1973c). In other studies we have shown that gonadotropin responses to GnRH are suppressed within 30 min if 17β-estradiol is infused to reach levels just above the normal male range. Since the releasing hormone was infused simultaneously with the estrogen in these studies, the data suggest that the site of negative estrogen feedback in the male is the pituitary. Conclusive evidence for a positive estrogen feedback mechanism at the pituitary level in males is lacking, although this has been suggested by some authors.

Large doses of testosterone propionate (100 mg/day i.m. for 4 to 6 days) in normal males result in suppression of basal gonadotropin levels but little change in the LH response to the releasing hormone, despite an elevation of circulating testosterone levels above the normal range. The FSH response is clearly reduced. Similar results have been reported by Von zur Mühlen and Köbberline (1973), who administered 100 mg testosterone enanthate weekly for 4 weeks. This treatment eventually diminished gonadotropin responses to the releasing hormone. The effects of testosterone may be due in part to the conversion of testosterone to estrogen, since systemic estrogen levels do not have to rise above the normal range to produce a negative feedback effect on the pituitary.

It seems likely that in males the feedback effects of testosterone on LH release in response to endogenous GnRH are mediated through conversion to estrogen. There may also be a direct effect of testosterone on basal gonadotropin levels by an action at the hypothalamic level; the diminishing response to GnRH over several weeks of testosterone administration may be due to a failure of releasing hormone synthesis in the hypothalamus, resulting in inadequate stores of releasable gonadotropin. The greater suppressive effect of testosterone (as well as of estrogen) on FSH secretion has been noted during administration of this hormone to normal males (Lee et al., 1972). It appears therefore that, although less time is required for FSH release than for LH, certain dose levels of estrogen or testosterone result in a greater percentage fall in FSH. Recovery from suppression was reported to be quicker for LH than FSH (Lee et al., 1972), although Von zur Mühlen and Köberling (1973) reported that there was no difference. (These conflicting results may be due to the fact that different doses of testosterone were used.)

Dihydrotestosterone (DHT) infusions over 48 hr reportedly suppress basal levels of LH and FSH (Stewart-Bentley et al., 1974), although the effect on the latter is small. DHT is not significantly converted to estrogen in the body. However, DHT infusions in supraphysiological doses have no effect on the pituitary responses to GnRH infusion (Mortimer et al., 1975a). This suggests that any gonadotropin-suppressing effect of DHT at the pituitary level is weak compared to estrogen, but DHT may act primarily at the hypothalamic level.

Apart from gonadal steroids, a substance often called "inhibin" has clear effects on FSH secretion. This substance is produced during the end stages of spermatogenesis and inhibits FSH secretion; it is probably a protein. During long-term GnRH therapy in patients with hypothalamic-pituitary disease, the FSH response to the releasing hormone diminishes as spermatogenesis is induced, while LH secretion remains unchanged. Since this occurs despite the presence of injected releasing hormone, it is clear that the site of inhibin feedback is the pituitary (Mortimer et al., 1974b). The differential feedback effects on LH and FSH occur despite the administration of the single synthetic decapeptide, suggesting pituitary responses can be modified differentially by gonadal steroids and inhibin.

The influence of gonadal steroids on pituitary responsiveness to the releasing hormone in females is less well understood. During a normal menstrual cycle LH and FSH secretion from the pituitary results in steroidogenesis in the ovaries. The usually accepted concept is that the induced rise in circulating estrogens results in a midcycle surge in GnRH secretion with subsequent LH and FSH peaks and ovulation. There is then a rise in progesterone with a fall in gonadotropin levels, although the latter remain higher than in the follicular phase.

Support for the concept of altered pituitary responsiveness by gonadal steroids is provided by Nillius and Wide (1972) and Yen et al. (1972). These authors showed that serial injections of the releasing hormone throughout the normal menstrual cycle resulted in a characteristic pattern. There was a relatively small response during the early follicular phase and a larger response in the luteal phase; but the greatest rise in both gonadotropins was seen at midcycle, coincident with the rise in plasma estradiol. This suggested that there was a positive feedback of estrogen at the pituitary level, enhancing the response to GnRH. However, the demonstration of a rise in circulating GnRH (up to 17 pg/ml) at midcycle suggests that there is also increased secretion and probably synthesis of the releasing hormone (Arimura et al., 1974a). The positive feedback effect of estrogens has also been demonstrated following intramuscular administration of 1 mg 17β-estradiol in normal females; after 48 to 72 hr there is a rise in LH but not FSH (Nillius and Wide, 1971). Larger doses of estrogens suppress gonadotropin levels, and the response to the releasing hormone may be suppressed in females taking oral contraceptives. The action of progesterone results in suppression of pituitary responsiveness to the releasing hormone in rats (Arimura and Schally, 1970) and in normal women. In part, this effect may be responsible for the modulation of gonadotropin secretion in the menstrual cycle.

Acromegaly

GnRH has been reported to cause the release of GH in acromegaly. This is further evidence of the nonspecificity of the pituitary cell receptor in this condition (Faglia et al., 1973c).

Hypogonadism

In clinical practice a routine test is comprised of giving 100 μg GnRH as an intravenous bolus. A normal range of response can be defined by sampling blood for LH and FSH over 60 min. Initial studies showed that the condition of isolated gonadotropin deficiency was in fact due to a hypothalamic deficiency of the releasing hormone rather than to pituitary cell dysfunction; these patients had both LH and FSH responses to exogenous GnRH (Marshall et al., 1972; Mortimer et al., 1973d). Patients who do not respond to a single 100-μg injection do respond after repeated administration of the releasing hormone. The use of the test in other forms of clinical hypogonadism has not been of great diagnostic value since it is not possible to distinguish consistently between hypothalamic and pituitary disease. An absent or impaired gonadotropin response to the releasing hormone generally suggests hypothalamic or pituitary dysfunction, although a normal response does not exclude underlying pathology. Exaggerated responses are seen in primary gonadal failure but may also occur in patients with hypothalamic or pituitary disease and are common in the galactorrhea-amenorrhea syndrome with hyperprolactinemia. The reason for this is uncertain but may be related to the fact that prolactin in high concentrations inhibits the action of gonadotropins on the ovary and testis, thereby reducing or preventing the normal cyclical variation in sex hormone levels. As a result, normal feedback mechanisms are not maintained (Mortimer et al., 1973d; McNatty et al., 1974; McNeilly, 1974; Thorner et al., 1974). There does not appear to be competition between gonadotropin and prolactin release at the pituitary level in humans (Mortimer et al., 1973a), although such competition may be present in rats (Ben David et al., 1971).

A review of 155 patients with hypothalamic-pituitary-gonadal dysfunction showed that although 137 were clinically hypogonadal at the time of testing all but nine had a rise in either LH or FSH when GnRH was injected (Mortimer et al., 1973d). Therefore although these patients were not secreting gonadotropins spontaneously, they had gonadotrops capable of being stimulated by GnRH. This suggested that although the test could not differentiate between hypothalamic and pituitary disease, the releasing hormone might have therapeutic potential.

The time course of the effects of GnRH is the same whether it is given intravenously, intramuscularly, or subcutaneously. There are no side effects after subcutaneous administration except for slight and brief discomfort at the injection site, and so this route has been used for long-term therapy. Although GnRH is absorbed via the nasal mucosa, much more material is required to produce the same effect as subcutaneous administration (London et al., 1973; Mortimer et al., 1974c).

Subcutaneous GnRH therapy has proved to be effective in male patients with clinical hypogonadism due to so-called isolated gonadotropin deficiency or to hypothalamic or pituitary tumors. Self-administration of 500 μg s.c. every 8 hr for up to 1 yr has been reported to induce continuing synthesis as well as release of the gonadotropins in the 12 patients so far reported (Mortimer et al., 1974*b*) and in 10 additional patients (*unpublished observations*). In five patients (two prepubertal boys with craniopharyngiomas and three adults: one with a craniopharyngioma, one with a diffuse hypothalamic tumor, and one with isolated gonadotropin deficiency) the initial pattern of gonadotropin response was similar to that reported in normal prepubertal patients: FSH responses were similar to those of adults, but the LH responses were smaller (Franchimont, 1972). After 4 to 6 weeks of therapy this pattern was changed and LH responses were greater than FSH responses. Prolonged therapy in the patients produced a rise in androgen levels and improved pubertal ratings in prepubertal subjects; in adults potency returned with improved virilization. However, the improved sexual function returned after only 3 to 16 days of treatment, before there was much rise in serum testosterone. This discrepancy between potency and circulating androgen levels prompted the suggestion that GnRH might have a direct effect on behavior separate from any endocrine-mediated actions. Effects of GnRH on sexual behavior have been reported in hypophysectomized and ovariectomized rats (Moss and McCann, 1973; Pfaff, 1973). Four patients (one acromegalic, one with craniopharyngioma, and two with isolated gonadotropin deficiency syndromes) have now been treated for more than a year, and spermatogenesis has occurred in each. Total sperm counts of 7.8 to 432×10^6 with a 40% to 70% motility have been recorded. An example is shown in Fig. 8–2.

A therapeutic trial involving the use of GnRH in 10 infertile males with normal external genitalia who clinically were considered to be endocrinologically normal (they had normal urinary gonadotropins measured by mouse bioassay) was carried out by Zarate et al. (1973*b*). Treatment with 500 μg b.i.d. for 6 months resulted in an increase in total sperm count in three of four patients with azoospermia. The maximum sperm count reached was 6 million. Three of six patients with oligospermia showed an increase from 1 to 5 million sperms to over 10 million in 3 months. The count then fell despite continued therapy. Three other patients with oligospermia had no significant improvement, although all had increased sperm motility. Releasing hormone therapy merits further evaluation in the therapy of hypogonadism due to organic causes, whereas its place in psychogenic impotence remains to be explored.

Attempts have been made to induce ovulation with GnRH. In 1972 Akande and his associates reported a series of studies in eight patients with secondary amenorrhea. One had anorexia nervosa, one thyrotoxicosis, one diabetes mellitis, and one amenorrhea after oral contraceptive therapy; the diagnosis was not recorded in four. The patients received various regimens, and although a rise in gonadotropins was recorded ovulation was produced

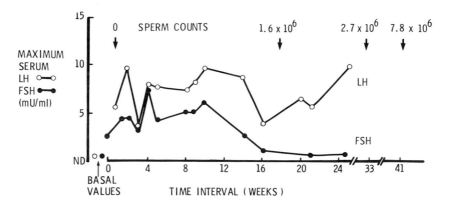

FIG. 8–2. Maximum serum LH and FSH levels following a therapeutic dose of GnRH 500 μg s.c. every 8 hr recorded over 25 weeks of therapy in a male with "isolated gonadotropin deficiency." Increasing total sperm counts are shown at the top. (From Mortimer et al., 1974b.)

in only one. This patient had ovulated spontaneously while basal sampling was being carried out over the preceding 28 to 35 days. Keller (1973) investigated the therapeutic possibility of GnRH, and although ovulation and pregnancy occurred in his series it was difficult to determine whether it was due to GnRH or the concomitant administration of clomiphene.

Breckwoldt et al. (1974) concluded that the synthetic decapeptide was not suitable for induction of ovulation since its value was too closely limited by pituitary responsiveness. Zanartu and associates (1973) produced ovulation in two of 16 women with secondary amenorrhea following depot medroxyprogesterone acetate or chlormadinone therapy for contraceptive purposes, but the possibility of spontaneous ovulation was not completely excluded. However, we produced ovarian steroidogenesis, apparent ovulation, and menstruation with GnRH in two of four patients with anorexia nervosa; they had had well-documented secondary amenorrhea for 5 to 7 yr. These patients were either at their ideal body weight or 3.5 to 5.8 kg below it, and each was unresponsive to clomiphene. Each received GnRH (500 μg s.c.) every 8 hr for 14 days, with human chorionic gonadotropin (HCG) 4,500 units i.m. on day 14 (Fig. 8–3). However, ovulation had apparently occurred due to releasing hormone therapy alone, since plasma progesterone had risen from undetectable levels to 6.4 and 9.9 ng/ml on day 14 prior to the HCG administration. Two further patients treated with GnRH had a return of clomiphene responsiveness together with ovulation and menstruation (Mortimer et al., 1975b). These studies also showed that despite the amenorrhea in treated anorexia nervosa, the pituitary contained adequate stores of gonadotropins. The gonadotropins were not being released presumably because of an acquired deficiency or availability of the endogenous releasing hormone. It is possible therefore that in anorexia nervosa there is a disturbance of the normal mechanisms involved in GnRH synthesis and

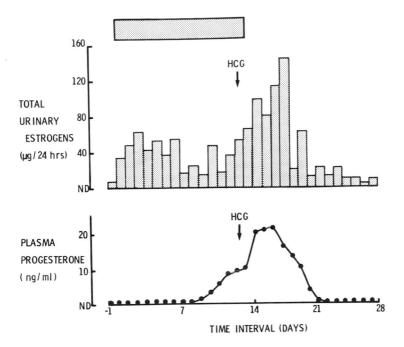

FIG. 8–3. GnRH therapy, 500 μg s.c. every 8 hr for 14 days (*horizontal bar*), in a female with anorexia nervosa. Human chorionic gonadotropin (HCG) 4,500 units i.m. was given on day 14.

secretion. Thus there may be a state of acquired GnRH deficiency secondary to psychogenic influences. This may be related in part to weight loss, since a return to ideal body weight often results in a return of menstruation. In four patients treated with GnRH on days 1 through 7 and then on days 12, 13, and 14, secondary and spontaneous rises in basal gonadotropins and estrogen were seen during the third and fourth weeks of the treatment cycle without additional therapy. This suggested that the induced rise in circulating estrogens resulted in a positive feedback at the hypothalamic level. In severe anorexia nervosa there may be impaired initial LH and FSH response to small doses of GnRH (Palmer et al., 1975). However, repeated administration may also prove to be of therapeutic value in these patients.

Assays for GnRH

Radioimmunoassays have been developed for GnRH, and a rise in circulating levels at midcycle was shown by Arimura et al. (1974a). Our unpublished observations show that this occurs in brief pulses that are not necessarily paralleled by changes in circulating gonadotropins. Further evidence for this discrepancy comes from infusion studies with the releasing hormone; these have shown asynchronous pulsatile release of LH and FSH despite rising, plateaued, or falling GnRH levels. The peripheral releasing hormone levels and gonadotropin levels were clearly not in phase (Mortimer et al., 1975b). Pulsatile releasing hormone levels measured by bioassay have also been noted in postmenopausal females (Seyler and Reichlin, 1973). In animals being used to produce anti-GnRH antiserum, there is gonadal atrophy; and administration of anti-GnRH to cycling rats on the morning of proestrous prevents the LH and FSH surge and ovulation in the afternoon (Arimura et al., 1973a,b; Koch et al., 1973).

The half-life of GnRH in the circulation is less than 5 min, and inactivation occurs rapidly due to the cleavage of pyro-Glu-His from the N-terminal end of the molecule (Redding et al., 1973).

Analogues of GnRH

Various analogues have been synthesized that have enhanced activity, due either to increased binding to pituitary cells or to their ability to resist enzymatic degradation. D-Ala^6-des-Gly^{10}-GnRH ethylamide and D-Leu^6-des-Gly^{10}-GnRH ethylamide have 15 to 60 times the activity of the decapeptide in rats on the release of gonadotropins (Arimura et al., 1974b; Vilchez-Martinez et al., 1974a). Clinical trials are now in progress with these superactive analogues. Inhibitory derivatives have also been synthesized and may someday provide a nonsteroidal form of contraception (Vilchez-Martinez et al., 1974b).

GROWTH HORMONE-RELEASING HORMONE

To date there is no authentic hypothalamic GH-releasing hormone (GRH) shown to be active in man, although clear evidence for its existence has been elicited in animals (Sandow et al., 1972). Since GnRH can be used to treat hypogonadotropic hypogonadism, there is great interest in obtaining a GRH that could be used to treat patients with small stature who are GH-deficient.

GROWTH HORMONE-INHIBITING HORMONE

The 14 amino acid polypeptide isolated from ovine hypothalami inhibits the release of GH from rat and human pituitary cells *in vitro* and from rats *in vivo* (Brazeau et al., 1973). The synthetic material either in the oxidized (cyclized) or reduced (linear) form has the full biological activity of the native peptide. Early work with this hormone showed that it inhibited GH secretion in humans during exercise, insulin-induced hypoglycemia, arginine infusions, sleep, and L-DOPA (Hall et al., 1973; Prange Hansen et al., 1973; Siler et al., 1973; Besser et al., 1974a; Mortimer et al., 1974d). Plasma GH was also reduced in patients with acromegaly following intravenous, intramuscular, and subcutaneous injections of GIH, as well as throughout infusions lasting 28 hr (Hall et al., 1973; Besser et al., 1974b). However, the effects after bolus injections or following infusions are transient, and there is a rapid rebound in plasma GH indicating that the biologically active half-life of GIH is extremely short (Fig. 8–4). This tetradecapeptide also inhibits the TSH and FSH responses to TRH (Hall et al., 1973; Yen et al., 1974) and was shown to lower the serum TSH in an acromegalic and thyrotoxic patient who was euthyroid on carbimazole therapy at the time of testing (Besser et al., 1974b). It does not affect the serum prolactin response to TRH or insulin-induced hypoglycemia in normal males, although levels have been reported to fall in acromegaly (Hall et al., 1973; Yen et al., 1974). The gonadotropin responses to GnRH and ACTH as well as the plasma

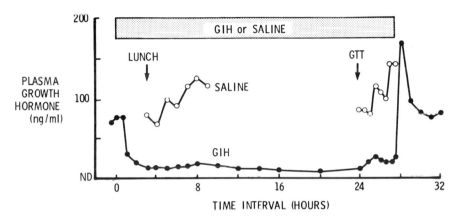

FIG. 8–4. Effects of a 28 hr infusion of GIH or saline on plasma GH levels in an acromegalic patient. GTT, oral glucose tolerance test. (From Besser et al., 1974b.)

corticosteroid responses during insulin-induced hypoglycemia are unaffected (Hall et al., 1973).

GIH acts on endocrine glands other than the pituitary. Administration of GIH inhibits insulin and glucagon secretion (Alberti et al., 1973; Alford et al., 1974; Mortimer et al., 1974d). Insulin release after tolbutamide is blocked (Gerich et al., 1974). Other actions include inhibition of the secretion of gastrin and gastric acid in the Zollinger-Ellison syndrome, vasoactive intestinal polypeptide (VIP), and gastric inhibiting peptide (GIP). It may also inhibit gut motility (Bloom et al., 1974). The wide variety of hormones affected by this polypeptide suggests that it interferes in some way with regulating mechanisms common to a variety of cells capable of hormone secretion. This appears to be by a direct action on the somatotrop and pancreas, and probably other secretory cells as well. During infusions lasting up to 28 hr, it does not seem to affect the synthesis of GH, insulin, or glucagon since a rapid rebound is seen when the infusion is stopped. The action of GIH on the cell may be due primarily to interference with exocytosis, although inhibition of the cyclic AMP system may be involved (Brazeau and Guillemin, 1974; Hertelendy et al., 1974).

GIH is found outside the hypothalamus. Recent work by Arimura et al. (1975) suggests that it is present in high concentration in the pancreas, stomach, and duodenum. Despite the suppression of so many different hormones, GIH treatment is associated with remarkably few side effects. Syncope after intravenous infusion, arousal from sleep, and cramps and diarrhea have been reported (Parker et al., 1974). We have not observed such effects, although with doses up to 10 μg/min some patients report sinking feelings in the chest. Impaired platelet function has been reported after prolonged and repeated infusions of linear GIH in baboons, but this remains to be confirmed in humans (Ricketts, 1975).

In view of its action, GIH may prove useful in the medical treatment of conditions associated with GH excess. GH secretion in acromegaly can be reduced in a dose-related manner. The minimum effective dose is approximately 1.3 μg/min (Besser et al., 1974a; Yen et al., 1974). However, this form of therapy may be superceded since it has been reported that the orally active ergot alkaloid bromocriptine lowers GH levels in acromegaly (Liuzzi et al., 1972). This compound appears to act as a dopaminergic agonist and during long-term therapy it lowers GH levels in acromegaly (Fig. 8–5) but not in normal subjects. The treatment leads to marked clinical improvement and amelioration of the associated diabetes mellitus (Thorner et al., 1975).

Many believe that GIH may prove beneficial in the management of diabetes mellitus. It is held that the inappropriately elevated GH levels seen in some diabetics may be etiologically important in the development of the angiopathic complications, and that oversecretion of GH and glucagon may contribute to the instability of brittle diabetes. If this is so then the combined GH release and glucagon release inhibiting activity of GIH should be beneficial. No work has yet been reported on the effects of GIH on diabetic angiopathy. Our studies and those of Gerich et al. (1974) showed that simultaneous administration of GIH and insulin enhances the glucose-lowering action of insulin (Fig. 8–6), but there is no evidence as yet that it produces better control of the blood glucose. Preprandial administration of a prolonged-action form of GIH such as the protamine zinc derivative (Besser et al., 1974b) may hold greater promise.

Administration of GIH may also prove effective in the diagnosis and treatment of glucagon-producing pancreatic tumors, since hormone levels are dramatically reduced and there is a fall in blood glucose levels (Mortimer et al., 1974d). Insulinomas may be similarly treated, and shorter courses of therapy may be useful in reducing gastrin, gastric acidity, and the pain and bleeding associated with gastric or duodenal ulceration (Bloom et al., 1974). This may provide valuable time for preoperative assessment and correction of

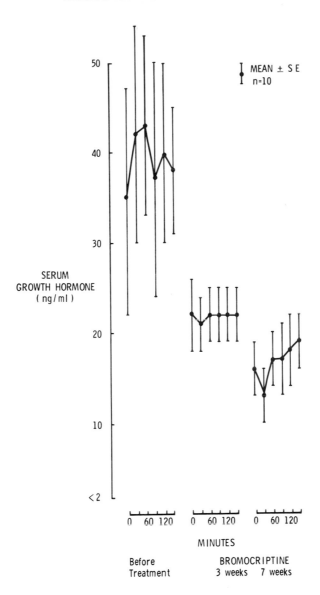

FIG. 8–5. Serum GH levels during oral glucose tolerance tests in 10 acromegalics before and after 3 and 7 weeks of therapy with bromocriptine. (From Thorner et al., 1975.)

electrolyte and blood loss especially in patients with the Zollinger-Ellison syndrome.

VIP levels were also reduced in a patient with the watery diarrhea syndrome of Verner and Morrison associated with a pancreatic tumor. Analogues less quickly destroyed than GIH are being sought for long-term

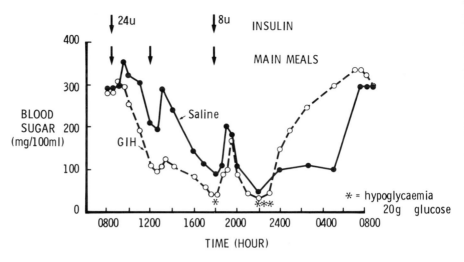

FIG. 8—6. Effects of a 24-hr infusion of GIH (*dashed line*) or saline (*solid line*) on blood sugar in an unstable diabetic. Glucose 20 g i.v. was given when hypoglycemia symptoms occurred at the points indicated by the asterisks.

therapy since the combination with protamine zinc, arachis oil, and 16% gelatin prolong the action of GIH for a maximum of only 5 hr. Apart from the wide-ranging therapeutic significance of GIH, it also provides a useful tool for exploration of hormonal factors controlling carbohydrate metabolism. Early work in this field suggests that glucagon may well play an important role in the maintenance of basal blood glucose levels (Alford et al., 1974).

Radioimmunoassays are currently being devised for assaying endogenous GIH, although in view of the short half-life (less than 5 min) it may prove difficult to measure the hormone in the circulation (Arimura et al., 1974c). However, it is clear that this release-inhibiting hormone has opened up a completely new field in understanding the regulation of GH secretion and may yet prove to be important in the physiological control of many other hormones.

CORTICOTROPIN-RELEASING HORMONE

The identity of corticotropin-releasing hormone (CRH) remains a mystery despite the fact that extracts of the median eminence and posterior pituitary were shown two decades ago to release ACTH (Saffran et al., 1955). The CRH secreted during stress in rats was differentiated from vasopressin by bioassay, although insufficient amounts have been available for the characterization of its structure (Anderson, 1966). A partial amino acid sequence has been described, but the exact nature of CRN is still unclear (Schally and

Bowers, 1964). Vasopressin certainly can act as a CRH, but it does not seem to act in concentrations that are likely to occur physiologically.

HYPOTHALAMIC HORMONES AFFECTING MELANOCYTE-STIMULATING HORMONE SECRETION

Melanocyte-stimulating hormone (MSH) is a pigment-regulating hormone found in the pars intermedia in lower animals, but recently considerable doubt has been cast on the concept that it exists at all in man (Bloomfield et al., 1974). The pigment hormone in humans appears to be ACTH, and the immunoreactive β-MSH-like activity previously ascribed to MSH appears to be due to the circulation of a lipotropin that contains a sequence identical to that which has been called β-MSH. Extracts of hypothalami from both light- and dark-adapted frogs inhibit MSH secretion from the pars intermedia of the dark-adapted frog. In 1971 Nair et al. prepared an extract of bovine hypothalami that consisted of two active peptides with MSH release-inhibiting (MIH) activity in frogs. The amino acid sequences of the MIH are different, although there is a unifying link between them in that they are all contained within the structure of oxytocin. There appears to be species specificity among related peptides with MIH activity. It has also been suggested that there is an MSH-releasing hormone (MRH). This is a pentapeptide consisting of the N-terminal amino acids of oxytocin except that the structure is linear instead of cyclic (Kastin et al., 1968, 1969). Although active in lower forms, MIH and MRH do not appear to be active in normal human subjects, and MIH has not yet been shown to be effective in controlling the hyperpigmentation associated with Nelson's syndrome.

PROLACTIN RELEASE-INHIBITING HORMONE

Prolactin is known to be predominantly under inhibitory control since isolation of the pituitary away from the hypothalamus resulted in the continuous secretion of prolactin (Desclin, 1950; Everett, 1954). Later, crude hypothalamic extracts were found to inhibit prolactin secretion from rat pituitary glands *in vitro* (Meites et al., 1963; Talwalker et al., 1963; Welsch et al., 1971). Using *in vitro* methods, PIH activity has been shown to be modified by a wide range of substances (Kragt and Meites, 1967). A decrease in activity occurs following the administration of estrogen, progesterone, testosterone, and cortisol. Drugs with central actions also reduce PIH activity *in vitro*, as well as *in vivo* in animals and man. In general dopamine-depleting agents (e.g., reserpine and dopamine receptor blocking drugs such as phenothiazines, the butyrophenones, metoclopramide, sulpiride, and pimozide) all reduce PIH activity and promote prolactin secretion (Thorner, 1975). An increase in PIH activity is seen with dopamine agonists, dopamine itself, L-DOPA, iproniazid, and prolactin itself. It had been thought that dopaminergic mechanisms promoted the release of PIH from the hypothalamus, but recent work throws some doubt on this. Schally and associates (1974) found that highly purified hypothalamic extracts with high PIH activity contained large amounts of dopamine but no polypeptide compounds. It seems possible that dopamine is itself the physiological PIH, although other hypothalamic substances with PIH activity may also exist (Chapter 6).

Clinically, dopaminergic agents may be used to lower normal or elevated circulating prolactin levels. Dopamine infusions or L-DOPA (which is converted to dopamine) lower prolactin, but the effects are too transient and inconsistent to be of much clinical use (Malarky et al., 1971). However, the ergot alkaloid 2-bromo-α-ergocryptine (bromocriptine, CB154), which has been shown to be a long-acting dopamine agonist, rapidly and consistently lowers prolactin levels by an action on the pituitary cells (Besser et al., 1972b; del Pozo et al., 1973).

The drug appears to be devoid of other actions on the pituitary except in acromegaly when GH levels are reduced as well (Liuzzi et al., 1972; Thorner et al., 1975). The majority of male or female patients with hyperprolactinemia are hypogonadal, whether the hyperprolactinemia is physiological during the postpartum period and the first 3 months of breast feeding or pathological due to pituitary or hypothalamic disease. Although it is generally stated that hyperprolactinemia is accompanied by gonadotropin deficiency, there is no evidence for this in humans. Thus gonadotropin levels are usually normal in hyperprolactinemia, and the LH and FSH responses to GnRH are usually normal or even excessive. In addition, reduction of prolactin levels with bromocriptine therapy results in the rapid return of normal gonadal function (Besser et al., 1972b; Mortimer et al., 1973d; Thorner et al., 1974). Human ovaries and testes appear to produce subnormal amounts of gonadal steroids in response to exogenous gonadotropin administration when prolactin levels are high (Besser and Thorner, 1975). These data together with in vitro evidence of an antigonadotropic action of prolactin at the gonadal level (Zarate et al., 1973a; McNatty et al., 1974) suggest that the hypogonadism associated with hyperprolactinemia is the result of the blockade of the actions of the gonadotropins by prolactin rather than any impairment of gonadotropin secretion. This provides an explanation for the rapid beneficial clinical response to the dopaminergic actions of bromocriptine when it lowers circulating prolactin levels. Not only does the galactorrhea disappear, but menstruation and fertility return within a very few weeks. A return of potency occurs in male patients.

PROLACTIN-RELEASING HORMONE

Although TRH has prolactin-releasing activity in addition to its effects on TSH, it is usually thought not to be the physiologically important prolactin-releasing hormone (PRH). The actions of TRH on the release of prolactin and TSH can be dissociated in many situations; examples include isolated TSH deficiency (Sachson et al., 1972) and normal subjects given GIH (Hall et al., 1973) and TRH (Mortimer et al., 1974a) infusions. It is possible, however, that the galactorrhea and hyperprolactinemia sometimes seen in primary hypothyroidism are the result of excessive TRH secretion (Edwards et al., 1971).

CONCLUSION

It is clear that there have been many major advances in the field of clinical neuroendocrinology since the isolation and synthesis of the three hypothalamic regulatory hormones TRH, GnRH, and GIH. Apart from adding to the elucidation of the complex physiological and neuropharmacological interrelationships of the endocrine glands of the body, of which the brain is merely one, the clinical application of these hormones has been of immense value in the diagnosis and treatment of a wide variety of conditions resulting from hormonal deficiency or excess. It is hoped that continued research will clarify and consolidate these early successes while we await the discovery and availability of further hormones.

REFERENCES

Akande, E. O., Carr, P. J., Dutton, A., Bonnar, J., Corker, C. S., McKinnon, P. C. B., and Robinson, D. (1972): Effect of synthetic gonadotrophin releasing hormone in secondary amenorrhoea. *Lancet*, 2:112–116.

Alberti, K. G. M. M., Christensen, N. J., Christensen, S. E., Prange Hansen, Aa., Iversen, J., Lundbaek, K., Seyer-Hansen, K., and Ørskov, H. (1973): Inhibition of insulin secretion by somatostatin. *Lancet*, 2:1299–1300.

Alford, F. P., Bloom, S. R., Nabarro, J. D. N., Hall, R., Besser, G. M., Coy, D. H., Kastin, A. J., and Schally, A. V. (1974): Glucagon control of fasting glucose in man. *Lancet*, 2:974–976.

Anderson, E. (1966): Adrenocorticotrophin-releasing hormone in peripheral blood: Increase during stress. *Science*, 152:379–380.

Arimura, A., and Schally, A. V. (1970): Progesterone suppression of LH-releasing hormone-induced stimulation LH release in rats. *Endocrinology*, 87:653–657.

Arimura, A., Sato, H., Kumasaka, J., Worobec, R. B., Debeljuk, L., Dunn, J., and Schally, A. V. (1973a): Production of antiserum to LH-releasing hormone (LH-RH) associated with gonadal atrophy in rabbits: Development of radioimmunoassay for LH-RH. *Endocrinology*, 93:1092–1113.

Arimura, A., Debeljuk, L., Shino, M., Rennels, E. G., and Schally, A. V. (1973b): Follicular stimulation by chronic treatment with synthetic LH-releasing hormone in hypophysectomised female rats bearing pituitary grafts. *Endocrinology*, 92:1507–1514.

Arimura, A., Kastin, A. J., Schally, A. V., Saito, M., Kumasaka, T., Yaoi, Y., Nishi, N., and Ohjura, K. (1974a): Immunoreactive LH-releasing hormone in plasma: Midcycle elevation in women. *J. Clin. Endocrinol. Metab.*, 38:510–513.

Arimura, A., Vilchez-Martinez, J. A., Coy, D. H., Coy, E. J. Hirotsu, Y., and Schally, A. V. (1974b): (D-Ala^6 Des-Gly-NH$_2$^{10})-LH-RH ethylamide: A new analogue with unusually high LH-RH/FSH-RH activity. *Endocrinology*, 95:174–177.

Arimura, A., Sato, H., and Coy, D. H. (1974c): A radioimmunoassay for GH-release inhibiting factor. *Endocrinology*, 94:212A (abstract).

Arimura, A., Sato, H., Dupont, A., Nishi, N., and Schally, A. V., (1975): Abundance of immunoreactive GH-release inhibiting hormone in the stomach and the pancreas of rat. *Fed. Proc.,* 34:273.

Ben David, M., Danon, A., and Sulman, F. G. (1971): Evidence of antagonism between prolactin and gonadotropin secretion: Effect of methalibure on perphenazine-induced prolactin secretion in ovariectomised rats. *J. Endocrinol.,* 51:719–725.

Besser, G. M., and Thorner, M. O. (1975): Prolactin. In: *Advanced Medicine,* edited by A. F. Lant. Pittman, London (*in press*)

Besser, G. M., McNeilly, A. S., Anderson, D. C., Marshall, J. C., Harsoulis, P., Hall, R., Ormston, B. J., Alexander, L., and Collins, W. P. (1972*a*): Hormonal responses to synthetic luteinizing hormone and follicle stimulating hormone releasing hormone in man. *Br. Med. J.,* 3:267–271.

Besser, G. M., Parke, L., Edwards, C. R. W., Forsyth, I. A., and McNeilly, A. S. (1972*b*): Galactorrhoea: Successful treatment with reduction of plasma prolactin levels by bromergocryptine. *Br. Med J.,* 3:699–672.

Besser, G. M., Mortimer, C. H., Carr, D., Schally, A. V., Coy, D. H., Evered, D., Kastin, A. J., Tunbridge, W. M. G., Thorner, M. O., and Hall, R. (1974*a*): Growth hormone release inhibiting hormone in acromegaly. *Br. Med. J.,* 1:352–355.

Besser, G. M., Mortimer, G. H., McNeilly, A. S., Thorner, M. O., Batistoni, G. A., Bloom, S. R., Kastrup, K. W., Hanssen, K. F., Hall, R., Coy, D. H., Kastin, A. J., and Schally, A. V. (1974*b*): Long term infusion of growth hormone release inhibiting hormone in acromegaly: Effects on pituitary and pancreatic hormones. *Br. Med. J.,* 4:622–627.

Bloom, S. R., Mortimer, C. H., Besser, G. M., Hall, R., Gomez-Pan, A., Roy, V. M., Russell, R. C. G., Coy, D. H., Kastin, A. J., and Schally, A. V. (1974): Inhibition of gastrin and gastric acid secretion by growth-hormone release inhibiting hormone. *Lancet,* 2:1106–1113.

Bloomfield, G. A., Scott, A. P., Lowry, P. J., Gilkes, J. J. H., and Rees, L. H. (1974): A reappraisal of human β MSH. *Nature (Lond.),* 252:492–493.

Bowers, C. Y., Currie, B. L., Johannson, K. N. G., and Folkers, K. (1973): Biological evidence that separate hypothalamic hormones release the follicle stimulating and luteinizing hormones. *Biochem. Biophys. Res. Commun.,* 50:20–23.

Brazeau, P., and Guillemin, R. (1974): Somatostatin: Newcomer from the hypothalamus. *N. Engl. J. Med.,* 290:963–964.

Brazeau, P., Vale, W., Burgus, R., Ling, N., Butcher, M., Rivier, J., and Gullemin, R. (1973): Hypothalamic polypeptide that inhibits the secretion of immunoreactive pituitary growth hormone. *Science,* 179:77–79.

Breckwoldt, M., Czygan, P. J., Lehmann, F., and Bettendorf, G. (1974): Synthetic LH-RH as a therapeutic agent. *Acta Endocrinol. (Kbh.),* 75:209–212.

Burgus, R., Dunn, T. F., Desiderio, D., Ward, D. N., Vale, W., and Guillemin, R. (1970): Characterisation of ovine hypothalamic hypophysiotropic TSH-releasing factor. *Nature (Lond.),* 226:321–325.

Burgus, R., Monahan, M., Rivier, J., Vale, W., Ling, N., Grant, G., Amoss, M., and Guillemin, R. (1973): Structure-biological activity relationships of thyrotrophin and luteinizing hormone releasing factor analogues. In: *Hypothalamic Hypophysiotrophic Hormones,* edited by C. Gual and E. Rosemberg, pp. 12–23. International Congress Series No. 263. Excerpta Medica, Amsterdam.

Carr, D., Gomez-Pan, A., Weightman, D., Roy, M. V., Hall, R., Besser, G. M., Thorner, M. O., McNeilly, A. S., Schally, A. V., Kastin, A. J., Coy, D. H. (1975): Growth hormone release inhibiting hormone actions on thyrotrophin and prolactin secretion after thyrotrophin releasing hormone. *Br. Med. J. (in press).*

Costom, B. H., Grumbach, M. M., and Kaplan, S. L. (1971): Effect of thyrotropin releasing factor on serum thyroid stimulating hormone: An approach to distinguishing hypothalamic from pituitary forms of idiopathic hypopituitary dwarfism. *J. Clin. Invest,* 50:2219–2225.

del Pozo, E., Brun de Re, R., Varga, L., and Friesen, H. (1973): The inhibition of prolactin secretion in man by CB 154 (2 brom α ergocryptine). *J. Clin. Endocrinol. Metab.,* 35:768–771.

CLINICAL NEUROENDOCRINOLOGY 249

Desclin, L. (1950): A propos du mecanisme d'action des estrogenes sur le lobe anterieur de l'hypophyse chez le rat. *Ann. Endocrinol.* (Paris), 11:656–659.
Edwards, C. R. W., Forsyth, I. A., and Besser, G. M. (1971): Amenorrhoea, galactorrhoea and primary hypothyroidism with high circulating levels of prolactin. *Br. Med. J.,* 3:462–464.
Evered, D., Young, E. T., Ormston, B. J., Menzies, R., Smith, P. A., and Hall, R. (1973): Treatment of hypothyroidism: A reappraisal of thyroxine therapy. *Br. Med. J.,* 3:131–134.
Everett, J. W. (1954): Luteotrophic function of autografts of the rat hypophysis. *Endocrinology,* 54:685–690.
Faglia, G., Peck-Peccoz, C., Ferrari, C., Ambrosi, B., Spada, A., and Travaglini, P. (1973a): Enhanced plasma thyrotrophin reponse to thyrotrophin releasing hormone following oestradiol administration in man. *Clin. Endocrinol. (Oxf.),* 2:207–210.
Faglia, G., Beck-Peccoz, C., Ferrari, C., Travaglini, P., Ambrosi, B., and Spada, A. (1973b): Plasma growth hormone reponse to thyrotropin-releasing hormone in acromegaly. *J. Clin. Endocrinol. Metab.,* 36:1259–1262.
Faglia, G., Beck-Peccoz, P., Ferrari, C., Travaglini, P., Parrachi, A., Spada, A., and Lewin, A. (1973c). Plasma growth hormone response to gonadotropin releasing hormone in patients with active acromegaly. *J. Clin. Endocrinol. Metab.,* 36:1259–1262.
Fairclough, P. D., Cryer, R. J., McAllister, J., Hawkins, L., Jones, A. E., McKendrick, M., Hall, R., and Besser, G. M. (1973): Serum TSH responses to intravenously and orally administered TRH after thyroidectomy for carcinoma of the thyroid. *Clin. Endocrinol. (Oxf.),* 2:351–359.
Fleischer, N., Lorente, M., Kirkland, J., Kirkland, R., Clayton, G., and Calderon, M. (1972): Synthetic thyrotropin releasing factor as a test of pituitary thyrotropin reserve. *J. Clin. Endocrinol. Metab.,* 34:617–624.
Folkers, K., Enzman, F., Boler, J., Bowers, C. Y., and Schally, A. V. (1969): Discovery of modification of the synthetic tripeptide sequence of the thyrotropin releasing hormone having activity. *Biochem. Biophys. Res. Commun.,* 37:123–126.
Franchimont, P. (1972): Thyrotrophin releasing hormone. In: *Frontiers in Hormone Research 1972,* Vol. 1, edited by R. Hall, I. Werner, and H. Holgate, pp. 139–140. Karger, Basel.
Geiger, R., Konig, W., Wissman, H., Geissen, K., and Enzman, R. (1971): Synthesis and characterisation of a decapeptide having LH-RH/FSH-RH activity. *Biochem. Biophys. Res. Commun.,* 45:767–773.
Gerich, J. E., Lorente, M., Scheider, V., and Forsham, P. (1974): Effect of somatostatin on plasma glucose and insulin responses to glucagon and tolbutamide in man. *J. Clin. Endocrinol. Metab.,* 39:1057–1060.
Gilbert, D. M., Besser, G. M., Bitensky, L., and Chayen, J. (1975): On the possibility of bioassaying TRH at sub-picogramme levels. *Nature (Lond.) (in press).*
Gual, C., Kastin, A. J., and Schally, A. V. (1972): Clinical experience with hypothalamic releasing hormones. I. Thyrotropin releasing hormone. *Recent Prog. Horm. Res.,* 28:173–200.
Guillemin, R. (1968): Hypothalamic control of concomitant secretion of ACTH and TSH. *Mem. Soc. Endocrinol.,* 17:19–26.
Haigler, E. D., Pittman, J. A., and Hershman, J. M. (1971): Direct evaluation of pituitary thyrotropin reserve utilizing synthetic thyrotropin releasing hormone. *J. Clin. Endocrinol. Metab.,* 33:573–581.
Haigler, E. D., Hershman, J. M., and Pittman, J. A. (1972): Response to orally administered synthetic thyrotropin-releasing hormone in man. *J. Clin. Endocrinol. Metab.,* 35:631–635.
Hall, R., Amos, J., Garry, R., and Buxton, R. L. (1970): Thyroid stimulating hormone response to synthetic thyrotrophin releasing hormone in man. *Br. Med. J.,* 2:274–277.
Hall, R., Besser, G. M., Ormston, B. J., Cryer, R. J., and McKendrick, M. (1972): The thyrotrophin releasing hormone test in diseases of the pituitary and hypothalamus. *Lancet* 1:759–763.
Hall, R., Anderson, J., Smart, G. A., and Besser, G. M. (1974): In: *Fundamentals of Clinical Endocrinology,* second ed., p. 82. Pitman Medical, Bath, England.
Hall, R., Besser, G. M., Schally, A. V., Coy, D. H., Evered, D., Goldie, D. J., Kastin,

A. J., McNeilly, A. S., Mortimer, C. H., Tunbridge, W. M. G., Phenekos, C., and Weightman, D. (1973): Growth hormone release inhibiting hormone: Its actions in normal subjects and in acromegaly. *Lancet*, 2:581–584.

Harris, G. W. (1950): Oestrous rhythm, pseudopregnancy and the pituitary stalk in the rat. *J. Physiol. (Lond.)*, 111:347–360.

Harris, G. W., and Johnson, R. T. (1950): Regeneration of the hypophyseal portal vessels after section of the hypophyseal stalk in the monkey (*Macacus rhesus*). *Nature (Lond.)*, 165:819–820.

Hertelendy, F., Yen, M., and Todd, H. (1974): Inhibition by somatostatin of prostaglandin stimulated growth hormone release and cyclic AMP accumulation in rat pituitary glands. *J. Int. Res. Commun.*, 2:1216.

Irie, M., and Tsushima, T. (1972): Increase in serum growth hormone concentration following thyrotropin-releasing hormone injection in patients with acromegaly or gigantism. *J. Clin. Endocrinol. Metab.*, 35:97–100.

Jacobs, L. S., Snyder, P. J., Wilber, J. F., Utiger, R. D., and Daughaday, W. H. (1971): Increased serum prolactin after administration of synthetic TRH in man. *J. Clin. Endocrinol. Metab.*, 33:996–998.

James, V. H. T., and Landon, J., editors (1968): *The Investigation of Hypothalamic Pituitary Adrenal Function*. Cambridge University Press, Cambridge, England.

Jeffcoate, S. L., and White, N. (1974): Use of benzamidine to prevent the destruction of thyrotrophin-releasing hormone (TRH) by blood. *J. Clin. Endocrinol. Metab.*, 38:155–157.

Kastin, A. J., Miller, M. C., and Schally, A. V. (1968): MSH activity in the rat pituitary after treatment with Nembutal and morphine: A new bioassay for MSH-release inhibiting factor (MIF). *Endocrinology*, 83:137–140.

Kastin, A. J., Schally, A. V., Viosca, S., and Miller, M. C. (1969): MSH activity in plasma and pituitaries of rats after various treatments. *Endocrinology*, 84:20–27.

Kastin, A. J., Ehrensing, R. H., Schalch, D. S., and Anderson, M. S. (1972): Improvement in mental depression with decreased thyrotropin response after administration of thyrotropin-releasing hormone. *Lancet*, 2:740–742.

Keller, P. J. (1973): Treatment of anovulation with synthetic luteinizing hormone-releasing hormone. *Am. J. Obstet. Gynecol.*, 116:698–705.

Koch, Y., Wilchek, M., Fridkin, M., Chobsieng, P., Zor, U., and Lindner, H. R. (1973): Production and characterization of antiserum to synthetic gonadotrophin-releasing hormone. *Biochem. Biophys. Res. Commun.*, 55:623–629.

Kragt, C. L., and Meites, J. (1967): Dose response relationships between hypothalamic PIF and prolactin release by rat pituitary tissue in vitro. *Endocrinology*, 80:1170–1173.

Lawton, N. F. (1972): Effects of TRH on thyroid hormone release. In: *Frontiers in Hormone Research 1972*, Vol. 1, edited by R. Hall, I. Werner, and H. Holgate, pp. 91–113. Karger, Basel.

Lee, P. A., Jaffe, R. R., Midgeley, A. R., Kohen, F., and Niswender, G. R. (1972): Regulation of human gonadotrophins: Suppression of serum LH and FSH in adult males following exogenous testosterone administration. *J. Clin. Endocrinol. Metab.*, 35:636–641.

Liuzzi, A., Chiodini, P. G., Botalla, L., Cremoscoli, G., Muller, E. E., and Silverstrini, F. (1972): Inhibitory effect of L-dopa on GH release in acromegalic patients. *J. Clin. Endocrinol. Metab.*, 35:941–943.

London, D. R., Butt, W. R., Lynch, S. S., Marshall, J. C., Owusu, S., Robinson, W. R., and Stephenson, J. M. (1973): Hormonal responses to intranasal luteinizing hormone-releasing hormone. *J. Clin. Endocrinol. Metab.*, 31:829–831.

Malarky, W. B., Jacobs, L. S., and Daughaday, W. H. (1971): Levodopa supression of prolactin in non-puerperal galactorrhoea. *N. Engl. J. Med.*, 285:1160–1163.

Marshall, J. C., Harsoulis, P., Anderson, D. C., McNeilly, A. S., Besser, G. M., and Hall, R. (1972): Isolated pituitary gonadotrophin deficiency: Gonadotrophin secretion after synthetic luteinizing hormone and follicle stimulating hormone. *Br. Med. J.*, 4:643–645.

McCann, S. M. (1962): A hypothalamic luteinizing releasing factor. *Ann. J. Physiol.*, 202:395–400.

McCann, S. M., and Dhariwal, A. P. S. (1966): Hypothalamic releasing factors and the neurosecretory link between the brain and anterior pituitary. *Neuroendocrinology,* 1:261–296.

McNatty, K. P., Sawers, R. S., and McNeilly, A. S. (1974): A possible role for prolactin in control of steroid secretion by the human graafian follicle. *Nature* [*New Biol.*], 250:653–655.

McNeilly, A. S. (1974): Prolactin and human reproduction. *Br. J. Hosp. Med.,* 12:57.

Meites, J., Nicoll, C. S., and Talwalker, P. I. C. (1963): The central nervous system and the secretion and release of prolactin. In: *Advances in Neuroendocrinology,* edited by A. V. Nalbandov, p. 238. University of Illinois Press, Urbana.

Mortimer, C. H., Besser, G. M., McNeilly, A. S., Tunbridge, W. M. G., Gomez-Pan, A., and Hall, R. (1973*a*): Interaction between secretion of the gonadotrophins, prolactin, growth hormone, thyrotrophin and corticosteroids in man: The effects of LH/FSH-RH, TRH and hypoglycaemia alone and in combination. *Clin. Endocrinol.,* 2:317–326.

Mortimer, C. H., Besser, G. M., McNeilly, A. S., Goldie, D. H., and Hook, J. (1973*b*): Asynchronous changes in circulating levels of LH and FSH during continuous infusions of the gonadotrophin releasing hormone. *Nature (Lond.),* 246:22–23.

Mortimer, C. H., Besser, G. M., McNeilly, A. S., and Goldie, D. (1973*c*): Asynchronous pulsatile LH and FSH responses during LH/FSH-RH and TRH infusions. *J. Endocrinol.,* 59:12–13.

Mortimer, C. H., Besser, G. M., McNeilly, A. S., Marshall, J. C., Harsoulis, P., Tunbridge, W. M. G., Gomez-Pan, A., and Hall, R. (1973*d*): The LH and FSH releasing hormone test in patients with hypothalamic-pituitary-gonadal dysfunction. *Br. Med. J.,* 4:73–77.

Mortimer, C. H., Besser, G. M., Goldie, D. J., Hook, J., and McNeilly, A. S. (1974*a*): The TSH, FSH and prolactin responses to continuous infusions of TRH and the effects of oestrogen administration in normal males. *Clin. Endocrinol.,* 3:97–103.

Mortimer, C. H., McNeilly, A. S., Murray, M. A. F., Fisher, R. A. F., and Besser, G. M. (1974*b*): Gonadotrophin releasing hormone therapy in hypogonadal males with hypothalamic pituitary dysfunction. *Br. Med. J.,* 4:617–621.

Mortimer, C. H., Besser, G. M., Hook, J., and McNeilly, A. S. (1974*c*): Intravenous, intramuscular, subcutaneous and intranasal administration of LH/FSH-RH: The duration of effect and occurence of asynchronous pulsatile release of LH and FSH. *Clin. Endocrinol.,* 3:19–25.

Mortimer, C. H., Carr, D., Lind, T., Bloom, S. R., Mallinson, C. N., Schally, A. V., Tunbridge, W. M. G., Yeomans, L., Coy, D. H., Kastin, A. J., Besser, G. M., and Hall, R. (1974*d*): Growth hormone release inhibiting hormone: Effects on circulating glucagon, insulin and growth hormone in normal diabetic, acromegalic and hypopituitary patients. *Lancet,* 1:697–701.

Mortimer, C. H., McNeilly, A. S., Murray, M. A. F., Anderson, D. C., Edwards, C. R. W., Benker, G., Liendo-Ch, P., and Besser, G. M. (1975*a*): Modulation of pituitary responses to LRH by 17β estradiol, dihydrotestosterone, testosterone and inhibin in males. *Endocrinology,* 96:74A.

Mortimer, C. H., Besser, G. M., and McNeilly, A. S. (1975*b*): Gonadotrophin releasing hormone therapy in the induction of puberty, potency, spermatogenesis and ovulation in patients with hypothalamic-pituitary gonadal dysfunction. In: *Hypothalamic Hormones: Chemistry, Physiology, Pharmacology, and Clinical Uses.* Academic Press, New York (*in press*).

Moss, R. L., and McCann, S. M. (1973): Induction of mating behaviour in rats by luteinizing hormone-releasing factor. *Science,* 181:177–179.

Mountjoy, C. Q., Price, J. S., Weller, M., Hunter, P., Hall, R., and Dewar, J. H. (1974): A double blind crossover sequential trial of oral thyrotrophin releasing hormone in depression. *Lancet,* 2:958–960.

Nair, R. M. G., Kastin, A. J., and Schally, A. V. (1971): Isolation and structure of hypothalamic MSH release inhibiting hormone. *Biochem. Biophys. Res. Commun.,* 43:1376–1381.

Nillius, S. J., and Wide, L. (1971): Induction of a mid-cycle-like peak of luteinizing hormone in young women by exogenous oestradiol 17β. *J. Obstet. Gynaecol. Br. Commonw.,* 78:822–827.

Nillius, S. J., and Wide, L. (1972): Variation in LH and FSH response to LH-releasing hormone during the menstrual cycle. *J. Obstet. Gynaecol. Br. Commonw.,* 79:865–873.

Noel, G. H., Suh, H. K., and Frantz, A. G. (1973): L-Dopa suppression of TRH stimulated prolactin release in man. *J. Clin. Endocrinol. Metab.,* 36:1255–1258.

Ormston, B. J. (1972): Clinical effects of TRH on TSH release after i.v. and oral administration in normal volunteers and patients with thyroid disease. In: *Frontiers in Hormone Research 1972,* Vol. 1, edited by R. Hall, I. Werner, and H. Holgate, pp. 45–75. Karger, Basel.

Ormston, B. J., Garry, R., Cryer, R. J., Besser, G. M., and Hall, R. (1971): Thyrotropin-releasing hormone as a thyroid function test. *Lancet,* 2:10–14.

Ormston, B. J., Alexander, L., Evered, D. C., Clark, F., Bird, T., Appleton, D., and Hall, R. (1973): Thyrotrophin response to thyrotrophin releasing hormone in ophthalmic Graves' disease: Correlation with other aspects of thyroid function, thyroid supressibility and activity of eye signs. *Clin. Endocrinol.,* 2:369–376.

Palmer, R. L., Crisp, A. H., MacKinnon, P. C. B., Franklin, M., Bonnar, J., and Wheeler, M. (1975): Pituitary sensitivity to 50 μg LH/FSH-RH in subjects with anorexia nervosa in acute and recovery stages. *Br. Med. J.,* 1:179–182.

Parker, D. C., Rossman, L. G., Siler, T. M., Rivier, J., Yen, S. S. C., and Guillemin, R. (1974): Inhibition of the sleep related peak in physiologic human growth hormone release by somatostatin. *J. Clin. Endocrinol. Metab.,* 38:496–499.

Patel, Y. C., and Burger, H. G. (1973): Serum thyrotropin (TSH) in pituitary and or hypothalamic hypothyroidism: Normal or elevated basal levels and paradoxical response to thyrotropin releasing hormone. *J. Clin. Endocrinol. Metab.,* 37:190–196.

Pfaff, D. W. (1973): Luteinizing hormone-releasing factor potentiates lordosis behaviour in hypophysectomised, ovariectomised female rats. *Science,* 182:1148–1149.

Pokroy, N., Epstein, S., Hendricks, S., and Pimstone, B. (1974): Thyrotrophin response to intravenous thyrotrophin-releasing hormone in patients with hepatic and renal disease. *Horm. Metab. Res.,* 6:132–136.

Prange, A. J., Wilson, I. C., Lara, P. P., Alltop, L. B., and Breese, G. R. (1972): Effects of thyrotrophin releasing hormone in depression. *Lancet,* 2:999–1002.

Prange Hansen, Aa., Ørskov, H., Seyer-Hansen, K., and Lundbaek, K. (1973): Some actions of growth hormone release inhibiting factor. *Br. Med. J.,* 3:523–524.

Redding, T. W., Kastin, A. J., Gonzalez-Barcena, B., Coy, D. H., Coy, E. J., Schalch, D. S., and Schally, A. V. (1973): The half-time, metabolism and excretion of tritiated luteinizing hormone-releasing hormone (LH-RH) in man. *J. Clin. Endocrinol. Metab.,* 37:626–631.

Rees, L., Butler, P. W. P., Gosling, C., and Besser, G. M. (1971): Adrenergic blockade and the corticosteroid and growth hormone response to methylamphetamine. *Nature (Lond.),* 228:565–566.

Ricketts, H. T., (1975): Somatostatin, hormone inhibitor. *JAMA,* 231:391–392.

Sachson, R., Rosen, S. W., Cuatrecasas, P., Roth, J., and Frantz, A. G. (1972): Prolactin stimulation by thyrotropin-releasing hormone in a patient with isolated thyrotropin deficiency. *N. Engl. J. Med.,* 287:972–973.

Saffran, M., Schally, A. V., and Benfey, B. G. (1955): Stimulation of the release of corticotropin from the adenohypophysis by a neurohypophysial factor. *Endocrinology,* 57:439–444.

Sandow, J., Arimura, A., and Schally, A. V. (1972): Stimulation of growth hormone release by anterior pituitary perfusion in the rat. *Endocrinology,* 90:1315–1319.

Schally, A. V., and Bowers, C. Y. (1964): Corticotropin releasing factor and other hypothalamic peptides. *Metabolism (Suppl.),* 13:1190–1205.

Schally, A. V., Arimura, A., Baba, Y., Nair, R. M. G., Matsuo, A., Redding, T. W., Debeljuk, L., and White, M. F. (1971): Isolation and properties of the FSH and LH releasing hormone. *Biochem. Biophys. Res. Commun.,* 43:393–399.

Schally, A. V., Arimura, A., Takahara, J., Redding, T. W., and Dupont, A. (1974): Inhibition of prolactin release in vitro and in vivo by catecholamines. *Fed. Proc.,* 33:237.

Seyler, L. E., and Reichlin, S. (1973): Luteinizing hormone releasing factor (LRF) in plasma of post menopausal women. *J. Clin. Endocrinol. Metab.,* 37:197–203.

Shenkman, L., Mitsuma, T., and Hollander, C. S. (1973): Modulation of pituitary responsiveness to thyrotropin-releasing hormone by tri-iodothyronine. *J. Clin. Invest.*, 52:205–209.

Sievertsson, H., Chang, J. K., Bogentoff, C., Currie, B. L., Folkers, K., and Bowers, C. Y. (1971): Synthesis of the luteinizing releasing hormone of the hypothalamus and its hormonal activity. *Biochem. Biophys. Res. Commun.*, 44:1566–1571.

Siler, T. M., VandenBerg, G., Yen, S. S. C., Brazeau, P., Vale, W., and Guillemin, R. (1973): Inhibition of growth hormone release in humans by somatostatin. *J. Clin. Endocrinol. Metab.*, 37:632–634.

Snyder, P. J., and Utiger, R. D. (1972): Response to thyrotropin-releasing hormone (TRH) in normal man. *J. Clin. Endocrinol. Metab.*, 34:380–385.

Snyder, P. J., and Utiger, R. D. (1973): Repetitive administration of thyrotropin-releasing hormone results in small elevations of serum thyroid hormones and in marked inhibition of thyrotropin response. *J. Clin. Invest.*, 52:2305–2312.

Spaulding, S. W., Burrow, G. N., Donabedian, R., and Van Woert, M. (1972): L-Dopa suppression of thyrotropin releasing hormone response in man. *J. Clin. Endocrinol. Metab.*, 35:182–185.

Stewart-Bentley, M., Odell, W., and Horton, R. (1974): The feedback control of luteinizing hormone in normal adult men. *J. Clin. Endocrinol. Metab.*, 38:545–553.

Talwalker, P. K., Ratner, A., and Meites, J. (1963): In vitro inhibition of pituitary prolactin synthesis and release by hypothalamic extract. *Am. J. Physiol.*, 205:213–218.

Thorner, M. O. (1975): Hypothesis: Dopamine is an important neurotransmitter in the autonomic nervous system. *Lancet* (*in press*).

Thorner, M. O., McNeilly, A. S., Hagen, C., and Besser, G. M. (1974): Long-term treatment of galactorrhoea and hypogonadism with bromocriptine. *Br. Med. J.*, 2:419–422.

Thorner, M. O., Chait, A., Aitken, M., Benker, G., Bloom, S. R., Mortimer, C. H., Sanders, P., Stuart Mason, A., and Besser, G. M. (1975): Successful treatment of acromegaly with bromocriptine. *Br. Med. J.*, 1:299–303.

Vilchez-Martinez, J. A., Coy, D. H., Arimura, A., Coy, E. J., Hirotsu, Y., and Schally, A. V. (1974a): Synthesis and biological properties of (Leu-6)-LH-RH and (D-Leu[6]-des Gly-NH$_2$10)-LH-RH ethylamide. *Biochem. Biophys. Res. Commun.*, 59:1226–1231.

Vilchez-Martinez, J. A., Schally, A. V., Coy, D. H., Coy, E. J., Debeljuk, L., and Arimura, A. (1974b): In vivo inhibition of LH release by a synthetic antagonist of LH releasing hormone (LH-RH). *Endocrinology*, 95:213–218.

Von zur Mühlen, A., and Köbberling, J. (1973): Effect of testosterone on the LH and FSH release induced by LH-releasing factor (LRF) in normal men. *Horm. Metab. Res.*, 5:266–270.

Von zur Mühlen, A., Hesch, R. D., Köbberling, J., and Emrich, D. (1971): Thyrotrophin releasing factor (TRF) in the diagnosis of thyroid disorders: Its application in different states of Graves' disease. *Acta Endocrinol. (Kbh.) (Suppl.)*, 155:6.

Weeke, J. (1974): The influence of the circadian thyrotropin rhythm on the thyrotropin response to thyrotropin-releasing hormone in normal subjects. *Scand. J. Clin. Lab. Invest.*, 33:17–20.

Welsch, C. W., Squiers, M. D., Cassell, E., Chen, C. L., and Meites, J. (1971): Median eminence lesions and serum prolactin: Influence of ovariectomy and ergocornine. *Am. J. Physiol.*, 221:1714–1717.

Yen, S. S. C., VandenBerg, G., Rebar, R., and Ehara, Y. (1972): Variation of pituitary responsiveness to synthetic LRF during different phases of the menstrual cycle. *J. Clin. Endocrinol. Metab.*, 35:931–934.

Yen, S. S. C., Siler, T. M., and De Vane, A. W. (1974): Effect of somatostatin in patients with acromegaly. *N. Engl. J. Med.*, 290:935–938.

Zanartu, J., Dabancens, A., Rodriguez-Bravo, R., and Schally, A. V. (1973): Induction of ovulation with synthetic gonadotrophin releasing hormone in women with constant anovulation induced by contraceptive steroids. *Br. Med. J.*, 1:605–608.

Zarate, A., Jacobs, L. S., Canales, E. S., Schally, A. V., de la Cruz, A., Soria, J., and Daughaday, W. H. (1973a): Functional evaluation of pituitary reserve in patients with the amenorrhoea-galactorrhoea syndrome utilizing luteinizing hormone-releasing hormone (LH-RH), l-dopa and chlorpromazine. *J. Clin. Endocrinol. Metab.*, 37:855–859.

Zarate, A., Valdes-Vallina, F., Gonzalez, A., Perez-Ubierna, C., Canales, E. S., and Schally, A. V. (1973*b*): Therapeutic effect of synthetic luteinizing hormone releasing hormone (LH-RH) in male infertility due to idiopathic azoospermia and oligospermia. *Fertil. Steril.*, 24:485–487.

Frontiers in Neuroendocrinology, Vol. 4,
edited by L. Martini and W. F. Ganong.
Raven Press, New York © 1976.

Chapter 9

Development of Hormonal Secretion by the Human Fetal Pituitary Gland

Selna L. Kaplan and Melvin M. Grumbach

Department of Pediatrics, University of California San Francisco, San Francisco, California 94143

Considerable evidence has been amassed during the past two decades, particularly in experimental animals, on the vital role of the fetal endocrine glands in the morphogenesis and functional maturation of the fetus (Jost, 1953; Jost and Picon, 1970). Data on the hormonal regulation of prenatal human development are limited. The capacity of the human fetal pituitary gland to secrete polypeptide hormones and of the hypothalamus to store releasing factors is established early in gestation. Maturation of the central nervous system (CNS) regulation of the hypothalamic pituitary complex occurs later. The chronology of the synthesis and secretion of human fetal pituitary growth hormone (Kaplan et al., 1972), prolactin (Grumbach and Kaplan, 1974; Aubert et al., 1975), FSH and LH (Kaplan et al., 1969; Grumbach and Kaplan, 1973; Kaplan and Grumbach, 1975), ACTH (Allen et al., 1973; Winters et al., 1974a), TSH (Fisher et al., 1970; Greenberg et al., 1970), and vasopressin (Skowsky and Fisher, 1973; Skowsky et al., 1973) is the subject of this review.

EMBRYONIC DEVELOPMENT

The anlage of the human fetal pituitary is first apparent at 4 to 5 weeks' gestational age as thickened cells along the inner wall of the pouch of Rathke, which joins to the wall of the diencephalon (Covell, 1927). The primordium of the posterior lobe appears at 7 weeks' gestation. Cytological differentiation of the fetal pituitary is apparent early, with the presence of basophilic cells by the seventh week of gestation and acidophilic cells by the ninth to 10th week (Daikoku, 1958; Falin, 1961; Conklin, 1968). Rapid cytological differentiation is accompanied by a sharp increase in pituitary weight. Between the 10th and 24th weeks the weight of the pituitary gland increases fourfold, and a further seven- to 10-fold over the mean weight at 24 weeks is observed at term (Fig. 9–1). The mean weight at 10 to 14 weeks is 3 mg, at 25 to 29 weeks 50 mg, and at term 99 mg (Kaplan et al., 1972). Coincident

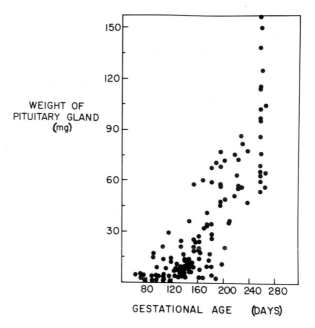

FIG. 9–1. Weight of the pituitary gland as a function of gestational age.

with the development of the pituitary gland, other developmental changes occur in the CNS. The first hypothalamic nuclei and the fibers of the supra-optic tract appear by 8 weeks' gestation (Weill and Bernfeld, 1954). Mono-amine fluorescence is first noted at 10 weeks in the hypothalamus and at 13 weeks in the median eminence (Hyyppa, 1972). Increased vascularization and capillary formation occur at 100 days of age, coincident with develop-ment of the primary plexus of the portal system (Espinasse, 1933; Niemi-neva, 1949). Further differentiation of the pars tuberalis, median eminence, and remainder of the hypothalamic nuclei occurs by the 16th week. The continuity of a primary and secondary plexus of the portal system and maturation of the hypothalamus are completed by the 19th to 21st week. Thus by midgestation the hypothalamic-pituitary unit has reached an ad-vanced stage of anatomical development.

Coincident with these morphological developments in the hypothalamic-pituitary system, secretory activity has also been documented. The presence of secretory granules in the human fetal pituitary gland has been substanti-ated by histochemical, electron microscopic, and immunofluorescence tech-niques (Grumbach, 1962; Ellis et al., 1966). The synthesis and secretion of most pituitary hormones has been confirmed by *in vitro* studies (Pasteels et al., 1963; Gitlin and Biasucci, 1969; Solomon et al., 1969; Gailani et al., 1970; Siler-Khodr et al., 1974). Sequential changes of the fetal pituitary hormones have been determined by both immunological and bioassay meth-ods (Grumbach and Kaplan, 1974).

HUMAN GROWTH HORMONE

The immunochemical and physicochemical characteristics of the growth hormone (GH) synthesized by the fetal pituitary gland are comparable to those of the child and adult in our studies (Kaplan et al., 1972). Serial dilutions of pituitary homogenates and sera from fetuses and pituitary homogenates of adults show a parallel displacement reaction to that of purified human growth hormone (hGH) in the immunoassay for growth hormone. By immunoelectrophoresis, the precipitin arc for the fetal pituitary homogenate when reacted with antisera to hGH is located in a slightly cathodal position. This is comparable to that seen with homogenates of pituitaries from children and adults. In contrast, purified pituitary hGH migrates to a more anodal position that the pituitary homogenates. Disk gel and starch gel electrophoresis show comparable mobility of the major bands of growth hormone in pituitary homogenates from fetuses, children, and adults.

Immunoreactive growth hormone can be demonstrated in the pituitary gland by 10 weeks' gestation (the youngest fetus available in our studies), at which time the content is 0.17 μg with a concentration of 0.04 $\mu g/mg$. The presence of immunoreactive growth hormone was demonstrated by Matsuzaki et al. (1971) in the pituitary glands from three of eight fetuses at 7 weeks' gestation and six of nine fetuses at 8 weeks' gestation. An incremental rise in the content and concentration of pituitary hGH occurs during gestation (Fig. 9–2). The peak concentration of hGH was attained by 25 to 29 weeks' gestation. The content and concentration were significantly different at gestational ages 10 to 14, 15 to 19, 20 to 24, and 25 to 29 weeks. In the pituitary glands of fetuses at term, the content and concentration of hGH is comparable to that in the pituitary gland of infants aged 1 month to 1 yr. There is a significant relationship of the content and concentration to gestational age, crown-rump length, and weight of the pituitary gland (Fig. 9–2).

Secretion of immunoreactive growth hormone by the fetal pituitary occurs as early as 70 days of gestation, at which time a serum concentration of 14.5 ng/ml has been observed. A brisk rise to peak levels is observed at 20 to 24 weeks, with a 60% decrement in serum concentration by term. The mean concentration of serum hGH at 10 to 14 weeks is 65.2 ± 9.6 ng/ml, at 20 to 24 weeks 119.3 ± 19.8 ng/ml, and at 30 to 34 weeks 26.5 ± 11.5 ng/ml (Fig. 9–3). The latter is not significantly different from the concentration in umbilical venous serum samples at delivery (33.5 ± 4.2 ng/ml). A significant negative correlation of the concentration of serum hGH with gestational age was demonstrated by our data. There was no correlation of the concentration of serum growth hormone with the pituitary content of growth hormone in matched serum and pituitary specimens from 17 fetuses. Matsuzaki et al. (1971) confirmed the brisk rise in serum hGH in the human fetus with peak levels at midgestation.

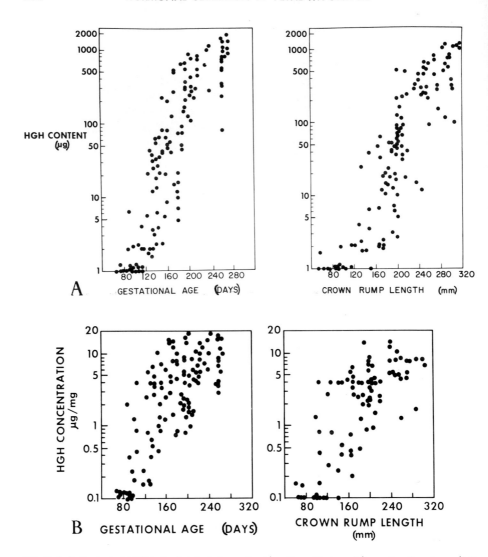

FIG. 9–2. *A:* Content of hGH in the fetal pituitary gland (semilogarithmic scale) as a function of age (*left panel*) and crown-rump length (*right panel*). Concentration of hGH in fetal pituitary gland (semilogarithmic scale) as a function of gestational age (*left panel*) and crown-rump length (*right panel*). (From Kaplan et al., 1972.)

The secretion of immunoreactive and biologically active growth hormone by human fetal pituitary glands in tissue culture has been shown at 14 to 24 weeks' gestational age by Pasteels et al. (1963), Gitlin and Biassuci (1969), Solomon et al. (1969), and Gailani et al. (1970), and at 7 to 12 weeks' gestational age by Siler-Khodr et al. (1974). Parlow (1973) reported bioassayable hGH concentrations of 0.2 IU/100 mg dry weight of glands at less

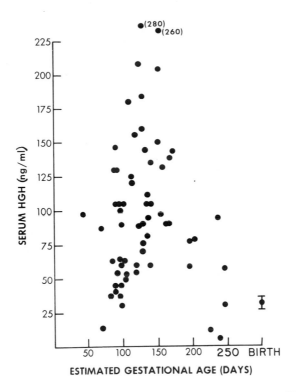

FIG. 9–3. Concentration of hGH in fetal serum as a function of gestational age. (From Kaplan et al., 1972.)

than 5 months' gestational age and 0.8 IU at 5 to 8 months in the human fetus.

Changes in the synthesis and secretion of hGH by the pituitary gland can be correlated with morphogenetic development of the pituitary and hypothalamus during gestation (Kaplan et al., 1972). The initial stage of growth hormone secretion early in gestation, before establishment of the portal system, may be a consequence of autonomous secretion by the pituitary or limited stimulation by growth hormone-releasing hormone (GRH). By midgestation secretion of GRH without secretion of growth hormone release-inhibiting hormone (GIH) or other inhibitory factors can lead to increased secretion by the fetal pituitary gland. We suggest that neuroinhibitory influences are established by late gestation partially as a consequence of maturation of the hypothalamic monoaminergic systems and the development of neurophysiological function.

The CNS regulation of hGH secretion does not attain a full functional state until the postnatal period. The elevated levels of serum hGH, the limited suppressability of hGH following glucose administration, and the absence of a sleep-induced hGH rise observed in the newborn but not in the 3-month-old infant suggests postnatal maturation of the regulatory control of GH secretion. It is unlikely that the secretory pattern of GH during gestation could be due to autonomous release of growth hormone with absent or deficient GRH. The low levels of serum hGH in the anencephalic fetus, despite the presence of functional pituitary tissue, does not support this possibility (Grumbach and Kaplan, 1974).

The stress of parturition, fetal distress, and other factors may be responsible for some of the elevations in the serum hGH concentration observed in the fetus at midgestation and at term (Turner et al., 1971). However, in our studies the concentration of hGH in serum of fetuses removed by hysterotomy was similar to that of spontaneously aborted fetuses. Delayed removal of hGH from the fetal circulation could contribute to elevated levels, but the disappearance rate of exogenously administered hGH in premature infants is comparable to that observed in the child and adult (Cornblath et al., 1965). Transplacental passage of growth hormone from the maternal circulation is negligible and does not contribute to the elevated fetal growth hormone levels (Gitlin et al., 1965).

PROLACTIN

Prolactin is secreted in high concentrations by pregnant women with the serum prolactin increasing from levels of 24 ng/ml at 10 weeks' gestation to 207 ng/ml at term. Amniotic fluid has a higher concentration of prolactin than the maternal circulation, ranging from 1.2 to 7 μg/ml at midgestation with a fall to 0.3 μg/ml by term (Tyson et al., 1972).

The presence of prolactin activity in human fetal pituitary glands was first demonstrated in cultures from 5- to 7-month-old fetuses by both histochemical and immunofluorescence techniques (Pasteels, 1967). Biologically active prolactin was observed by Levina (1968) in pituitary glands from human fetuses at 18 to 40 weeks' gestation.

In studies of immunoreactive prolactin in sera and pituitary glands from human fetuses (Aubert et al., 1975), we used a heterologous radioimmunoassay for human prolactin in which neither hGH nor human chorionic sommatomammotropin (hCS) cross react (Aubert et al., 1974). Serial dilutions of serum and pituitary homogenates from fetuses give parallel displacement of the tracer when compared with the purified human prolactin standard. Prolactin is present as early as 68 days' gestation. In contrast to the results with hGH, only 7 of 31 pituitary glands had detectable prolactin ($>$ 2 ng/pituitary) between 68 and 110 days' gestation, but prolactin was consistently present in pituitaries of fetuses older than 110 days (Fig. 9–4). There was a rapid rise in content from 4.1 $\pm$ 1.4 ng for the 10th to 14th week to 2,039 $\pm$ 459 ng during the latter third of gestation (Table 9–1). There is a significant positive correlation between prolactin and growth hormone content

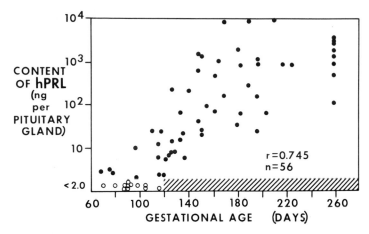

FIG. 9–4. Prolactin (hPRL) content in the fetal pituitary gland (semilogarithmic scale) as a function of gestational age. (From Grumbach and Kaplan, 1974.)

throughout gestation with a growth hormone/human prolactin ratio of 125:1 during early gestation and a further rise to 290:1 at term.

The secretion of prolactin by the human fetal pituitary is confirmed by its presence in the fetal circulation. Immunoreactive prolactin was present in serum at a concentration of 5.7 ng/ml at 88 days' gestation, the youngest fetus studied. The secretory pattern of prolactin secretion is biphasic, with a relatively constant level between 88 to 160 days' gestation at a mean concentration of 19.5 ng/ml. During the last trimester there is a sharp incremental rise in concentration to peak levels of 167.8 ± 14.2 ng/ml at term (Fig. 9–5). This is in contrast to the concentration of 118.8 ± 14.2 ng/ml in matched specimens of maternal sera at term.

The concentration of serum prolactin in anencephalic infants at term is comparable to that of normal newborns. The administration of thyrotropin-releasing hormone (TRH) to anencephalic infants induced a fourfold rise in

TABLE 9–1. Prolactin content of human fetal pituitary glands

Weeks of gestation	No. of glands	Prolactin (ng Lewis 203–1 hPRL)		
		Mean ± SE		Range
10–14	5	4.1 ±	1.4	2.1– 9.7
15–19	13	14.8 ±	4.6	2.4– 65.6
20–24	14	405 ±	142	5.8–1,540
25–29	10	542 ±	204	24 –1,947
30–34	2	872		856 – 887
35–40	7	2,039 ±	459	493 –3,689
1–2 mo	4	5,429 ± 2,275		233 –9,855

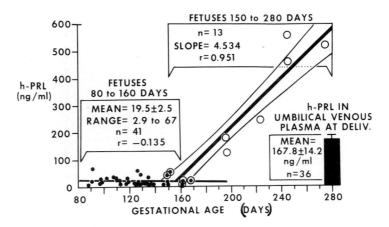

FIG. 9–5. Concentration of serum hPRl as a function of gestational age. The linear regression lines are indicated for gestational days 80 to 160 and 150 to 280. The mean value for hPRL in umbilical venous plasma is indicated by the solid bar on the right. (From Grumbach and Kaplan, 1973.)

prolactin, thus confirming that prolactin is secreted and stored in the pituitary remnants of such infants (Aubert et al., 1975). The secretory pattern of TSH differs in the anencephalic fetuses; the basal level of plasma TSH is undetectable (Allen et al., 1974), but there is an appropriate exaggerated response to TRH (Grumbach and Kaplan, 1974).

These findings suggest that a specific stimulatory agent for the release of pituitary prolactin is not essential. The elevated levels of fetal prolactin do not appear to be the consequence of increased TRH secretion during gestation (Aubert et al., 1975) but correlate directly with the rapid rise of estrogen during the latter part of gestation and its stimulatory effect on the pituitary secretion of prolactin (Shutt et al., 1974).

FETAL TSH

The development of secretory activity of the fetal thyroid gland can be correlated with the development of TSH secretion by the human fetal pituitary gland. According to the studies of Shepard (1967), the development of the thyroid gland occurs in three phases. It first appears at 16 to 17 days' gestation and descends to the anterior neck position by 32 days. During the precolloid phase (47 to 72 days' gestation) the thyroid gland increases in size and thyroglobulin synthesis is present but not dependent on TSH secretion.

Immunoreactive TSH is first detectable in low concentration in the pituitary and serum of human fetuses by 12 to 14 weeks (Gitlin and Biasucci, 1969; Fukuchi et al., 1970; Gailani et al., 1970; Siler-Khodr et al., 1974), coincident with the appearance of radioiodine uptake, synthesis of iodothyronines, and colloid development. At 20 to 24 weeks there is a marked increase in pituitary and serum immunoreactive TSH with subsequent increases in serum thyroxine-binding globulin (TBG), protein-bound thyroxine, and free thyroxine (Fisher et al., 1970; Greenberg et al., 1970). Thereafter the TSH levels remain relatively constant. Bioassayable TSH is not detectable in the human fetal pituitary gland until 14 weeks (Mitskevitch, 1950; Fukuchi et al., 1970). The content is 2 mIU at 14 weeks, 25.9 at 24 weeks, and 40 mIU at 32 weeks.

From midgestation to term, serum TSH and free thyroxine (T_4) levels are approximately threefold greater in the fetal than in the maternal circulation. There is a secondary rise in TSH, from levels of 9.5 μU/ml in cord blood to 86 μU/ml within 30 min after delivery, with a comparable increase in serum T_4 and triiodothyronine (T_3) concentrations (Fisher and Odell, 1969). By 48 hr of age, serum TSH decreases rapidly to levels comparable to those seen in older infants. The neonatal thyroidal hyperactivity is sustained until 2 to 3 weeks postnatally.

TRH has been detected in the brain of human fetuses by 4.5 weeks' gestational age. At 8 weeks significant TRH concentrations are present in the hypothalamus (11.3 pg/mg) with a further rise by midgestation (Winters et al., 1974b).

These data support the contention that TSH secretory activity of the fetal pituitary is evident early in gestation with a hypersecretory state attained from mid to late gestation. The mediation of this hypersecretory stage by stimulation of TRH release is supported by the low levels of TSH demonstrable in anencephalic fetuses. The presence of a functional feedback system during midgestation is suggested further by clinical evidence of goiter formation in newborns whose mothers were treated with goitrogens. The postnatal TSH surge is believed to be the consequence of cord clamping and stimulation of adrenergic mechanisms (Sack et al., 1975).

FETAL ACTH

The essentiality of the hypothalamic-pituitary system for the development of the fetal adrenal has been inferred from the observation of small or atrophied adrenal glands lacking a fetal cortex in infants with anencephaly or aplasia of the pituitary gland (Benirschke, 1956).

In the normal fetus the adrenal gland is first apparent at 4 weeks' gestation. There is a twofold increase in the weight of the adrenal gland between the 24th and 32nd weeks of gestation and a threefold increase thereafter to term. This rapid increase in size is attributable principally to a more rapid increase of the fetal zone of the adrenal cortex during the latter half of gestation. Thus the peak weight of the adrenal gland is attained just before birth, at which time the fetal zone represents 80% of the gland and the neocortex the remainder. During the first postnatal week there is a 40% reduction in the weight of the gland primarily due to a decrease in the fetal zone of the adrenal gland.

The weight of the adrenal gland of the anencephalic fetus is comparable to the normal fetus until 20 weeks' gestation. Thereafter in the anencephalic fetus there is no further growth, and eventual involution of the adrenal gland is apparent at birth. This difference in adrenal size of the anencephalic fetus is the consequence primarily of a decrease in the fetal cortex, since the three distinctive though narrow zones of the neocortex can be identified (Benirschke, 1956). Fetal ACTH appears essential for normal growth of the fetal and neocortical zones of the adrenal. In addition to ACTH, other factors have been suggested as critical for growth of the adrenal (Winters et al., 1974a).

The concentration of immunoreactive plasma ACTH is markedly elevated in the human fetus by 12 to 19 weeks' gestation, with a mean level of 249 ± 65.7 pg/ml (Winters et al., 1974a). A gradual decrease in the concentration occurs by 35 to 42 weeks (to 143 ± 7.0 pg/ml) and a further decrease during the first postnatal week (to 120 ± 8.3 pg/ml). These levels are significantly higher than those in older children and adults, in whom the mean is 43 ± 3.7 pg/ml (Allen et al., 1973). The ACTH level in the plasma of anencephalic infants is 20% that found in normal infants of similar age.

Bioassayable ACTH is present in the human fetal pituitary gland by 9 to 10 weeks' gestational age with a content of 1 to 1.5 mU (Skebelskaya, 1965; Pavlova et al., 1968). By 17 to 19 weeks the mean concentration is 12.3 ± 2.4 mU/mg dry weight; at 20 to 22 weeks it is 30.9 ± 2.0 mU/mg; and at 26 to 27 weeks it is 256 mU/mg, which is comparable to the ACTH content in the pituitary gland of the newborn (117 ± 10.8 mU/mg). Parlow (1973) found lower concentrations of bioassayable ACTH in human fetal pituitaries; his values were 45 mU/100 mg dry weight at 5 to 8 months and 83 mU/100 mg dry weight at 8 to 9 months' gestation.

Plasma cortisol in the fetus, a presumed secretory product of the fetal adrenal gland, is detectable at 12 to 18 weeks' gestation at levels of 7 ng/ml. There is a threefold rise by term (Murphy, 1973). The inverse relationship of the plasma cortisol and immunoreactive ACTH levels may be due to a functional feedback system, but it could also be due to decreased activity of cortisol-synthesizing enzymes independent of ACTH secretion. The concentration of plasma cortisone is greater than cortisol at all gestational ages; the cortisone is derived principally from transplacental passage of maternal cortisol, which is converted to cortisone (Murphy, 1973). Although plasma cortisol in the fetus increases significantly with the onset of labor and is higher after a spontaneous than a cesarean delivery, Winters et al. (1974a) could not demonstrate a higher ACTH level in infants born by spontaneous delivery.

That the transplacental passage of ACTH is limited with little or no maternal contribution to the measurable ACTH levels in the fetus is substantiated by the facts that the ACTH level is higher in cord than in maternal plasma during a normal gestation, the ACTH levels are low in cord samples of anencephalic infants, and there is a marked discrepancy in the maternal and cord plasma ACTH levels (20:1) in a patient with Nelson's syndrome (Allen et al., 1973). Furthermore, infusion of ACTH into the maternal circulation at delivery induced a fall rather than a rise in the ACTH level in venous cord samples (Miyakawa et al., 1974).

A relationship between increased fetal ACTH secretion and initiation of parturition has been demonstrated in sheep. Fetal hypophysectomy and/or adrenalectomy results in prolongation of gestation in this species. In the rhesus monkey fetal hypophysectomy (but not adrenalectomy) is associated with delayed parturition. In the human, anencephaly and pituitary aplasia are often associated with a prolonged gestation, whereas primary adrenal hypoplasia in the human fetus is not. However, administration of high concentrations of long-acting corticoids to human fetuses (Liggins et al., 1973) or dexamethasone to pregnant women near term (Anderson and Turnbull, 1973) failed to induce premature delivery. Present evidence does not support the view that ACTH secretion by the human fetus plays a significant role in the initiation of parturition.

FETAL FSH AND LH

The studies of Pearse (1953), Falin (1961), Mitskevich and Levina (1965), and Volodina (1966) provide histochemical evidence of gonadotropin-containing cells in the pituitary of the human fetus early in gestation (at 8 to 9 weeks). There is a gradual increase in the basophilic cell complement with a high proportional representation by the 28th week of gestation. The secretory activity of these pituitary cells has been established by the *in vitro* organ culture studies of Gitlin and Biasucci (1969), Groom et al. (1971), Hartemann et al. (1973), and Siler-Khodr et al. (1974).

The presence of immunoreactive human luteinizing hormone (hLH[1]) and human follicle-stimulating hormone (hFSH[1]) has been demonstrated in the pituitary of the human fetus in our studies (Kaplan et al., 1969; Grumbach and Kaplan, 1974; Kaplan and Grumbach, 1975) as early as 68 days' gestation. (This was the youngest fetus we studied.) The content and concentration of pituitary hLH and hFSH show a sharp increment by midgestation, with an apparent decrease in concentration by term (Figs. 9–6 and 9–7).

There was a significant sex difference in the pituitary content and concentration of hLH and hFSH, with higher levels in the female than in the male (Table 9–2). Sex differences in the pituitary hLH and hFSH contents are similar to those reported by Levina (1970), who noted that biologically

---

[1] All values are expressed in terms of a purified pituitary standard: LER-960 for hLH and LER-869 for hFSH.

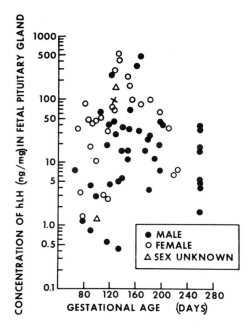

FIG. 9–6. Concentration of hLH in the fetal pituitary gland (semilogarithmic scale) as a function of gestational age. The values for hLH are expressed in terms of pituitary standard LER-960. (From Kaplan and Grumbach, 1975.)

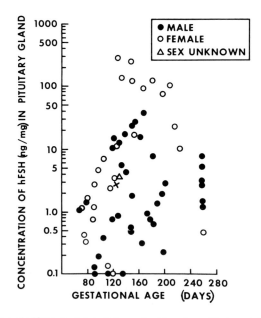

FIG. 9–7. Concentration of hFSH in the fetal pituitary gland (semilogarithmic scale) as a function of gestational age. The values for hFSH are expressed in terms of pituitary standard LER-869. (From Kaplan and Grumbach, 1975.)

TABLE 9-2. Mean content and concentration of LH and FSH in the pituitary gland of female and male fetuses

Gestational age (days)	No.	Sex	LH content[a] (ng/pituitary)	LH conc. (ng/mg)	FSH content[b] (ng/pituitary)	FSH conc. (ng/mg)	FSH/LH content
68–104 (10–14 wk)	9	F	88.2 ± 44.2	32.7 ± 9.1	7.4 ± 5.2	1.6 ± 0.5	0.08 ± 0.02
	5	M	21.0 ± 11.5	3.3 ± 1.2	1.8 ± 0.7	0.6 ± 0.3	0.32 ± 0.2
105–139 (15–19 wk)	11	F	797.0 ± 274.7	153.1 ± 57.3	315.8 ± 216.0	49.6 ± 32.8	0.22 ± 0.09
	12	M	165.3 ± 56.0	39.2 ± 19.2	13.0 ± 4.4	5.8 ± 2.1	0.35 ± 0.2
140–174 (20–24 wk)	4	F	3,940 ± 1,846	129.9 ± 35.6	3,725.6 ± 2,105.9	119.5 ± 47.0	0.87 ± 0.23
	10	M	489.4 ± 148.3	114.5 ± 57.1	51.2 ± 18.6	11.5 ± 4.4	0.07 ± 0.02
175–209 (25–29 wk)	3	F	4,983.8 ± 1,128.4	75.4[c]	5,788.6 ± 1,460.7	101.8[c]	1.17 ± 0.18
	9	M	1,222.0 ± 389.6	22.3 ± 5.2	149.5 ± 69.1	2.2 ± 0.9	0.11 ± 0.09
210–244 (30–34 wk)	3	F	2,353.5 ± 1,165.5	42.1 ± 17.4	2,010.2 ± 908.3	67.7 ± 22.2	2.54 ± 1.05
245–280 (35–40 wk)	9	M	1,590.2 ± 484.3	15.0 ± 4.9	360.5 ± 122.3	3.1 ± 0.9	0.54 ± 0.25

[a] Mean ± SE (LER-960).
[b] Mean ± SE (LER-869).
[c] Mean of two samples.

active pituitary hFSH was present in the female at 13 to 14 weeks and in the male human fetus at 20 to 21 weeks. Bioassayable pituitary hLH was detected in females only from 18 to 28 weeks of gestation, but was demonstrable by immunoassay (hemagglutination-inhibition method) at 13 weeks in both sexes, with higher levels in female than in male fetuses. Parlow (1973) reported the presence of bioassayable pituitary hLH (but not hFSH) in the human fetus at midgestation but did not observe a sex difference.

Not only synthesis and storage, but secretion, of hLH and hFSH by the human fetal pituitary gland were found throughout gestation (Kaplan et al., 1969; Grumbach and Kaplan, 1974; Kaplan and Grumbach, 1975). Early in gestation (84 days) the concentration of hFSH was 11 ng/ml and rose at midgestation to mean levels of 16.2 ± 5 ng/ml at 20 to 24 weeks. During early to midgestation, the levels of serum hFSH were comparable to those observed in the castrate adult. A decrease in serum hFSH was noted during late gestation and at term, with levels of 1.7± 0.05 ng/ml at 30 to 34 weeks and 1.08 ± 0.2 ng/ml in cord samples at term. The mean concentration in maternal serum at term was 1.2 ± 0.1 ng/ml. Serum hFSH was generally higher in the female than male fetuses at all stages of gestation (Fig. 9–8). Reyes et al. (1974) reported significantly higher levels of serum hFSH in females than in male human fetuses from 11 to 20 weeks' gestational age. There was no correlation between the pituitary content or concentration of hLH or hFSH and the serum concentration of the respective hormone in 15 matched specimens (Grumbach and Kaplan, 1974).

Measurement of immunoreactive hLH in fetal serum has been hampered by the inability of most anti-hLH and anti-hCG sera to discriminate between hLH and the placental gonadotropin, human chorionic gonadotropin (hCG) (Grumbach and Kaplan, 1974; Reyes et al., 1974). By using antisera to the

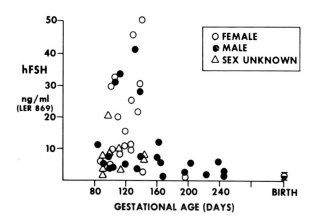

FIG. 9–8. Concentration of hFSH in fetal serum as a function of gestational age. Mean concentration (±SE) at birth is indicated.

β-subunit of hLH (Vaitukaitis et al., 1972*a*) and of hCG (Vaitukaitis et al., 1972*b*), we attempted to distinguish between these two hormones in the serum of human fetuses throughout gestation. Peak levels were attained at 110 to 160 days; they gradually decreased by late gestation, and at term the mean levels were less than 1 ng/ml. The hLH levels in fetal sera were comparable to those of castrated adults. In the presence of elevated levels of α-LH in fetal sera, cross reaction could occur in this assay system. This possibility has not been excluded in our studies. Cross reaction of hCG in the β-LH assay was observed only at the high concentrations present in some maternal sera.

Peak concentrations of serum hCG were present in the fetus by 90 to 110 days' gestation and decreased to a mean concentration of 268.5 ± 16.1 mIU/ml in cord sera at term. There was a significant negative correlation between serum hCG values and gestational age. The mean concentration of maternal hCG at term was $5,400 \pm 200$ mIU/ml.

In six anencephalic infants the concentration of serum hFSH and hLH was less than 1 ng/ml at term, whereas the mean serum hLH-hCG was 12.3 ng/ml.

Limited data are available on the storage and synthesis of LH-releasing hormone (LRH) in the human fetus. Hypothalamic fragments from human fetuses at midgestation can stimulate the release of hLH and hFSH by human fetal pituitary glands as demonstrated by an *in vitro* system (Levina, 1970). This activity is present by 19 weeks in the female but not until the 24th week in the male fetus. During the late gestational period, hypothalamic fragments show decreased or absent activity in this assay system.

Radioimmunoassayable LRH was present in homogenates of whole brain at 4.5 weeks of age in the human fetus at a concentration of 0.52 pg/mg (Winters et al., 1974*b*). The concentration of LRH in the hypothalamus was significantly higher by 8 weeks' gestation (9.52 pg/mg) with concentrations of 3.04 to 65.77 pg/mg between 12 to 22 weeks.

Maturational changes in the hypothalamic regulation of fetal hLH and hFSH secretion with the development of the inhibitory pituitary gonadal feedback system can be inferred from the above data. We suggest that during the early gestational period, when the hypothalamus and the hypophyseal portal system are not fully functional, fetal hLH and hFSH may be released autonomously. The secretion of castrate levels of hLH and hFSH by midgestation may be induced by increased LRH stimulation and/or autonomous secretion. The decreased release of hLH and hFSH into the fetal circulation is consistent with the development of inhibitory feedback restraint by the fetal hypothalamus, which leads to decreased LRH secretion.

The negative feedback system for sex steroids has not fully matured at birth. In the human neonate the rapid fall in sex steroids of placental origin may result in decreased inhibition of hypothalamic LRH. As a result there is a brisk rise from the low levels of plasma hLH and hFSH present at birth to peak levels by 2 weeks of age (Faiman and Winter, 1971; Forest et al.,

1974). In the male infant plasma testosterone rises with peak levels at 3 months of age (Faiman and Winter, 1971; Forest et al., 1974); there is a less pronounced rise in plasma estradiol in female infants (Bidlingmaier et al., 1973). Thus the increased sensitivity of the prepubertal gonadostat to feedback by sex steroids (Grumbach et al., 1974) is not attained until late infancy or early childhood.

The onset and progression of sexual differentiation in the male fetus is dependent on the secretion of testicular testosterone (Jost, 1965). The development of synthetic and secretory activity of the fetal testis (Siiteri and Wilson, 1974) is temporally related to the high concentration of fetal serum hCG early in gestation and later with the peak secretory activity of the fetal pituitary (Grumbach and Kaplan, 1973, 1974). Fetal pituitary gonadotropins are not essential for male sex differentiation in the human, but their secretion may be critical for growth of the testes and external genitalia of the male. Underdevelopment of the external genitalia occurs in male anencephalic fetuses (Bearn, 1968) as well as in male infants with apituitarism or hypothalamic hypopituitarism (Blizzard and Alberts, 1956; Goodman et al., 1968; Lovinger et al., 1975). Fetal pituitary gonadotropins may affect ovarian development since anencephalic female fetuses have decreased follicular development and hypoplastic ovaries (Ch'in, 1938; Grumbach and Kaplan, 1973, 1974; Ross, 1974).

VASOPRESSIN

Considerable data are available concerning renal function and control of fluid balance in the neonate. However, information is limited concerning the secretory pattern of vasopressin and its control in the fetus. Neurosecretory material is present in the supraoptic and paraventricular nuclei of the human fetus (Benirschke and McKay, 1953) and in the neurohypophysis by 23 to 28 weeks' gestation (Rodeck and Caesar, 1956; Raiha and Hjelt, 1957). Skowsky and Fisher (1973), utilizing a sensitive radioimmunoassay method, demonstrated the presence of arginine vasopressin (AVP) and arginine vasotocin (AVT) in the pituitary gland of the human fetus. AVP and AVT are present at 12 weeks of age. The AVT concentration is greater than that of AVP early in gestation. There is a steady increase until 18 weeks, at which time the concentrations of the two hormones are equivalent (AVP 2.8 mU/mg/pituitary and AVT 2.9 mU/mg/pituitary). The vasopressin content in the pituitary gland of the newborn is 350 to 400 mU (Heller and Zaimis, 1949).

In the past plasma AVP values were invariably low owing to the unrecognized presence of a vasopressinase. Currently, bio- and immunoassay methods ensure inhibition of the action of this enzyme and prevent inactivation of AVP. Utilizing a bioassay method, Hoppenstein et al. (1968) reported elevated concentrations of plasma AVP at birth. The levels were higher in infants born by vaginal delivery (35 μU/ml) than in those born by cesarean section (0.83 μU/ml). AVP concentration in matched maternal samples was 2 μU/ml. Plasma levels of AVP decreased rapidly during the first day of life. Chard and associates (1971) obtained similar results using a radioimmunoassay procedure. In venous cord plasma AVP levels were 80 μU/ml in infants born by vaginal delivery and 21 μU/ml in cesarean section infants. These differences in AVP concentration were attributed to the stress of vaginal delivery and indicate the responsiveness of the newborn hypothalamoneurohypophyseal complex. The presence of high levels of urinary vasopressin in the newborn (Ames, 1953) and the infant's ability to respond appropriately to a water load (Smith, 1959) and to an infusion of isotonic dextran or hypertonic saline provide further evidence of functional volume and osmoreceptor systems at birth (Fisher et al., 1963). Thus the decreased concentrating ability of the newborn may be the result of decreased renal function rather than blunted responsiveness to or decreased secretion of vasopressin.

A developmental change in the secretion of a hypothalamoneurohypophyseal factor that stimulates the synthesis of arginine vasopressin and neurophysin has been reported in the guinea pig. Pearson et al. (1975) demonstrated that arginine vasopressin is present in the hypothalamoneurohypophyseal complex of the guinea pig by 30 to 35 days, increases to peak levels at 40 to 55 days, and continues to rise until term. The stimulatory factor is present only between 40 to 55 days of gestation and is not detectable either before or after this period. This is the interval during which the neurosecretory neurons undergo the most rapid period of synthesis and storage of vasopressin. Similar studies have not been carried out in the human fetus.

CONCLUSIONS

We reviewed the evidence for the ontogenesis of pituitary hormones in the human fetus. Based on limited available data, we propose that the maturation of the hypothalamic pituitary system proceeds from a state of hyperactivity with uncontrolled secretion of hypothalamic releasing hormones early in gestation to a partially controlled regulation by CNS inhibitory influences during late gestation. At birth this process is still incomplete and continues for a variable period postnatally.

Studies in the anencephalic fetus provide supportive evidence for the essential role of the hypothalamic releasing hormones in the secretion of fetal pituitary hormones. It is apparent that other hormones and factors in the fetal circulation also affect the secretion of fetal pituitary hormones. Fetal estrogens may directly or indirectly stimulate the release of prolactin by the pituitary as implied by the elevated levels of plasma prolactin in the anencephalic infant and in the normal newborn. A major deficit in our understanding of the ontogenesis of CNS control mechanisms during gestation is the limited information available on the pattern of synthesis and secretion of the hypothalamohypophysiotropic hormones and of the biogenic amines by the human fetus. There is a paucity of data as well on the morphogenetic development of the hypothalamus and hypothalamic pituitary portal system.

ACKNOWLEDGMENTS

We acknowledge the valuable assistance of Dr. Thomas Shepard in the collection of specimens and the cooperation of the late Dr. Dorothy Anderson, as well as Doctors Cynthia Barrett, William Blanc, Delbert Fisher, Mitchell Golbus, Arnold Klopper, Abraham Rudolph, and Lotte Strauss in the collection of pituitaries and blood specimens from fetuses. Angeles Jardiolin and Gail Doherty provided technical assistance, and Kathleen Hayward secretarial assistance. We thank the National Pituitary Agency for the purified hGH, LH, FSH, and βhCG standards; Dr. H. G. Friesen and Dr. U. J. Lewis for the purified hPRL; Dr. Rudi Lequin for the purified βLH and antiserum to βLH; and Organon Company for the purified hCG.

This work was supported in part by grants from the National Institute of Child Health and Human Development and the National Institute of Arthritis, Metabolism, and Digestive Diseases, N.I.H., U.S.P.H.S.

REFERENCES

Allen, J. P., Cook, D. M., Kendall, J. W., and McGilvra, R. (1973): Maternal-fetal ACTH relationship in man. *J. Clin. Endocrinol. Metab.* 37:230–234.

Allen, J. P., Greer, M. A., McGilvra, R., Castro, A., and Fisher, D. A. (1974): Endocrine function in an anencephalic infant. *J. Clin. Endocrinol. Metab.*, 38:94–98.

Ames, R. G. (1953): Urinary water excretion and neurohypophysial function in full term and premature infants shortly after birth. *Pediatrics,* 12:272–282.

Anderson, A. B. M., and Turnbull, A. C. (1973): Comparative aspects of factors involved in the onset of labour in ovine and human pregnancy. *Mem. Soc. Endocrinol.,* 20:141–162.

Aubert, M. L., Grumbach, M. M., and Kaplan, S. L. (1974): Heterologous radioimmunoassay for plasma human prolactin (hPRL); values in normal subjects, puberty, pregnancy and in pituitary disorders. *Acta Endocrinol. (Kbh.),* 77:460–476.

Aubert, M. L., Grumbach, M. M., and Kaplan, S. L. (1975): The ontogenesis of human fetal hormones. III. Prolactin. *J. Clin. Invest.,* 56:155–164.

Bearn, J. G. (1968): Anencephaly and the development of the male genital tract. *Acta Paediatr. Acad. Sci. Hung.,* 9:159–180.

Benirschke, K. (1956): Adrenals in anencephaly and hydrocephaly. *Obstet. Gynecol.,* 8:412–425.

Benirschke, K., and McKay, D. B. (1953): The antidiuretic hormone in fetus and infant. *Obstet. Gynecol.,* 1:638–649.

Bidlingmaier, F., Wagner-Barnack, M., Butenandt, O., and Knorr, D. (1973): Plasma estrogens in childhood and puberty under physiologic and pathologic conditions. *Pediatr. Res.,* 7:901–907.

Blizzard, R. M., and Alberts, M. (1956): Hypopituitarism, hypoadrenalism and hypogonadism in the newborn infant. *J. Pediatr.,* 48:782–792.

Chard, T., Hudson, C. N., Edwards, C. R. W., and Boyd, N. R. H. (1971): Release of oxytocin and vasopressin by the human foetus during labour. *Nature (Lond.),* 234: 352–354.

Ch'in, K. Y. (1938): Endocrine glands of anencephalic foetuses: Quantitative and morphologic study of 15 cases. *Chin. Med. J. (Suppl.)*, 2:63–90.

Conklin, J. L. (1968): A histochemical study of mucoid cells in the pars distalis of the human hypophysis. *Anat. Rec.*, 160:59–78.

Cornblath, M., Parker, M. L., Reisner, S. H., Forbes, A. E., and Daughaday, W. H. (1965): Secretion and metabolism of growth hormone in premature and full-term infants. *J. Clin. Endocrinol. Metab.*, 25:209–218.

Covell, W. P. (1927): Growth of the human prenatal hypophysis and the hypophyseal fossa. *Am. J. Anat.*, 38:379–422.

Daikoku, S. (1958): Studies on the human foetal pituitary. I. Quantitative observations. *Tokushima J. Exp. Med.*, 5:200–213.

Ellis, S. T., Beck, J. S., and Currie, A. R. (1966): The cellular localization of growth hormone in the human fetal adenohypophysis. *J. Pathol.*, 92:179–184.

Espinasse, P. G. (1933): The development of the hypophysioportal system in man. *J. Anat.*, 68:11–18.

Faiman, C., and Winter, J. S. D. (1971): Sex differences in gonadotropin concentrations in infancy. *Nature (Lond.)*, 232:130.

Falin, L. I. (1961): The development of human hypophysis and differentiation of cells of its anterior lobe during embryonic life. *Acta Anat. (Basel)*, 44:188–205.

Fisher, D. A., and Odell, W. D. (1969): Acute release of thyrotropin in the newborn. *J. Clin. Invest.*, 48:1670–1677.

Fisher, D. A., Pyle, H. R., Porter, J. C., Beard, A. C., and Panos, T. C. (1963): Studies of the control of water balance in the newborn. *Am. J. Dis. Child.*, 106:137–146.

Fisher, D. A., Hobel, C. J., Garza, R., and Pierce, C. A. (1970): Thyroid function in preterm fetus. *Pediatrics*, 46:208–216.

Forest, M. G., Sizonenko, P. C., Cathiard, A. M., and Bertrand, J. (1974): The hypophysogonadal function in human during the first year of life: Evidence for testicular activity and feedback mechanism in early infancy. *J. Clin. Invest.*, 53:819–828.

Fukuchi, M., Inoue, T., Abe, H., and Kumahara, Y. (1970): Thyrotropin in human fetal pituitaries. *J. Clin. Endocrinol. Metab.*, 31:565–569.

Gailani, S. D., Nussbaum, A., McDougall, W. J., and McLimans, W. F. (1970): Studies on hormone production by human fetal pituitary cell cultures. *Proc. Soc. Exp. Biol. Med.*, 134:27–32.

Gitlin, D., and Biasucci, A. (1969): Ontogenesis of immunoreactive growth hormone, follicle-stimulating hormone, thyroid stimulating hormone, luteinizing hormone, chorionic prolactin and chorionic gonadotropin in the human conceptus. *J. Clin. Endocrinol., Metab.*, 29:926–935.

Gitlin, D., Kumate, J., and Morales, C. (1965): Metabolism and maternofetal transfer of human growth hormone in the pregnant woman at term. *J. Clin. Endocrinol. Metab.*, 25:1599–1608.

Goodman, H. G., Grumbach, M. M., and Kaplan, S. L. (1968): Growth and growth hormone. II. A comparison of isolated growth hormone deficiency and multiple pituitary hormone deficiencies in 35 patients with idiopathic hypopituitary dwarfism. *N. Engl. J. Med.*, 278:57–68.

Greenberg, A. H., Czernichow, P., Reba, R. C., Tyson, J., and Blizzard, R. M. (1970): Observations on the maturation of thyroid function in early fetal life. *J. Clin. Invest.*, 49:1790–1803.

Groom, G. V., Groom, M. A., Cooke, I. D., and Boyns, A. R. (1971): The secretion of immuno-reactive luteinizing hormone and follicle-stimulating hormone by the human foetal pituitary in organ culture. *J. Endocrinol.*, 49:335–344.

Grumbach, M. M. (1962): Intracellular detection of hormones by immunochemical means: growth hormone. In: *Immunoassay of Hormones*, Vol. 14, edited by G. E. W. Wolstenholme and M. Cameron, pp. 373–374. Ciba Foundation Colloquium on Endocrinology.

Grumbach, M. M., and Kaplan, S. L. (1973): Ontogenesis of growth hormone, insulin, prolactin, and gonadotropin secretion in the human fetus. In: *Foetal and Neonatal Physiology*, pp. 462–487. Proceedings of Sir Joseph Barcroft Centenary Symposium. Cambridge University Press, London.

Grumbach, M. M., and Kaplan, S. L. (1974): Fetal pituitary hormones and the maturation of central nervous system regulation of anterior pituitary function. In: *Modern Perinatal Medicine*, edited by L. Gluck, pp. 247–271. Year Book Medical Publishers, Chicago.

Grumbach, M. M., Roth, J. C., Kaplan, S. L., and Kelch, R. P. (1974): Hypothalamic-pituitary regulation of puberty: evidence and concepts derived from clinical research. In: *The Control of the Onset of Puberty*, edited by M. M. Grumbach, G. D. Grave, and F. Mayer, pp. 115–166. Wiley, New York.

Hartemann, P., Malaprade, D., Lemoine, D., Grignon, G., Nabet, P., and Pierson, M. (1973): Mise en évidences des éléments morphologiques et des activités sécrétoires STH et LH sans l'hypophyse de foetus humain au cours du développement. *C. R. Soc. Biol. [D] (Paris)*, 167:105–110.

Heller, H., and Zaimis, E. J. (1949): The antidiuretic and oxytocic hormones in the posterior pituitary glands of newborn infants and adults. *J. Physiol. (Lond.)*, 109: 162–169.

Hoppenstein, J. M., Miltenberger, F. W., and Moran, W. H. (1968): The increase in blood levels of vasopressin in infants during birth and surgical procedures. *Surg. Gynecol. Obstet.*, 127:966–974.

Hyyppa, M. (1972): Hypothalamic monoamines in human fetuses. *Neuroendocrinology*, 9:257–266.

Jost, A. (1953): Problems of fetal endocrinology: The gonadal and hypophyseal hormones. *Recent Prog. Horm. Res.*, 8:379–418.

Jost, A. (1965): Gonadal hormones in sex differentiation of the mammalian fetus. In: *Organogenesis*, edited by P. L. de Hann and H. Vesprung, pp. 611–628. Holt Rinehart & Winston, New York.

Jost, A., and Picon, L. (1970): Hormonal control of fetal development and metabolism. *Adv. Metab. Disord.*, 4:123–184.

Kaplan, S. L., and Grumbach, M. M. (1975): The ontogenesis of human fetal hormones. II. Luteinizing hormone (LH) and follicle stimulating hormone (FSH). *Acta Endocrinol. (Kbh.) (in press)*.

Kaplan, S. L., Grumbach, M. M., and Shepard, T. H. (1969): Gonadotropins in serum and pituitary of human fetuses and infants. *Pediatr. Res.*, 3:512.

Kaplan, S. L., Grumbach, M. M., and Shepard, T. H. (1972): The ontogenesis of human fetal hormones. I. Growth hormone and insulin. *J. Clin. Invest.*, 51:3080–3093.

Levina, S. E. (1968): Endocrine features in development of human hypothalamus, hypophysis and placenta. *Gen. Comp. Endocrinol.*, 11:151–159.

Levina, S. E. (1970): Regulation of secretion of hypophyseal gonadotropins in human embryogenesis. *Probl. Endokrinol. (Mosk.)*, 16:53–59.

Liggins, G. C., Fairclough, R. J., Grieves, S. A., Kendall, J. Z., and Knox, B. S. (1973): The physiological mechanisms controlling the initiation of ovine parturition. *Recent Prog. Horm. Res.*, 29:111–150.

Lovinger, R. D., Kaplan, S. L., and Grumbach, M. M. (1975): Congenital hypopituitarism associated with neonatal hypoglycemia and microphallus: Four cases secondary to hypothalamic hormone deficiencies. *J. Pediatr. (in press)*.

Matsuzaki, F., Irie, M., and Shizume, K. (1971): Growth hormone in human fetal pituitary glands and cord blood. *J. Clin. Endocrinol. Metab.*, 33:908–911.

Mitskevitch, M. S. (1950): The time of discovery of thyrotropic action of the foetal hypophysis in man and some agricultural animals. *C. R. Acad. Sci. [D] (Paris)*, 70:165–167.

Mitskevitch, M. S., and Levina, S. E. (1965): Investigation on the structure and gonadotropic activity of the anterior pituitary in human embryogenesis. *Arch. Anat. Microsc. Morphol. Exp.*, 54:129–144.

Miyakawa, I., Ikeda, I., and Maeyama, M. (1974): Transport of ACTH across human placenta. *J. Clin. Endocrinol. Metab.*, 39:440–442.

Murphy, B. E. P. (1973): Does the human fetal adrenal play a role in parturition. *Am. J. Obstet. Gynecol.*, 115:521–525.

Niemineva, K. (1949): Observations on the development of the hypophysial-portal system. *Acta Paediatr. Scand.*, 39:366–377.

Parlow, A. F. (1973): Human pituitary growth hormone, adrenocorticotropic hormone, follicle stimulating hormone and luteinizing hormone concentrations in relation to age and sex, as revealed by biological assays. In: *Advances in Human Growth Hormone Research*, edited by S. Raiti, pp. 658–669. DHEW Publication No. (NIH) 74–612.

Pasteels, J. L. (1967): Hormone de croissance et prolactine dans l'hypophyse humaine. *Ann. Endocrinol. (Paris)*, 28:117–126.

Pasteels, J. L., Brauman, H., and Brauman, J. (1963): Etude comparée de la sécrétion d'hormone somatotrope par l'hypophyse humaine in vitro et san activité lactogenique. *C. R. Acad. Sci. [D] (Paris)*, 256:2031–2033.

Pavlova, E. B., Pronina, T. S., and Skebelskaya, Y. B. (1968): Histostructure of adenohypophysis of human fetuses and contents of somatotropic and adrenocorticotropic hormones. *Gen. Comp. Endocrinol.*, 10:269–276.

Pearse, A. G. E. (1953): Cytological and cytochemical investigations on the foetal and adult hypophysis in various physiologic and pathologic states. *J. Pathol.*, 65:355–370.

Pearson, D. B., Goodman, R., and Sachs, H. (1975): Stimulated vasopressin synthesis by a fetal hypothalamic factor. *Science*, 187:1081–1082.

Raiha, N., and Hjelt, L. (1957): The correlation between the development of the hypophysial portal system and the onset of neurosecretory activity in the human fetus and infant. *Acta Paediatr. Scand.*, 46:610–616.

Reyes, F. I., Boroditsky, R. S., Winter, J. S. D., and Faiman, C. (1974): Studies on human sexual development. II. Fetal and maternal serum gonadotropins and sex steroid concentrations. *J. Clin. Endocrinol. Metab.*, 38:612–617.

Rodeck, H., and Caesar, R. (1956): Zur entwicklung des neurosekretorischen systems bei saugern und mensche and der regulationsmechanismusdes wasserhaushaltes. *Z. Zellforsch.*, 44:666–691.

Ross, G. T. (1974): Gonadotropins and preantral follicular maturation in women. *Fertil. Steril.*, 25:522–543.

Sack, J., Beaudry, M., DeLamater, P., Oh, W., and Fisher, D. (1975): Umbilical cord cutting triggers hypertriiodinemia and non-shivering thermogenesis in newborn lamb. *J. Pediatr. (in press)*.

Shepard, T. H. (1967): Onset of function in the human fetal thyroid: Biochemical and radioautographic studies from organ culture. *J. Clin. Endocrinol. Metab.*, 27:945–958.

Shutt, D. A., Smith, L. D., and Shearman, R. P. (1974): Oestrone, oestradiol-17β, and oestriol levels in human foetal plasma during gestation and at term. *J. Endocrinol.*, 60:333–341.

Siiteri, P. K., and Wilson, J. D. (1974): Testosterone formation and metabolism during male sex differentiation in human embryo. *J. Clin. Endocrinol. Metab.*, 38:113–125.

Siler-Khodr, T. M., Morgenstern, L. L., and Greenwood, F. C. (1974): Hormone synthesis and release from human fetal adenohypophyses in vitro. *J. Clin. Endocrinol. Metab.*, 39:891–905.

Skebelskaya, Y. B. (1965): Adrenocorticotropic activity of the human fetal hypophysis. *Probl. Endokrinol. (Mosk.)*, 11:77–82.

Skowsky, R., and Fisher, D. A. (1973): Immunoreactive arginine vasopressin (AVP) and arginine vasotocin (AVT) in the fetal pituitary of man and sheep. *Clin. Res.*, 21:205.

Skowsky, W. R., Bashore, R. A., Smith, F. G., and Fisher, D. A. (1973): Vasopressin metabolism in the foetus and newborn. In: *Foetal and Neonatal Physiology*, pp. 439–447. Proceedings of Sir Joseph Barcroft Centenary Symposium. Cambridge University Press, London.

Smith, C. A. (1959): *The Physiology of the Newborn Infant*. Charles C Thomas, Springfield, Ill.

Solomon, I. L., Grant, D. B., Burr, I. M., Kaplan, S. L., and Grumbach, M. M. (1969): Correlation between immunoreactive growth hormone and prolactin activity in human and simian pituitary cell cultures. *Proc. Soc. Exp. Biol. Med.*, 132:505–508.

Turner, R. C., Schneeloch, B., and Paterson, P. (1971): Changes in plasma growth hormone and insulin of the human foetus following hysterotomy. *Acta Endocrinol. (Kbh.)*, 66:577–586.

Tyson, J. E., Hwang, P., Guyda, H., and Friesen, H. G. (1972): Studies of prolactin secretion in human pregnancy. *Am. J. Obstet. Gynecol.*, 113:14–20.

Vaitukaitis, J. L., Ross, G. T., Reichert, L. E., Jr., and Ward, D. N. (1972a): Immunologic basis for within and between species cross-reactivity of luteinizing hormone. *Endocrinology,* 91:1337–1342.

Vaitukaitis, J. L., Braunstein, G. D., and Ross, G. T. (1972*b*): A radioimmunoassay which specifically measures human chorionic gonodatropin in the presence of human luteinizing hormone. *Am. J. Obstet. Gynecol.,* 113:751–758.

Volodina, E. P. (1966): Concerning the histochemical characteristics of the cells of the anterior lobe of hypophysis in man during ontogenesis. *Probl. Endokrinol. (Mosk.),* 12:16–20.

Weill, J., and Bernfeld, J., editors (1954): *Le Syndrome Hypothalamique.* Masson & Cie, Paris.

Winters, A. J., Oliver, C., Colston, C., MacDonald, P. C., and Porter, J. C. (1974*a*): Plasma ACTH levels in the human fetus and neonate as related to age and parturition. *J. Clin. Endocrinol. Metab.,* 39:269–273.

Winters, A. J., Eskay, R. L., and Porter, J. C. (1974*b*): Concentration and distribution of TRH and LRH in the human fetal brain. *J. Clin. Endocrinol. Metab.,* 39:960–963.

Subject Index

Acetylcholine (ACh)
  CRH secretion and, 200-202,
    205-207, 219
    steroids and, 213-220
  distribution in hypothalamic
    nuclei, 12-14
  microphoretically applied, PO
    neurons and, 114-117
Acromegaly
  GIH and, 148
  GH secretion and, somatostatin
    and, 146
  GnRh-induced GH release and,
    235
  monoaminergic control of GH
    release and, 157
  TRH-induced GH secretion and,
    143-144, 231
ACTH, see also ACTH secretion
  GH secretion and, 144
  Nelson's syndrome, GIH and, 146
ACTH secretion, 132
  catecholamines and, 206-207
  corticosteroid feedback mecha-
    nisms, 211-220
  CRH and, 245
  by fetal pituitary gland, 263-265
  5-hydroxytryptamine and,
    202-203
  noradrenergic neuroinhibitory
    control of, 206-207
  parturition and, 265
  pentobarbital and, 154
  PGs and, 78-79
  vasopressin and, 32-33, 39, 41, 53
Addison's disease
  in euthyroid patients, and TSH
    response to TRH, 230-231
  GH secretion and, 136
Adenohypophysis
  cyclic AMP, prostaglandins and,
    76-77

hypothalamic regulatory hormone
  mode of action in, 63-87
  neurophysiological correlates of
    function of, 99-102
Adenomas
  ACTH secreting, GIH and, 148
  GH secreting, 157-158
  pancreatic delta cell, and GIH, 148
Adenosine 3,5′-monophosphate, see
  Cyclic AMP
Adolescents, GH secretion patterns
  in, 130
Adrenal glands
  ascorbic acid, prostaglandins and,
    79
  fetal development of, 263-265
  PGs and, 75
Adrenalectomy
  bilateral sham, corticotropic
    response to, 217
  catecholamine levels and, 17, 19-20
  hypersecretion after stress and,
    212-213
  vasopressin in zona externa and, 32
α-Adrenergic blocking agents, and
  GH secretion, 138, 155
β-Adrenergic blocking agents, and GH
  secretion, 138
Age, and GH secretion patterns, 130
Amino acids
  GH secretion and, 131, 138,
    143-145
  of neurophysins of different species,
    28
  putative, as neurotransmitters in
    CRH release in vitro, 207-209
γ-Aminobutyric acid (GABA)
  ACh-induced CRH release in vitro
    and, 207-209
  CRH secretion and, 201, 206,
    209-210

distribution in hypothalamic
nuclei, 14
Amygdala
functions of, 152
GH secretion and, 150-152
GIH localization in, 141-142, 148
regulation of ovulation and, 47, 49
Anencephaly, 271
and serum prolactin, 261-262
Anesthesia
electrophysiological research and,
102
GH secretion and, 133, 137
microelectrophoresis and,
117-118
Angiopathy, diabetic, and GIH
therapy, 242
Anorexia nervosa, and GnRh therapy,
238-239
Anterior hypothalamic (AH)
nucleus, acetylcholine in, 12
Anterior pituitary
brain areas involved in hormone
release from, 1
cyclic AMP, and hypothalamic
regulatory hormones, 63-66
evidence for neural link in control
of, 97-99
LH and FSH release, LRH effect
on, 71-73
link between hypothalamus and,
97-98
neural activity related to function
of, 108-117
PGs and, 75-86
Antibodies, to bovine serum albumin,
26
Antidromic identification, 95
localization of GIH, 149
neural connection between hypothalamic nuclei and median
eminence, 102-108
Antisera
to brain antigens, and immunocytochemical methods, 26-27
cross-species, in immunocytochemical studies on neurophysin
distribution, 28

estrogen, LH secretion and, 70-71
to LRH, PG-induced LH release
and, 84
Apomorphine
GH secretion and, 138, 155-156
PRL secretion and, 181-183
Arcuate neurons
electrical stimulation of PO-AH
area and, 105-106
electrochemical stimulation of PO
region and, 102
electrophoretically applied NE and
DA and, 111-113
LRH release and, 119
unit responses in, anterior
pituitary function and, 95-119
Arcuate (ARC) nucleus, 98
AVP in, 14
choline acetyltransferase
activity in, 14
dopamine levels in, 10
histamine in, 12
LRH in, 15, 43-46
PNMT activity and deafferentation
of hypothalamus, 10
serotonin levels, 11
somatostatin in, 16
TRH in, 16
Arcuate-ventromedial (ARC-VM)
complex
electrophysiological identification
of neurons in, 104-105
LRH release and, 98
neural connections to PO-AH
areas, 106-107
ARC-VM complex, *see* Arcuate-ventromedial complex
Arginine, GH secretion and, 143,
157
Arginine vasotocin (AVT), in fetal
in fetal pituitary gland, 270-271
distribution in hypothalamic
nuclei, 14
Arginine vasotocian (AVT), in fetal
pituitary gland, 270-271
Aspartate, CRH release and, 208
Aspirin, ovulation and, 80

Assays, of immunoreactive hLH in
  fetal serum, 268-269; *see also*
  Bioassays; Immunoassays
Atropine
  ACH-stimulated CRH release *in
    vitro* and, 202
  5-HT-induced CRH secretion and,
    204-205

Baboons
  GH secretion in, 135
  LRH distribution in, 46
Bethanacol, CRH release and, 202
Bioassays, *see also* Immunoassays
  compared with immunoassays of
    GIH levels in hypothalamic
    nuclei, 16-17
  GRH and, 142-143
  of plasma AVP at birth, 270-271
Biogenic amines, neurosecretion and,
  52-53; *see also* Catecholamines;
  Dopamine; Histamine;
  Norepinephrine; Serotonin
Blocking agents, and plasma prolactin
  levels in ovariectomized,
  estrogen-treated rats, 180-181;
Bovine serum albumin (BSA), anti-
  bodies to, 26
Brain
  distribution of GIH in, 148-149
  removal of hypothalamic nuclei
    from, 1, 2-4
Brain antigens, localization of, 26
Brainstem, GIH in, 149
Brattleboro strain rats, vasopressin
  and oxytocin assays in, 33,
  35-41
Breast enlargement, tranquilizers and,
  175

Catecholamines, *see also* Dopamine;
  Epinephrine; Norepinephrine
  ACTH secretion and, 206-207
  direct inhibition of PRL secretion
    and, 172-174
  effect of suckling on, 185
  and estrogens, 185-186
  haloperidol and, 177-179

  localization in hypothalamic nuclei,
    4-7
  neuroendocrine control mechanisms
    and, 17, 19-20
  neurosecretion and, 52-53
  PRL secretion and, 171-181
  stress and, 17, 18
Caudal median eminence, LRH in, 42
Central nervous system (CNS)
  histamine in, 11-12
  5-HT implantation in, 203-204
  neurosecretory neurons and, 95-119
  regulation of hGH secretion in fetal
    pituitary gland and, 259-260
Cerebellum, GIH in, 149
Cerebral cortex, GIH in, 148
Cerebrospinal fluid
  and ependymal neurophysin, 34-35
  hypothalamic hormones, 25
  LRH transport and, 54
  neurophysin, 34-35
p-Chlorophenylalanine, GH secretion
  and, 157
Chlorpromazine
  sleep-associated GH secretion
    and, 136, 138
  GIH inhibition of GH secretion
    and, 145
Cholera enterotoxin GRH, GH
    secretion and, 144
Choline acetyltransferase
  ACh level determinations and, 12-14
  localization in rat hypothalamus, 9
Cholinergic nerves, termination of, 14
Cold stress, catecholamines and, 17
Compound S, *see* 11-Deoxycortisol
Contraception, LRH analogues and,
  64, 73-75
Coronal cuts, GH release and, 152
Corticomedical amygdaloid, electrical
  stimulation of, 154
Corticosterone (CS)
  CRH release *in vitro* and, 211-220
  GH secretion and, 134
  microphoretically applied, PO
    neurons and, 114-117
Corticotropin-releasing hormone (CRH),
  33, 34

ACTH secretion and, 41
assays in hypothalamus *in vitro*,
    199-200
clinical applications of, 244-245
neurons, 195
PGs and, 79
Corticotropin-releasing hormone
    secretion *in vitro*, 195-222
ACh and, 200-202
5-hydroxytryptamine and, 202-205
interactions with norepinephrine,
    GABA, and melatonin, 209-210
model of neurotransmitters involved
    in, 210-211
monoamines and, 205-207
nature of CRH and, 221
negative feedback control of,
    211-220
neurotransmitter regulation of,
    200-210
and preparation of hypothalamic
    tissue for, 196-200
putative amino acid neurotrans-
    mitters and, 207-209
Cortisol, and CRH release *in vitro*,
    213-214
Cow
    hypothalamus, vasopressin in, 14
    and TRH-induced GH secretion in,
        144
^{51}Cr-ethylenediaminetetraacetic acid
    (EDTA), 199
Cropsac bioassays, 169
Cushing's syndrome
    GH secretion and, 136
    TSH response to TRH and, 230
Cyclic AMP
    adenohypophyseal, PGs and, 76-77
    in anterior pituitary, effect of
        hypothalamic regulatory hor-
        mones on, 63-66
    GH release and, 144
    GIH and, 146, 241-242
    LH and FSH release and, 75
    LRH action and, 63-64
    pituitary hormone action and,
        86-87
    PRL and, 87

DA, *see* Dopamine
D1 rats, *see* Brattleboro rats
Deafferentation of basal hypothal-
    amus
    dopamine and norepinephrine
        levels and, 10
    phenylethanol-*N*-methyltrans-
        ferase activity, 10
    serotonin levels and, 11
Delayed feedback, and CRH secretion,
    211-216
11-Deoxycortisol, and CRH release
    in vitro, 213-214, 219
18-H-Deoxycorticosterone (DOC),
    and CRH release *in vitro*, 219
Dexamethasone, and CRH release
    in vitro, 214
Diabetes
    GIH therapy and, 242
    with hyperglucagonemia, and
        GIH, 148
Diabetes insipidus, and localization
    of specific neurophysins in
    rats, 35-37
Diencephalon, distribution of hypo-
    thalamic hormones and
    neurotransmitters within, 1-20
Dihydrotestosterone (DHT), and LH
    and FSH levels, 234
11β-17α-Dihydroxyprogesterone,
    and CRH release *in vitro*, 214
Dopamine (DA)
    CRH release *in vitro* and, 205
    distribution in hypothalamic
        nuclei, 4-5
    GH secretion and, 155-158
    hypothalamic hormone release
        and, 129
    localization in hypothalamic
        nuclei, 8-10
    microelectrophoretically applied
        PO neurons and, 114-117
    tuberoinfundibular neurons
        and, 110-113
    PIH and, 188-189
    pimozide and, 179-181
    pituitary glands from perphen-
        azine-treated rats and, 176-177

PRL secretion and, 172-174
turnover, estrogens and, 185
Dopamine-β-hydroxylase
  endocrine manipulations and,
    17, 20
  localization in rat hypothalamus, 9
  neuroendocrine control mechan-
    isms and, 17, 19-20
  norepinephrine and, 7
Dopaminergic cell bodies, 10
Dorsomedial hypothalamic nucleus
  choline acetyltransferase activity
    in, 14
  dopamine levels in, 10
  histamine in, 12
  norepinephrine localization in, 7
  TRH in, 16
Duodenum, GIH in, 242

EDTA, see [53]Cr-ethylenediamine-
  tetraacetic acid, 199
Electrical stimulation studies,
  see also Electrochemical
    stimulation studies
  of brain regions, GH release and,
    150-155
  of hypothalamus, GH release and,
    139-140, 141-142, 145
  of neurosecretory neurons
    hormone release and, 95-119
    in vivo, see Antidromic identi-
      fication technique
  of PO-SCH region, 99
Electrochemical stimulation studies,
  102
Electroencephalography (EEG),
  99-102
Electrolyte balance of hypothalamus
  in vitro, 198
Electrophysiological recording
  techniques, 95
  GIH-containing neurons and, 149
  link between hypothalamus and
    endocrine system and, 99-102
  neural correlates of endocrine
    function and, 102
  neurosecretion and, 53, 95-119

Endocrine glands
  electrophysiological studies of its
    neural correlates, 102
  GIH and, 147-148, 241-242
Enzymatic-isotropic assay, 12
Enzymes (see also under specific
    names)
  and neurotransmitter synthesis in
    rat hypothalamus, 9
  released from hypothalamic tissue
    in vitro, 196
Ependymal cells of lamina terminalis,
  LRH in, 98-99
Epinephrine
  localization in hypothalamic
    nuclei, 4-5, 9, 10
  multiunit activity of median
    eminence and, 102
Ergocorine, PRL secretion and,
  182-183
Ergot alkaloids, PRL secretion and,
  182-183
17-β-estradiol, LRH secretion and, 72
Estrogen, see also Estrogen-stimulated
    neurophysin
  feedback, neural circuit for, 109
  gonadotropin levels and, 235
  LRH release and, 71
  microphoretically applied, and
    PO neurons, 114-117
  in portal vein blood of monkeys,
    32-33
  preovulatory surge of LH and,
    70-72
  prolactin secretion and, 185-186
  tanycytes and, 46
Estrogen-stimulated neurophysin
  (ESN), 27, 38, 51-52
Estrous cycle
  correlation between single-cell
    activity and stages of, 99-100
  multiunit electrophysiological
    studies, 101
  prolactin release during, 185
Ethinyl estradiol, GnRH and, 233-234
Euthyroid, and Addison's disease,
  TSH response to TRH and,
    230-231

Exercise, GH secretion and, 154
Exocytosis, GIH and, 241-242

False-negative immunocytochemical
tests, 26
False-positive immunocytochemical
tests, 26
Fast feedback, and CRH release
in vitro, 216-220
Fasting, GH secretion and, 131
Feedback control, of GH secretion,
154-155
Fetal brain
LRH in, 269
TRH in, 263
Fetal pituitary gland
ACTH secretion, 263-265
development of hormonal
secretion in, 255-272
embryonic development of,
255-256
FSH and LH content of, 265-270
gonadotropins in, sexual develop-
ment and, 269
growth hormone secretion by,
257-260
PRL activity in, 260-262
TSH secretion in, 262-263
vasopressin secretion in, 270-271
Fluorescence histochemical
techniques
localization of neurotransmitters
in hypothalamic nuclei and, 4, 7
visualization of 5-HT and, 10-11
Flurazepam, and GH secretion during
SWS, 136
Follicle stimulating hormone (FSH)
secretion
cyclic AMP and, 64
GnRH and, 233
PGs and, 79-85
TRH and GIH inhibition of, 241
Follicular rupture, indomethacin
and, 80-81
Formalin stress, catecholamines and,
17
Free fatty acids (FFA), and growth
hormone regulation, 131

Frogs, MSH activity in, 245
Functional somatostatin receptors,
in GH-, TSH-, and PRL-secreting
cells, 66-70

Galactorrhea
nonpuerperal, ergots and, 183
tranquilizers and, 175
Galactorrhea-amenorrhea, prolactin
response to, TRH in, 231
Gastric inhibiting peptide (GIP),
GIH inhibition of, 241
Gastrin secretion, GIH and, 67,
147-148
Glucagon secretion
and GH release, 138, 144
GIH inhibition of, 147, 241
Glucocorticoids, inhibition of
tyrosine hydroxylase by, 52
Glucose, GH secretion and, 131, 136
Glutamate
CRH release and, 208
microelectrophoretically applied
and PO neurons, 114-117
tuberoinfundibular neurons,
and, 110-113
Glutamic acid decarboxylase, γ-amino-
butyric acid synthesis and, 14
Goat, milk yields in, serum prolactin
levels and, 183
Gomori stains, 25
Gonadectomy, catecholamine levels
and, 17, 19-20
Gonadotropin, binding sites for LRH
on, 72; *see also* Gonadotropin
release; Gonadotropin releasing
hormone
Gonadotropin release
fetal, 269
GnRH and, 233-234
PGs and, 81-85
Gonadotropin-releasing hormone
acromegaly and, 235
analogues, 240
anorexia nervosa and, 238-239
assays for, 239-240
clinical applications for, 232-240

hypogonadism therapy and,
236-239
in normal subjects, 233-235
Graves' disease, TSH response to
TRH in, 229
Growth hormone, *see* Growth hormone secretion
Growth hormone-release-inhibiting
hormone (GIH), *see*
Somatostatin
Growth hormone-releasing hormone
(GRH), 129, 240
amygdaloid lesions and, 151
cyclic AMP and, 78
existence of, 147
GH secretion and, 142-143
hypothalamic stimulation and,
139-142
Growth hormone secretion
brain regulation of, 129, 139-149
extrahypothalamic regulation of,
149-154
functional GIH receptors in cells
for, 67-68
GIH and, 67, 145-147
GnRH and, acromegaly and, 235
GRH and, 142-143
hypothalamic regulatory factors
for, 142-158
inhibition of cyclic AMP and, 65-66
monoaminergic control of, 155-158
neural regulation of, 138-149
patterns of, 130-138
peptides and, 143-145
PGs and, 77-78
pharmacological stimuli for,
137-138
rebound, 146-147
short-loop feedback control of,
147, 154-155
sleep-associated, 134-137
somatomedin and, 154-155
Spirometra mansonoides tapeworm
and, 154-155
stress and, 137
TRH and, in acromegaly, 231
Gut motility, GIH inhibition of, 241

Halasz-type knife cuts
deafferentation of hypothalamus
and, LRH in organum vasculosum and, 7
of lamina terminalis, 47
Haloperidol
catecholamines and, 177-179
ergot alkaloid inhibition of PRL
secretion and, 182-183
Hexamethonium
ACh-stimulated CRH release
in vitro and, 202
5-HT-induced CRH secretion and,
204-205
Hippocampus
electrical stimulation of, 151,
153-154
electrochemical stimulation of, 102
functions of, 152
Histamine
CRH release *in vitro* and, 205
distribution in hypothalamic
nuclei, 8, 11-12
Histaminergic nerves, 11-12
Histidine decarboxylase, 11
Histochemical techniques, *see*
Fluorescence histochemical
techniques
Human fetal pituitary gland, *see*
Fetal pituitary gland
Human follicle-stimulating hormone
in fetal pituitary gland, 265-270
Human growth hormone (hGH)
secretion, 130*ff*, of fetal
pituitary gland, 257-260
Humans
hormone-specific neurophysins in,
27-28
PRL levels and GIH in, 70
6-Hydroxydopamine, and dopamine
and norepinephrine levels,
15-16
5-Hydroxytryptamine (5-HT), *see*
Serotonin
Hyperglucagonemia, in diabetics,
GIH therapy and, 148
Hyperglycemia, GH secretion and,
131

Hyperprolactinemia, galactorrhea
    and, 183
Hyperthyroidism, TRH and, 186,
    229-230
Hypoglycemia, GH secretion and, 131,
    138, 146, 156
Hypogonadism, and GnRH, 236-239
Hypophysiotropins, secretion by
    parvicellular system, 26
Hypophysiotropic area of
    hypothalamus, 98
  catecholamines and, 172
Hypophysis
  connection between median
    eminence and, 169
  portal capillaries of, neurophysin
    around, 32-34
  portal plasma LRH activity
    in, and electrical stimulation
    of PO-SCH region, 99
Hypothalamic disease, TSH response
    to TRH and, 230
Hypothalamic extracts
  in vivo inhibitory effects on
    prolactin secretion, 170-171
  PIH activity in, 173-174
Hypothalamic hormones (*see also
    under specific names*)
  clinical applications of, 227-247
  cyclic AMP accumulation in an-
    terior pituitary, 63-66
  distribution within diencephalon,
    1-20
  GH secretion and, 129, 138-158
  influence on neural activity
    related to anterior pituitary
    function, 108-117
  localization by immunocyto-
    chemical techniques, 25-54
  mode of action in adenohypophysis,
    63-87
  paired secretion of, 39
  role of PGs in secretion and
    action of, 75-86
Hypothalamic neurons, *see*
    Neurosecretory neurons
Hypothalamic nuclei
  ACh in, 12-14

γ-aminobutyric acid in, 14
biologically active peptides in, 14
catecholamines in, 17-20
dopamine in, 8-10
epinephrine in, 10
GIH in, 16-17
histamine in, 11-12
localization of neurophysins in,
    27-41
localization of neurotransmitters
    in, 4-14
microdissection of, 2-4
neural connection between median
    eminence and, 102-108
norepinephrine in, 7-8
releasing hormones and release-
    inhibitory hormones in, 15-20
serotonin in, 10-11
TRH in, 15, 16
Hypothalamic prolactin-releasing
    hormone (PRH), 171
Hypothalamus, *see also* Hypothalamic
    nuclei; Hypothalamus *in vitro*;
    Neurosecretory neurons
  deafferentation of, *see* Deafferenta-
    tion of hypothalamus
  enzymes of, and neurotransmitter
    synthesis, 9
  GIH in, 50-51, 149
  link between anterior pituitary
    gland and, 97-98
  LRH as secretory product of,
    43
  noradrenergic innervation to, 8
  oxytocin in, 37-39
  role in prolactin secretion,
    169-171
  vasopressin in, 37-39
Hypothalamus *in vitro*
  advantages and disadvantages of,
    195-196
  CRH assay methods and, 199-200
  CRH secretion and, 195-222
  functional ability of, 200-220
  histological examination of, 197
  neurotransmitter regulation of
    CRH secretion in, 200-210
  preparation of, 196-197
  viability studies of, 198-199

Hypothalamoneurophypophyseal
    factor, and AVP and neuro-
    physin synthesis, 271
Hypothalamoneurophypophyseal
    system 96-97
    electrical stimulation of, 95
Hypothyroidism
    TRH test, 186, 229-230
    TSH levels, ergotryptamine and, 183

Imipramine, and GH secretion during
    SWS, 136
Immobilization stress, and
    catecholamines, 17, 18
Immunoassays, compared with bio-
    assays of GIH levels in hypo-
    thalamic nuclei, 16-17
Immunocytochemical techniques
    false-positive and false-negative
        results, 26
    on general distribution of neuro-
        physins, 28
    localization of hypothalamic
        hormones by, 25-54
    LRH localization and, 44, 46
Immunoelectron microscopy
    GIH localization, 43
    neurophysin localization, 28, 32
Immunoenzyme techniques, 26
Immunohistochemical techniques,
    localization of GIH, 141
Immunohistological studies, of LRH
    distribution in hypothalamic
    nuclei, 15
Immunoperoxidase technique
    localization of oxytocin and
        vasopressin in human hypo-
        thalamus, 37-39, 43
    localization of specific neuro-
        physins, 35-36
    pineal gland LRH assays, 49-50
Immunoreactive growth hormone,
    fetal pituitary gland secretion
    of, 257
Immunoreactive human luteinizing
    hormone (hLH), in fetal pitui-
    tary gland, 265-267
Immunoreactive prolactin, in fetal
    pituitary gland, 261

Immunostaining, 46
Indomethacin, and prevention of
    ovulation, 79-81
Infertility, and GnRH therapy,
    237-238; *see also* Ovulation
Inhibitin, and FSH secretion, 234-235
Insulin
    GIH inhibition of, 67, 147, 241
    -induced hypoglycemia, and GH
        secretion, 138, 146
Iponiazid, and dexamethasone
        inhibition of CRH release
        in vitro, 207
Isoproterenol, Gh secretion and, 138

Lactation, prolactin secretion
        and, 66
Lamina terminalis, LRH in, 98-99
Laron dwarf, 154
L-DOPA
    GH secretion and, 138, 145-146,
        155, 156-158
    PRL secretion and, 174-175, 188
        246
    PRL and TSH responses to TRH
        and, 231
    reserpine-induced pseudopregnancy
        and, 175
Lesions
    amygdaloid, and GH secretion,
        150-152
    hypothalamic
        GH secretion and, 138-139,
            142
        plasma ACTH and, 199
        PNMT level and, 10
        PRL secretion and, 171
    locus ceruleus, 7
    VMN, and GH rebound secretion,
        146-147
Leucine, and GH secretion, 143-145
Leucine 4,5-^{3}H, incubation of
    pituitary glands with, 172-173
Light-dark cycle, and GH secretion,
    134
Light microscopy, and localization of
    vasopressin and oxytocin in
    human hypothalamus, 37-39

Limbic regions, GH secretion and, 152-153
Lipids, GH secretion and, 131
Locus ceruleus
    function of, 152-153
    GH release and, 152
    lesions, and norepinephrine levels in hypothalamic nuclei, 7
Long-loop feedback, and CRH secretion, 211-220
Luteinizing hormone (LH)
    distribution of, 1
    exogenous, and ARC multiunit activity, 102
    release
        cyclic AMP and, 64
        GnRH and 233
        LRH analogues and, 73-75
        PGs and, 75, 79-85, 89
Luteinizing hormone-releasing hormone (LRH)
    analogues of, contraception and, 73-75
    in arcuate nucleus, 43-46
    changes in pituitary sensitivity to, 70-72
    cyclic AMP as mediator of, 63-64, 66
    determination of levels of, 118-119
    localization of, 15-16, 41-43, 44, 46, 53-54, 98-99
    microphoretically applied, 114-117
    in organum vasculosum of lamina terminalis, 26, 46-49
    oxytocin and, 39
    in pineal gland, 49-50
    in PO-SCH region, 101
    steroids and, 52
    tanycytes in, 46
Luteinizing hormone-releasing hormone secretion, 99
    electrical stimulation of PO-SCH region and, 99
    hypothalamic neurons and, 119
    by hypothalamus in vitro, 195
    and PO area and SCH region, 98, 108
Lysine, GH secretion and, 143

Magnocellular system
    cross-reaction of antihuman and antibovine antisera in, 28
    immunocytochemical studies of, 25-54
    neurophysin in, 28-32
    oxytocin and vasopressin secretion and, 25-26
    projection into portal bed, 32-33
    vasopressin in, 43-44
Mammary tumors, ergot-suppression of PRL-induced growth stimulation of, 183
Mass fragmentographic technique, 12
Maternal deprivation syndrome, and GH secretion, 136, 137
MBH, see Mediobasal hypothalamus
Medial forebrain bundle
    dopamine levels in, 10
    transection, histamine levels and, 11
    norepinephrine levels in, 7
    serotonin in, 11
Medial preoptic nucleus, LRH in, 15
Median eminence
    arginine vasopressin in, 14
    choline acetyltransferase activity in, 12-13
    dopamine levels in, 10
    effect of ACh on in vitro secretion of CRH in, 200-202
    GIH activity in, 16, 53-54, 141
    histamine in, 12
    of hypothalamus in vitro, 197, 198
    lesions, GH secretion and, 138
    LRH in, 15, 53-54
    multiunit activity of, 102
    neural connection between hypothalamic nuclei and, 102-108, 159
    norepinephrine in, 7
    PNMT activity and deafferentation of hypothalamus, 10
    prostaglandin-induced LH release and, 84
    release of releasing hormones into, 98
    serotonin levels, 11
    TRH in, 16

tyrosine hydroxylase, and endocrine manipulations, 20
zona externa of, *see* Zona externa of median eminence
Mediobasal hypothalamic neurons, *see* Peptidergic neurons
Mediobasal hypothalamus (MBH), 98
electrical stimulation of, GH secretion and, 139
GH secretion and, 150, 152
innervation of, 170
neural circuit for estrogen feedback in, 109
Medroxyprogesterone, GH secretion in SWS and, 136
Melanocyte-stimulating hormone, 173
clinical applications, 245
α-Melanocyte-stimulating hormone (α-MSH) GH secretion and, 144
Melatonin
CRH release *in vitro* and, 206-210
GH secretion and, 156
Menstrual cycle, ultrastructure of tanycytes and, 46
Mental depression, THR and, 232
Mesencephalic knife cuts, and dopamine-β-hydroxylase levels, 7
α-Methyl-p-tyrosine, GH secretion and, 157
α-Methyldopa, and reserpine-induced pseudopregnancy, 175
Microdissection
compared with immunocytochemical techniques, 25
localization of neurotransmitters in hypothalamic nuclei, 2-14
Microelectrophoresis, 95
action of hormones and neurotransmitters on hypothalamic neurons, 109-117
problems of, 117-118
of putative neurotransmitters and hormones, 110
Microrecording methods, 99
serum prolactin levels and, 183
TRH therapy and, 232

Monoamines
CRH release from hypothalamus *in vitro* and, 205-207
GH secretion and, 155-158
Morphine
ACTH response to prostaglandins and, 79
GH secretion and, 138, 145
Mouse, LRH distribution in, 46
MSH, *see* Melanocyte-stimulating hormone
Multiunit recording techniques, proestrus and, 101
Murine arcuate nucleus, LRH localization in, 44

Naps, GH secretion and, 135
Narcoleptics, GH secretion in sleep and, 135
NE, *see* Norepinephrine
Negative feedback
control of CRH secretion *in vitro* and, 211-220
for sex steroids, 269-270
TSH secretion and, 228
Nelson's syndrome
GH secretion and, 136
GIH and, 146
Neoplastic tissue, GRH activity, 145
Neuroendocrine control mechanisms, and catecholamine levels, 17, 19-20
Neuroendocrine function, and organum vasculosum of lamina terminalis, 26
Neuroendocrinology, clinical applications of, 227-247
Neurohumoral hypothesis, 98-102
Neurophysin
biogenic amines and, 52-53
ependymal, and cerebrospinal fluid, 34-35
hormone-specific, in humans, 27-28
fetal synthesis of, 271
around hypophyseal portal capillaries, 32-34

in hypothalamic nuclei, 14,
26-41
intracellular distribution of,
28-32, 53
steroid hormones and, 51-52
in suprachiasmatic nucleus, 39-41
Neurosecretion
biogenic amines and, 52-53
steroid hormones, 51-52
Neurosecretory neurons
anterior pituitary function and,
95-119
GH secretion and, 129, 138-149
Neurotransmitters, *see also* Catecholamines
CRH release and, model of, 210-211
distribution within diencephalon,
1-20
hypothalamic levels of enzymes
involved in, 9
influence on neural activity
related to anterior pituitary
function, 108-117
localization in hypothalamic nuclei,
4-14
putative amino acid, 207-209
and regulation of CRH secretion
200-210
role in CRH regulation, 195
TRH as, 16
Nicotine-stimulated neurophysin (NSN),
27, 38
in portal vein blood of monkeys,
32-33
Noradrenergic axons, dopamine in, 10
Norepinephrine (NE)
CRN secretion and, 201, 205-210
GH secretion and, 152, 155-158
hypothalamic hormone release
and, 129
localization in hypothalamic
nuclei, 4-5, 7-8
microelectrophoretically applied
PO neurons and, 114-117
tuberoinfundibular neurons
and, 110-113
multiunit activity of median
eminence and, 102

NSN, *see* Nicotine-stimulated neurophysin

One-cell-one-hormone theory, 39
Organum vasculosum of lamina
terminalis (OVLT)
GIH in, 51
LRH in, 15, 46-49, 54, 98-99
neuroendocrine function and, 26
Ovariectomy
effect of intrapituitary injection
of PGs on gonadotropin
release, 83-84
hypothalamic norepinephrine
turnover and, 186
plasma LH levels after electrochemical stimulation of hippocampus, 102
PRL secretion and, 171, 185
Ovaries, *see also* Ovariectomy
indomethacin blocking of ovulation
and, 80
Ovulation
ESN and, 27
GnRH therapy and, 237-238
hypothalamic neuronal activity
and, 99
indomethacin and, 79-81
intraventricular prostaglandins and, 83
LH and, 70-72
pentobarbital and, 154
preoptic area and, 49
regulation of, 47, 49
Oxytocin
adenohypophyseal function
and, 39
distribution in hypothalamic
nuclei, 14, 35-41, 53
microphoretically applied,
115-116
neurophysin associated with,
27
secretion studies, 25-26, 95-96

Pancreas, GIH in, 50-51, 147-148,
242
PAP technique, *see* Peroxidase antiperoxidase technique

Parachlorophenylalanine (pCPA),
and 5-HT-induced CRH
secretion, 209
Paraventricular nucleus (PVN)
arginine vasopressin in, 14
dopamine levels, 10
fields of, 32
neurophysin, 36-37, 39
neurosecretory nerve cells, *see*
Neurosecretory paraventricular
neurons
oxytocin in, 14
unit recording techniques and, 53
Parenchyma of hypothalamus, histamine levels in, 12
Pars intermedia, MSH, 245
Parturition, ACTH secretion and,
265
Parvicellular system, hypophysio-
tropin secretion by, 26
Pentobarbital
GH secretion and, 138
GIH inhibition of GH secretion
and, 145
hormone secretion and, 154
intraventricular prostaglandins
and gonadotropin release and,
82-83
neuroendocrine effects of, 154
PG effect on ACTH secretion
and, 78-79
PG effect on GH secretion and,
77-78
Peptidergic neurons, and synthesis
and release of GRH and
GIH, 129
Perikarya, LRH in, 43
Periventricular hypothalamic
nucleus
dopamine level, 10
electrical stimulation of PO-AH
areas and, 105-106
GIH in, 16
localization of in, 7
TRH in, 16
Peroxidase-antiperoxidase (PAP)
technique, 26, 34
Perphenazine, and prolactin secretion,
175-177, 182-183

Phenobarbital GH secretion in SWS
and, 136
Phentolamine
GABA inhibition of CRH
release and, 210
GH secretion and, 138, 155
norepinephrine inhibition of
CRH release *in vitro* and, 207
Phentothiazine derivatives, prolactin
secretion and, 175-177
Phenylalanine, GH secretion and, 143
Phenylethanol-*N*-methyltransferase
epinephrine levels and, 10
Phenylethanolamine *N*-methyl-
transferase, *see* Epinephrine
Picrotoxin, and GABA effect on
ACh-induced CRH release
in vitro, 207-209
Pig, GH regulation in, 131
Pimozide, PRL secretion, and
179-181, 182-183
Pineal gland
CRH release and, 209
GIH in, 149
LRH in, 49-50
Pituitary gland
ACTH release and, 5-HT and
hypothalamic extracts and, 204
disease, TSH response to
TRH and, 230
fetal, *see* Fetal pituitary gland
hormonal reserve test, 232
incubation with leucine 4,5-^{3}H,
172-173
isolation of hypothalamus from,
169-170
lactotrophs, catecholamines and,
173
pimozide implant in, 179-180
sensitivity to LRH, 71-72
releasing hormones, neural activity
and, 95-119
stalk section, GH secretion and,
138
tumors, PRL-secreting, 183-185
Plasma
ACTH, in basal hypothalamic-
lesioned animals, 199
corticosterone, PGs and, 78-79

GH, 77-78, 130-138
LH
  PRL and, 101
  PGs and, 81-82
  response to LRH, 71-73, 97
  peripheral, neurophysin in, 27
  TSH response to TRH in
    thyroidectomized rats, 85
Polyacrylamide electrophoresis, pro-
    lactin secretion studies and, 169
Portal blood, pituitary, GRH activity
    in, 142
Portal system, and suprachiasmatic
    axon terminations, 40-41
"Portal vessel-chemotransmitter
    hypothesis," see Neurohumoral
    hypothesis
Posterior hypothalamic nucleus,
    serotonin levels, 11
Prednisolone, 214-215
Pregnancy, and ESN, 27
Pregnant mare's serum gonadotropin
    (PMS), and LH excretion and
    indomethacin, 79-80
Premammillary nuclei, serotonin
    levels, 11
Preoptic-anterior hypothalamic
    (PO-AH) areas
  electrical stimulation of, 105-106
  neural connections to ARC-VM
    complex, 106-107
Preoptic (PO) area
  electrical stimulation of, GH secre-
    tion and, 139
  electrochemical stimulation of, 102
  GIH localization in, 141-142, 148
  ovulation and, 47, 49
  serotonin levels, 11
Preoptic area neurons
  ARC-VM complex and, 107-108
  LRH secretion and, 108
  pharmacological sensitivity of,
    114-117
  unit responses in, anterior pituitary
    function and, 95-119
Preoptic-suprachiasmatic region, 98
  electrical stimulation of, 99
  LRH release and, 98, 101, 119

neural circuit for estrogen feedback
    in, 109
  single-cell activity in, 101
PRH, see Prolactin-releasing hormone
Primates
  factors inhibiting GH secretion in,
    134
  factors stimulating GH secretion
    in, 133
Proestrus, electrical activity studies,
    101
Progesterone
  ARC multiunit activity and, 102
  CRH release in vitro and, 214
Prolactin release-inhibiting hormone
  clinical applications, 245-246
  in hypothalamic extracts, 173-174
  L-Dopa and, 174-175
  neurons, apomorphine and, 182
  perphenazine and, 177
Prolactin-releasing hormones (PRH),
    186-187, 189
  clinical applications, 246-247
Prolactin-secreting cells, functional
    TRH receptors in, 66-68
Prolactin (PRL) secretion, 132-133
  apomorphine and, 181-183
  catecholamines and, 171-181
  cyclic AMP and, 87
  dopamine and, 172-174
  ergot alkaloids and, 182-183
  estrogens and, 185-186
  by fetal pituitary glands, 260-262
  GIH and, 67-68, 70
  hypothalamus and, 169-171
  pentobarbital and, 154
  PGs and, 86
  pimozide and, 179-171
  by pituitary tumors, 183-185
  and PRH and TRH, 186-187, 189
  regulation of, 169-189
  short-loop negative feedback for,
    185
  tranquilizers and, 175-179
  TSH and, 231
Propranolol, GH secretion and, 138
Propylthiouracil, TRH-induced
    prolactin release in rats, 186

Prostaglandin synthetase inhibitors,
LH and FSH secretion, 79-81
Prostaglandins (PGs)
ACTH secretion and, 78-79
adenohypophyseal cyclic AMP and,
76-77
GH secretion and, 77-78
gonadotropin release and, 81-82,
83-85
LH release and anti-LRH serum, 84
and LH and FSH secretion, 79-85
PRL secretion and, 86
role in secretion and action of
hypothalamic hormones, 75-86
TSH secretion and, 85-86
Protamine zinc somatostatin, see PZ
somatostatin
Protein kinase, 66
Pseudopregnancy, reserpine-induced,
172, 175
Putative neurotransmitters
determinations of concentrations
of, 118-119
influence on hypothalamic
neurons, 109-117
PZ somatostatin, and GH secretion, 148

Radioimmunoassays
for GIH, 244
for GnRH, 238-240
for GRH, 142-143
for neurophysins, 27
in PRL secretion studies, 169
synthetic peptides and, 1
for TRH, 232
Raphe nucleus
electrochemical stimulation of,
102
GH secretion and, 152
serotonin,and, 11
SWS and, 153
Rat
GH inhibition in, 142
GH regulation in, 131-134
LRH distribution in, 46
microdissection of hypothalamic
nuclei of,

PMS-treated, indomethacin blocking of ovulation in, 79-81
with Spirometra mansonoides
infestation, GH secretion and,
154-155
REM sleep, GH secretion and, 135
Retrochiasmatic nucleus
arginine vasopressin in, 14
norepinephrine localization in, 7
Reproductive functions
relation between single and multiunit activity in hypothalamus
and, 102
tanycytes and, 46
Renal failure, TSH-induced GH
secretion and, 143-144
Reserpine
PRL secretion and, 175
pseudopregnancy and, 172
Rhesus monkeys
fetal hypophysectomy and delayed
parturition in, 265
GH secretion in, 133, 136-317
LRH distribution in, 46
nicotine and ESN in, 28
Ruminants, and role of FFA in GH
regulation in, 131

Serotonin
CRH secretion and, 202-207
GH secretion and, 152, 155-158
hypothalamic hormone release, 129
localization in hypothalamic
nuclei, 8, 10-11
microphoretically applied, 114-117
stimulation of
hypothalamus by, 199-200
Serum
prolactin
in anencephalic infants, 261-262
milk yields in goats and, 183
TSH levels, in hypothyroidism, 183
triiodothyronine, and TRH injections in normal subjects, 228
Sex differences
in fetal pituitary hLH and HFSH
content, 265-267

in pituitary response to GnRH, 234-235
in TSH responses to TRH, 228
Sexual differentiation, fetal, 270
"Sham rage," 152
Sheehan's syndrome, TSH response to TRH and, 231
Short-loop feedback, CRH release *in vitro* and, 220
Single-unit electrophysiological recording techniques, 99-102
Sleep, *see also* Naps; REM sleep; Slow-wave sleep
GH secretion and, 131, 146
Slow-wave sleep (SWS), GH release and, 134-137
raphe nuclei and, 153
Somatomedin, GH secretion and, 154-155
Somatostatin (GIH)
analogues, 87
clinical applications, 240-244
cyclic AMP accumulation in anterior pituitary gland, 64-65
diabetes with hyperglucagonemia and, 148
distribution in brain, 148-149
distribution in hypothalamic nuclei, 16-17
endocrine gland function and, 147-148
functional receptors for, 66-70
GH release and, 67, 145-147
hyperglucagonemia and, 148
hypothalamic stimulation and, 139-142
insulin and glucagon secretion and, 147
interaction between TRH and, 68-72
localization in hypothalamus, 43, 50-51, 53-54,
in organum vasculosum of lamina terminalis, 26
in protamine zinc, *see* PZ somatostatin
radioimmunoassays, 244
synthesis and release of, 129

TRH-induced GH release in acromegaly and, 144
Species variability
effects of stress on GH and, 137
in GH response to pharmocological agents, 156
role of FFA in GH regulation, 131
Spinal cord, GIH in, 149
Spirometra mansonoides, 154-155
Squirrel monkey, GH release in, 138
Steroids, *see also* Estrogen
CRH secretion *in vitro* and, 213-220
fetal, negative feedback system, 2629-70
GH secretion and, 136
gonadal, pituitary response to GnRH and, 234-235
neurophysin and, 52
neurosecretion and, 51-52
Stomach, GIH, 161, 242
Stress
catecholamines and, 17, 18
corticosteroid hypersecretion and, adrenalectomy and, 212-213
GH secretion and, 137
Subcommissural organ, GIH in, 51
Suckling, and plasma prolactin, 185
Suprachiasmatic nucleus (SCN)
adrenal rhythms and, 40
arginine vasopressin in, 14
catecholamines in, 52
dopamine in, 10
neurophysin and vasopressin in, 39-41
serotonin levels, 11
terminations of, 40-41
Supraoptic nucleus (SON)
AVP in, 14
fields of, 32
localization of oxytocin and vasopressin in, 37
neurophysin content in Brattleboro rats, 36-37
neurophysin in perikarya of, 28
oxytocin in, 14, 53
vasopressin in, 14, 53

Surgical stress
    corticotropic response to, 217
    GH secretion and, 137
Synaptosomes
    histamine in, 11-12
    isolated sheep, SRH release from,
        201
Systemic lupus erythematosus, GH
        secretion and, 136

Tanycytes, 35, 46
Testosterone propionate, and LH
        response to GnRH, 234
Tibial epiphyseal assay, as measure
        of GH activity, 142
Thalamus, GIH in, 149
Theophylline, and pituitary hormone
        release, 63
Thiamylal anesthesia, and plasma LH
        and PGs, 81-82
Thyroid
    carcinoma, TSH therapy and, 232
    disease, TRH and, 229-230
    hormones, TRH-induced
        prolactin release and, 186
Thyroid-stimulating hormone (TSH)
    clinical applications in pituitary
        and hypothalamic disease, 230
    cyclic AMP and, 64, 65-66
    distribution of, 1
    in fetal pituitary gland, 262-263
    interaction between GIH and,
        68-72
    and pentobarbital, 154
    PGs and, 85-86
    -producing cells, 66-72
    TRH and, 68, 146, 227-229, 241
Thyroidectomy
    catecholamine levels and, 17-20
    plasma TSH response to TRH, 85
Thyrotoxicosis, TSH response and,
        231
Thyrotropin, see Thyroid-stimulating
        hormone
Thyrotropin-releasing hormone (TRH)
    analogues, 228-229
    anencephalic infants and, 261-262

clinical applications
    in normal subjects, 227-229
    in primary thyroid disease,
        229-230
cyclic AMP and, 64, 66
distribution in hypothalamus, 15, 16
and dopamine inhibition of pro-
        lactin secretion, 189
in fetal brain, 263
FSH and TSH responses to, 241
functional receptors for, 66-68
and GH secretion in acromegaly,
        143-144
-induced TSH release, GIH and, 146
interactions with other hormones,
        231
localization of, 51
microphoretically applied, 114-117
PRL secretion and, 186-189, 231
radioimmunoassays, 232
secretion by hypothalamus in vitro,
        195
therapeutic value of, 232
TSH response to, in pituitary and
        hypothalamic disease, 230
Thyrotrophs, GIH and TRH receptors
        for, 69-70
Tranquilizers, prolactin secretion and,
        175-179
Tryptophan hydroxylase
    endocrine manipulation and, 17,
        20
    localization in rat hypothalamus, 9
    serotonin levels in hypothalamus
        and, 11
Tuberoinfundibular neurons, 171
    effect of microelectrophoretically
        applied norepinephrine,
        dopamine, and glutamate
        on, 110-113
    electrical stimulation of, GH
        secretion and, 140
    PRL injection and, 184
    recurrent neural circuit in, 105
Tumors
    hypothalamic, and GH secretion,
        136
    lung, GRH activity in, 145

mammary, prolactin-induced
growth and, 183
pancreatic, GIH therapy and,
242-243
pituitary, *see* Pituitary gland,
tumors
Tyrosine hydroxylase, 7
inhibition by glucocorticoids, 52
localization in rat hypothalamus, 9
neuroendocrine control
mechanisms and, 17, 19-20

Unit recording techniques, 53, 95-119;
Urethane anesthesia
PG effects on GH secretion and, 78
single-cell studies and, 101
GH secretion and, 156-157

Vasoactive intestinal polypeptide,
GIH inhibition of, 241-243
Vasopressin
ACTH release and, 32-33, 39, 41,
53
assays, CRH assays and, 199-200
cerebrospinal fluid transport of,
34-35
and electrical stimulation along
hypothalamo-neurohypophyseal
tract, 95
GH release and, 138, 144
GRH activity and, 143
localization of, 35-41, 53
in LRH, 42
in magnocellular perikarya, 43-44
neurophysin associated with, 27,
32

PGs and, 84
secretion studies, 25-26
in suprachiasmatic nucleus, 39-41
Ventral bundle lesions, 20
Ventral premammillary, GIH in, 16
Ventricular cerebrospinal fluid, LRH
and, 99
Ventromedial nucleus (VMN)
choline acetyltransferase activity
in, 14
dopamine levels, 10
electrical stimulation of, GH
secretion and, 139-142
GIH in, 16
GRH activity in, 141
histamine in, 12
lesions, GH secretion and, 138-139
TRH in, 16
Ventromedial nucleus-arcuate complex,
GH secretion and, 150
"VMH syndrome," 152-153
VMN, *see* Ventromedial nucleus

Watery diarrhea syndrome, and GIH
therapy, 243

Zollinger-Ellison syndrome, GIH
therapy and, 241, 243
Zona externa of median eminence
GIH in, 50
LRH in, 41-43
hormone release and, 25
Zona interna of median eminence,
neurophysin in, 32